Cutting-Edge Topics in
Dry Eye Disease

Cutting-Edge Topics in Dry Eye Disease

Editor

Kyung Chul Yoon

MDPI • Basel • Beijing • Wuhan • Barcelona • Belgrade • Manchester • Tokyo • Cluj • Tianjin

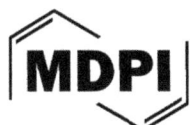

Editor
Kyung Chul Yoon
Department of Ophthalmology,
Chonnam National University
Medical School and Hospital
Korea

Editorial Office
MDPI
St. Alban-Anlage 66
4052 Basel, Switzerland

This is a reprint of articles from the Special Issue published online in the open access journal *Journal of Clinical Medicine* (ISSN 2077-0383) (available at: https://www.mdpi.com/journal/jcm/special_issues/Dry_Eye_Disease).

For citation purposes, cite each article independently as indicated on the article page online and as indicated below:

LastName, A.A.; LastName, B.B.; LastName, C.C. Article Title. *Journal Name* **Year**, *Volume Number*, Page Range.

ISBN 978-3-0365-0768-2 (Hbk)
ISBN 978-3-0365-0769-9 (PDF)

© 2021 by the authors. Articles in this book are Open Access and distributed under the Creative Commons Attribution (CC BY) license, which allows users to download, copy and build upon published articles, as long as the author and publisher are properly credited, which ensures maximum dissemination and a wider impact of our publications.

The book as a whole is distributed by MDPI under the terms and conditions of the Creative Commons license CC BY-NC-ND.

Contents

About the Editor vii

**Preface to "Cutting-Edge Topics in
Dry Eye Disease"** ix

**Motoko Kawashima, Masakazu Yamada, Chika Shigeyasu, Kazuhisa Suwaki, Miki Uchino,
Yoshimune Hiratsuka, Norihiko Yokoi, Kazuo Tsubota and for the DECS-J Study Group**
Association of Systemic Comorbidities with Dry Eye Disease
Reprinted from: *J. Clin. Med.* **2020**, *9*, 2040, doi:10.3390/jcm9072040 1

**Mamunur A.K.M. Rashid, Zhang Zhe Thia, Calesta Hui Yi Teo, Sumaiya Mamun, Hon Shing
Ong and Louis Tong**
Evaluation of Strip Meniscometry and Association with Clinical and Demographic Variables in
a Community Eye Study (in Bangladesh)
Reprinted from: *J. Clin. Med.* **2020**, *9*, 3366, doi:10.3390/jcm9103366 11

Sachiko Inoue, Motoko Kawashima, Reiko Arita, Ai Kozaki and Kazuo Tsubota
Investigation of Meibomian Gland Function and Dry Eye Disease in Patients with Graves'
Ophthalmopathy [†]
Reprinted from: *J. Clin. Med.* **2020**, *9*, 2814, doi:10.3390/jcm9092814 19

Reiko Arita, Shima Fukuoka and Motoko Kawashima
Proposed Algorithm for Management of Meibomian Gland Dysfunction Based on Noninvasive
Meibography
Reprinted from: *J. Clin. Med.* **2021**, *10*, 65, doi:10.3390/jcm10010065 31

**Shima Fukuoka, Reiko Arita, Takanori Mizoguchi, Motoko Kawashima, Shizuka Koh, Rika
Shirakawa, Takashi Suzuki, Satoshi Sasaki and Naoyuki Morishige**
Relation of Dietary Fatty Acids and Vitamin D to the
Prevalence of Meibomian Gland Dysfunction in Japanese Adults:
The Hirado–Takushima Study
Reprinted from: *J. Clin. Med.* **2021**, *10*, 350, doi:10.3390/jcm10020350 43

Reiko Arita, Shima Fukuoka, Takanori Mizoguchi and Naoyuki Morishige
Multicenter Study of Intense Pulsed Light for Patients with Refractory Aqueous-Deficient Dry
Eye Accompanied by Mild Meibomian Gland Dysfunction
Reprinted from: *J. Clin. Med.* **2020**, *9*, 3467, doi:10.3390/jcm9113467 61

**Gysbert-Botho van Setten, Christophe Baudouin, Jutta Horwath-Winter, Daniel Böhringer,
Oliver Stachs, Ebru Toker, Sultan Al-Zaaidi, Jose M. Benitez-del-Castillo, Ria Beck, Osama
Al-Sheikh, Berthold Seitz, Stefano Barabino, Herbert A. Reitsamer and Wolfgang G.K.
Müller-Lierheim**
The HYLAN M Study: Efficacy of 0.15% High Molecular Weight Hyaluronan Fluid in the
Treatment of Severe Dry Eye Disease in a Multicenter Randomized Trial
Reprinted from: *J. Clin. Med.* **2020**, *9*, 3536, doi:10.3390/jcm9113536 75

**Gysbert-Botho van Setten, Oliver Stachs, Bénédicte Dupas, Semra Akkaya Turhan, Berthold
Seitz, Herbert Reitsamer, Karsten Winter, Jutta Horwath-Winter, Rudolf F. Guthoff and
Wolfgang G.K. Müller-Lierheim**
High Molecular Weight Hyaluronan Promotes Corneal Nerve Growth in Severe Dry Eyes
Reprinted from: *J. Clin. Med.* **2020**, *9*, 3799, doi:10.3390/jcm9123799 101

Zhaolin Liu, Ming Jin, Ying Li, Jun Liu, Xianghua Xiao, Hongsheng Bi, Zhiqiang Pan, Huijun Shi, Xiaofeng Xie, Minglian Zhang, Xuemin Gao, Lei Li, Weijie Ouyang, Liying Tang, Jieli Wu, Yiran Yang, Jiaoyue Hu and Zuguo Liu
Efficacy and Safety of *Houttuynia* Eye Drops Atomization Treatment for Meibomian Gland Dysfunction-Related Dry Eye Disease: A Randomized, Double-Blinded, Placebo-Controlled Clinical Trial
Reprinted from: *J. Clin. Med.* **2020**, *9*, 4022, doi:10.3390/jcm9124022 . . . . **115**

Hyeon-Jeong Yoon, Jonghwa Kim and Kyung Chul Yoon
Treatment Response to Gabapentin in Neuropathic Ocular Pain Associated with Dry Eye
Reprinted from: *J. Clin. Med.* **2020**, *9*, 3765, doi:10.3390/jcm9113765 . . . . **129**

Hyeon Jeong Yoon, Jonghwa Kim, Jee Myung Yang, Edward T. Wei, Seong Jin Kim and Kyung Chul Yoon
Topical TRPM8 Agonist for Relieving Neuropathic Ocular Pain in Patients with Dry Eye: A Pilot Study
Reprinted from: *J. Clin. Med.* **2021**, *10*, 250, doi:10.3390/jcm10020250 . . . . **139**

About the Editor

Kyung Chul Yoon MD, PhD is a Professor of the Department of Ophthalmology, Chonnam National University Medical School, Gwangju, South Korea. Following his residency at the Chonnam National University Hospital, he completed a fellowship at the Keio University School of Medicine, Japan, in 2004, and the Cullen Eye Institute of the Baylor College of Medicine, Houston, USA, in 2006–2007. Dr. Yoon specializes in tear film and ocular surface disorders, especially dry eye disease. He is one of the pioneers in the field of clinical and experimental dry eye research and has published 340 scientific papers as well as 10 book chapters. Dr. Yoon is a committee member of the Tear Film and Ocular Surface Society DEWS II and Asia Dry Eye Advisory Board, and holds the position of director of the Korean Dry Eye Society, Korean Cornea Society, and Korean Society of Cataract and Refractive Surgery.

Preface to "Cutting-Edge Topics in Dry Eye Disease"

This Special Issue is dedicated to tear film abnormalities, including dry eye disease and Meibomian gland dysfunction, which are the most common ocular diseases. The Special Issue introduces new diagnostic and therapeutic approaches for these diseases and presents original articles that provide information on a new proposed algorithm for the management and prevention of Meibomian gland dysfunction, strip meniscometry, topical agents, and the use of intense pulsed laser treatment for dry eye disease. Specifically, novel treatment methods for neuropathic ocular pain associated with dry eye disease, such as oral gabapentin and TRPM8 agonists, are introduced.

Kyung Chul Yoon
Editor

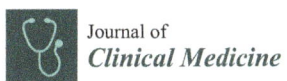

Article

Association of Systemic Comorbidities with Dry Eye Disease

Motoko Kawashima [1,*], Masakazu Yamada [2], Chika Shigeyasu [2], Kazuhisa Suwaki [3], Miki Uchino [1], Yoshimune Hiratsuka [4], Norihiko Yokoi [5], Kazuo Tsubota [1] and for the DECS-J Study Group

1. Department of Ophthalmology, Keio University School of Medicine, Tokyo 1608582, Japan; uchinomiki@yahoo.co.jp (M.U.); tsubota@z3.keio.jp (K.T.)
2. Department of Ophthalmology, Kyorin University School of Medicine, Tokyo 1818611, Japan; yamadamasakazu@ks.kyorin-u.ac.jp (M.Y.); shigeyasu@eye-center.org (C.S.)
3. Department of Japan Medical Affairs, Santen Pharmaceutical Co., Ltd., Osaka 5308552, Japan; kazuhisa.suwaki@santen.com
4. Department of Ophthalmology, Juntendo University Graduate School of Medicine, Tokyo 1138431, Japan; yoshi-h@tkf.att.ne.jp
5. Department of Ophthalmology, Kyoto Prefectural University of Medicine, Kyoto 6020841, Japan; nyokoi@koto.kpu-m.ac.jp
* Correspondence: motoko-k@a3.keio.jp; Tel.: +81-3-3353-1211; Fax: +81-3-3359-8302

Received: 2 June 2020; Accepted: 23 June 2020; Published: 29 June 2020

Abstract: We investigated the association between dry eye disease and systemic comorbidities, including dry eye subtype, quality of life (QOL) and health utility among patients with dry eye disease. This cross-sectional, observational study enrolled 449 patients with dry eye disease (386 females; mean age, 62.6 ± 15.7 [range, 21–90] years). Ophthalmic examination findings included tear film break-up time (TBUT), Schirmer I value and keratoconjunctival staining score. QOL and health utility were evaluated using the Dry Eye-Related Quality-of-Life Score (DEQS) and Human Utility Index Mark 3 (HUI-3), respectively. Background information, including systemic comorbidities, was obtained. Prevalence of systemic comorbidities was 48.8% (219/449). No significant difference occurred between DEQS and systemic comorbidity. However, patients with dry eye disease and systemic comorbidities (depression and insomnia) exhibited significantly worse ocular surface parameters, particularly regarding TBUT, than those without. Dry eye disease with insomnia or depression comorbidity significantly correlated with friction-related diseases (including conjunctivochalasis or lid wiper epitheliopathy). A high prevalence of several systemic comorbidities occurred in patients with dry eye disease. This study shows an association between ocular signs and systemic comorbidities, particularly depression and insomnia. Ophthalmologists should be aware of patients' systemic comorbidities in the diagnosis and management of dry eye disease.

Keywords: cross-sectional study; dry eye disease; systemic comorbidity

1. Introduction

Dry eye disease is a common disease caused by numerous factors including ocular surface problems, environmental factors such as humidity and wind, and systemic conditions. In addition, a variety of systemic medications can also induce dry eye disease [1–4]. Although it is widely recognized as an ocular surface disease, associated systemic conditions are not negligible, as they can negatively impact ocular health. Such systemic conditions include rheumatoid arthritis, vitamin A deficiency, bone marrow transplantation and postmenopausal estrogen therapy. Besides these causal relationships, epidemiological studies have also reported the association of dry eye disease with systemic diseases, including ischemic heart disease and hyperlipidemia. Depression, antidepressant use and insomnia are also reported to be associated with dry eye disease. Schein et al. reported that elderly individuals with systemic comorbidities are likely to have symptoms of dry eye disease [5]. These findings from statistical approaches and epidemiological studies should be carefully interpreted, as dry eye disease is a common disease and the elderly tend to be affected by multiple comorbidities.

Previous studies have demonstrated aging as the most clearly documented risk factor for dry eye disease [6]. Accordingly, the prevalence of this disease is increasing particularly in modern age societies like Japan. However, most previous studies reporting on the prevalence of dry eye disease and systemic comorbidities [4,7,8] have been based on epidemiological questionnaires. Therefore, the relationship between ocular parameters and systemic comorbidities has not been well investigated. For example, a previous study by Wang et al. revealed that a number of systemic diseases correlate with dry eye disease, but since the authors did not include any ocular examination, the relationship of specific dry eye parameters to these other conditions was not determined [9]. Therefore, we investigated the association between dry eye disease and systemic comorbidities, as part of the clinic-based Dry Eye Cross-Sectional Study (DECS-J) in Japan.

2. Materials and Methods

2.1. Ethics

This study was conducted in accordance with the guidelines of the World Medical Association, Declaration of Helsinki and the Ethical Guidelines for Medical and Health Research Involving Human Subjects in Japan. Subjects received full explanation of the procedures and provided written informed consent before enrollment. The study protocol was approved by the Institutional Review Board of the Clinical Study, Ryogoku Eye Clinic, Tokyo, Japan. The study was registered in a public registration system (University Hospital Medical Information Network registry no. UMIN 000015890) [10].

2.2. Study Population

We collected data from the DECS-J, which was an observational study conducted in 10 eye clinics in Japan. All investigators were specialists in ocular surface disorders and dry eye disease and belonged to the Japanese Dry Eye Society. To ensure the quality of the survey, two investigators' meetings were held prior to the start of patient enrollment to discuss the study protocols and examination procedures.

We consecutively enrolled outpatients who were at least 20 years old and were newly or previously diagnosed with dry eye disease. The criteria for diagnosis was as follows: (1) at least one abnormal tear examination result [Schirmer I test ≤ 5 mm, tear film break-up time (TBUT) ≤ 5 s]; (2) abnormal results in ocular surface vital staining tests (fluorescein keratoconjunctival staining score ≥ 3); and (3) presence of dry eye symptoms [11]. Subjects who met two or all three criteria were considered to probably or definitely have dry eye disease, respectively, and were included in the study. Up to 50 patients were enrolled at each of the 10 study sites from 1 December 2014 to 28 February 2015.

A total of 449 patients with an average age of 62.6 ± 15.7 years were included in this study. Of these, 386 (86.0%) were females. Table 1 shows the age distribution of the patients in this study.

Table 1. Age and sex distribution of the patients in this study.

Age (Years)	Sex		Total (n (%))
	Male (n (%))	Female (n (%))	
<40	7 (11.11)	37 (9.59)	44 (9.8)
40–64	21 (33.33)	139 (36.01)	160 (35.63)
≥65	35 (55.56)	210 (54.4)	245 (54.57)
Total	63 (100)	386 (100)	449 (100)

2.3. Systemic Comorbidities and Oral Medicine

Patients were asked to provide information regarding systemic comorbidities and oral medicine. Hypertension, insomnia and depression were defined as having hypertension or taking an antihypertensive medication; as having insomnia or taking a sedative; and as having depression or taking an antidepressant, respectively.

2.4. Quality of Life (QOL) and Health Utility Assessment

QOL and health utility among patients with dry eye disease were evaluated using the DEQS [12] and the Human Utility Index Mark 3 (HUI-3) questionnaires [13], respectively. The DEQS consists of 15 questions and is scored using an overall summary scale. The score derived from this questionnaire is considered to be a quantitative measure of dry eye symptoms, in which 0 indicates the best and 100 indicates the worst. Test/retest reliability and discriminant validity of the DEQS were confirmed in a previous study, showing that the score was significantly higher in patients with dry eye disease than in healthy controls (33.7 vs. 6.0) [9].

The HUI-3 is a standard method for assessing the utility value. It is a multi-attribute utility classification system for preferences associated with generic health states. It consists of 15 questions assessing eight health attributes: vision, hearing, speech, ambulation, dexterity, emotion, cognition and pain. Individual sets of answers were converted to utility values, using the method described by Furlong et al. [14]. A utility value representing the overall health state was derived by applying a weighted scoring algorithm, in which utility is defined on a continuous scale from 0 to 1, where 0 corresponds to the worst possible QOL outcome (equal to death) and 1 corresponds to the best possible one (equal to perfect health). Patients were asked to fill out the questionnaires at home and return them by post.

2.5. Ophthalmic Evaluation

Ophthalmic examinations included assessment of conjunctival and corneal vital staining with fluorescein sodium, measurement of the TBUT and the Schirmer I test.

Test strips containing fluorescein sodium (Fluores Ocular Examination Test Paper, Ayumi Pharmaceutical Co., Tokyo, Japan) were used for vital staining and TBUT measurement. After the tip of a wet test strip had been applied to the inferior temporal tear meniscus, patients were asked to blink several times to ensure adequate mixing of the fluorescein dye with the tears. The time interval between the last complete blink and the appearance of the first corneal dark spot was timed using a stopwatch. The average of three measurements was recorded as the TBUT. Corneal and conjunctival epithelial damage was then evaluated via corneal fluorescein staining, according to the National Eye Institute grading system [15]. Briefly, corneal staining was graded with a score of 0–3, assigned to each of five corneal zones (superior, nasal, central, inferior and temporal), with a maximum total score of 15. The fluorescein staining score of the keratoconjunctival was determined according to the modified grading system of van Bijsterveld [16], according to which each eye is divided into three sections (temporal conjunctiva, cornea and nasal conjunctiva) and scored from 0 to 3. The final score ranged from 0 (minimum) to 9 (maximum). The Schirmer I test was performed without topical anesthesia after all other examinations had been completed. A Schirmer test strip (Ayumi Pharmaceutical Co.) was placed on the outer one third of the temporal lower conjunctival fornix for 5 min. The strip was then removed, and the length of the wet filter paper was recorded in millimeters. To avoid any effect of keratoconjunctival staining on the Schirmer I test, the tests were performed 15 min apart, at minimum.

For each patient, the eye that met the most criteria for dry eye diagnosis was included in the study. If both eyes met the same number of criteria, the eye with the higher fluorescein staining score and the shorter TBUT was included. If these values were the same for both eyes, the right eye was used.

2.6. Classification of Dry Eye Subgroups

2.6.1. Aqueous-Deficient (AD)/sTBUT

We classified the subjects into aqueous-deficient (AD) and short TBUT dry eye subgroups. The AD dry eye group was comprised of subjects who fulfilled the following criteria: (1) the presence of dry eye symptoms and (2) decreased tear production (Schirmer value ≤ 5 mm). The short TBUT dry eye subgroup included subjects who met the following conditions: (1) the presence of dry eye symptoms, (2) abnormal tear stability (TBUT ≤ 5 s), (3) no abnormality in tear production (Schirmer value > 5 mm), and (4) no abnormality in the ocular surface vital staining test (keratoconjunctival score < 3) [17].

2.6.2. Meibomian Gland Function (MGD+/−)

We evaluated meibomian gland function (MGD in the central one-third of the upper eyelid using slit-lamp biomicroscopy. The patient was instructed to look down while the investigator gently and partially everted the upper lid to examine the lid margin. Typical pictures of the following signs/findings were distributed to each investigator to aid in the examination: (1) one or more abnormal findings around the meibomian gland orifices, such as vascular engorgement, anterior or posterior displacement of the mucocutaneous junction or irregularity of the lid margin (2) orifice obstruction, such as plugging, pouting and ridges [18]; and (3) hypersecretion or hyposecretion of the meibum [19]. We diagnosed MGD when all the signs and findings listed in the criteria were present [17].

2.6.3. Friction-Related Diseases (FRD+/−)

We considered that subjects had friction-related conditions when any of the following conditions were present: lid wiper epitheliopathy (in the upper and lower lids), conjunctivochalasis (at the central site of the lower eyelid) or superior limbic keratoconjunctivitis [17,20–22].

2.7. Statistical Methods

We used one eye from each subject for the analysis, as explained above (Section 2.5). Data for all parameters are presented as the mean ± standard deviation. We performed all statistical analyses using SAS software, version 9.4 (SAS Inc., Cary, NC, USA). For comparisons between groups, we used Fisher's exact test for dichotomous variables and Student's *t*-test for continuous variables. We performed a linear model analysis to adjust for the effects of age. To estimate the association between a given independent variable and the outcome after adjustment for age, multiple linear regression was used for continuous variables and multiple logistic regression was used for binary outcomes. We considered a *p*-value lower than 0.05 as statistically significant for all analyses.

3. Results

The prevalence of systemic comorbidities was 48.8% (219/449 cases). The most prevalent comorbidity was hypertension in 108 cases (24.1%), followed by insomnia in 67 cases (14.9%) and depression in 20 cases (4.5%). The 113 cases categorized as "others" included hyperlipidemia (15), Sjogren's syndrome (7), abnormal thyroid function (7), hypercholesteremia (7), angina (4), arrhythmia (4) and so on. Ninety-eight patients (21.8%) were taking anti-hypertensives and 55 (12.2%) were taking sedatives (Table 2).

Table 2. Prevalence of systemic comorbidities and oral medicine use.

		Cases	%	Age (Average ± SD)	Female (%)	Male (%)
Total		449		62.6 ± 15.6	386 (86.0)	63 (14.0)
Systemic comorbidity *1	(−)	230	51.2	56.3 ± 16.1	195 (84.8)	35 (15.2)
	(+)	219	48.8	69.2 ± 12.1	191 (87.2)	28 (12.8)
Details *2	Hypertension	108	24.1	73.1 ± 10.8	91 (84.3)	17 (15.7)
	Insomnia	67	14.9	71.0 ± 11.3	59 (88.1)	8 (11.9)
	Depression	20	4.5	64.9 ± 13.5	19 (95.0)	1 (5.0)
	DM	16	3.6	70.6 ± 11.6	14 (87.5)	2 (12.5)
	RA	15	3.3	70.4 ± 8.4	15 (100.0)	0 (0.0)
	Others	113	25.2	68.1 ± 12.4	105 (92.9)	8 (7.1)
Oral medicine *2	Antihypertensive	98	21.8	73.2 ± 11.1	82 (83.7)	16 (16.3)
	Sedative	55	12.2	70.9 ± 11.1	48 (87.3)	7 (12.7)
	Antidepressant	20	4.5	64.9 ± 13.5	19 (95.0)	1 (5.0)
	Others	147	32.7	68.5 ± 12.4	134 (91.2)	13 (8.8)

DM, diabetes mellitus; RA, rheumatoid arthritis; SD, standard deviation. *1: (+) indicates more than one comorbidity selected among hypertension, insomnia, depression, DM, RA or others. *2: multiple answers allowed.

Patients with dry eye disease who had any systemic comorbidities exhibited a significantly lower Schirmer value ($p = 0.004$), shorter TBUT ($p = 0.002$), higher keratoconjunctival staining score ($p = 0.0002$) and lower utility value estimated by HUI-3 ($p = 0.003$) than those without systemic comorbidities (Table 3). After adjustment for age, differences in TBUT, keratoconjunctival staining score and HUI-3 utility value remained statistically significant ($p = 0.011$, $p < 0.001$ and $p = 0.03$, respectively). Patients who in addition to dry eye disease also had hypertension or depression exhibited a significantly lower Schirmer value than those without ($p = 0.008$ and $p = 0.04$, respectively), while those who had insomnia or depression exhibited a significantly shorter TBUT than those without ($p = 0.01$ and $p = 0.04$, respectively). The DEQS score was lower in patients with dry eye disease and hypertension ($p = 0.003$). After adjustment for age, the TBUT in patients with depression or insomnia remained significantly shorter ($p = 0.04$ and $p = 0.04$, respectively).

Regarding oral medicine use, patients with dry eye disease who were prescribed antidepressants had a significantly lower Schirmer value ($p = 0.04$) and lower TBUT ($p = 0.04$), while those who used anti-hypertensives had a significantly lower Schirmer value ($p = 0.009$) and lower DEQS score ($p = 0.03$) than those who did not receive such medications. After adjustment for age, antidepressant use remained significantly different for both the Schirmer value and TBUT ($p = 0.05$ and $p = 0.04$, respectively; Table 4).

We examined the relationship between dry eye disease subtypes and systemic comorbidities. We found that patients with hypertension and insomnia had a significantly higher prevalence of MGD (hypertension: odds ratio [OR] 2.65, 95% confidence interval [CI] 1.64–4.28, $p < 0.01$; insomnia: OR 1.94, 95% CI 1.10–3.42, $p = 0.02$). Patients with dry eye disease and hypertension, insomnia or depression had a significantly higher prevalence of FRD (hypertension: OR 1.56, 95% CI 1.00–2.44, $p = 0.05$; insomnia: OR 2.66, 95% CI 1.57–4.51, $p < 0.01$; depression: OR 4.92, 95% CI 1.85–13.08, $p < 0.01$). After the OR was adjusted for age, insomnia and depression, comorbidities with dry eye disease were significantly associated with FRD (insomnia: OR 2.16, 95% CI 1.26–3.72, $p < 0.01$; depression: OR 4.89, 95% CI 1.81–13.22, $p < 0.01$; Table 5).

Table 3. Systemic comorbidities and dry eye parameters.

		No. of Cases	Schirmer Test (mm) (Mean ± SD)	TBUT (s) (Mean ± SD)	Keratoconjunctival Staining Score (Points) (Mean ± SD)	DEQS (Mean ± SD)	HUI (Mean ± SD)
Systemic comorbidity	+	219	8.38 ± 8.20	2.49 ± 1.59	3.16 ± 1.86	25.15 ± 20.69	0.72 ± 0.23
	−	230	10.98 ± 10.39	2.94 ± 1.51	2.47 ± 1.99	28.35 ± 20.50	0.79 ± 0.20
	p-value		0.004 *	0.002 *	0.0002 *	0.104	0.003 *
	Age-adjusted p-value		0.656	0.011 *	<0.001 *	0.411	0.030 *
Hypertension *	+	108	7.61 ± 7.19	2.66 ± 1.65	2.96 ± 1.75	21.71 ± 18.68	0.73 ± 0.24
	−	341	10.36 ± 9.99	2.74 ± 1.54	2.75 ± 2.02	28.40 ± 20.98	0.76 ± 0.21
	p-value		0.008	0.645	0.334	0.004 *	0.275
	Age-adjusted p-value		0.694	0.820	0.347	0.406	0.897
Insomnia *	+	67	8.63 ± 8.96	2.31 ± 1.55	2.81 ± 1.80	26.31 ± 19.59	0.74 ± 0.19
	−	382	9.88 ± 9.53	2.80 ± 1.56	2.80 ± 1.99	26.87 ± 20.83	0.76 ± 0.22
	p-value		0.318	0.018	0.993	0.84	0.516
	Age-adjusted p-value		0.698	0.044 *	0.960	0.249	0.938
Depression *	+	20	5.50 ± 5.85	2.03 ± 1.84	2.15 ± 1.90	26.05 ± 18.05	0.725 ± 0.213
	−	429	9.89 ± 9.54	2.76 ± 1.55	2.83 ± 1.96	26.82 ± 20.76	0.756 ± 0.215
	p-value		0.042 *	0.043 *	0.127	0.874	0.55
	Age-adjusted p-value		0.056	0.049 *	0.125	0.993	0.598

TBUT, tear film break up time; DEQS, Dry Eye-Related Quality-of-Life Score; HUI, health utilities index; * $p \leq 0.05$; "+": presence; "−": absence.

Table 4. Oral medicine and dry eye parameters.

		No. of Cases	Schirmer Value (mm)	TBUT (s)	Fluorescein Staining Score	DEQS	HUI
Antihypertensive	(+)	98	7.50 ± 6.84	2.74 ± 1.68	2.92 ± 1.73	21.39 ± 18.95	0.73 ± 0.25
	(−)	351	10.31 ± 9.99	2.72 ± 1.53	2.77 ± 2.02	28.33 ± 20.86	0.76 ± 0.20
	p		0.009 *	0.901	0.514	0.003 *	0.272
	Age-adjusted		0.626	0.413	0.548	0.342	0.853
Sedative	(+)	55	8.64 ± 9.13	2.38 ± 1.61	2.93 ± 1.82	27.54 ± 20.16	0.74 ± 0.20
	(−)	394	9.84 ± 9.49	2.77 ± 1.55	2.79 ± 1.98	26.69 ± 20.72	0.76 ± 0.22
	p		0.378	0.078	0.619	0.779	0.485
	Age-adjusted		0.741	0.149	0.649	0.138	0.837
Antidepressant	(+)	20	5.50 ± 5.85	2.03 ± 1.84	2.15 ± 1.90	26.05 ± 18.05	0.73 ± 0.21
	(−)	429	9.89 ± 9.54	2.76 ± 1.55	2.83 ± 1.96	26.82 ± 20.76	0.76 ± 0.22
	p		0.042 *	0.043 *	0.127	0.874	0.55
	Age-adjusted		0.056	0.049 *	0.125	0.993	0.598

TBUT: tear film break up time; DEQS: Dry Eye-Related Quality-of-Life Score; HUI: Health Utilities Index. * $p < 0.05$. Mean ± SD; "+": presence; "−": absence.

Table 5. Association between dry eye subtype and systemic comorbidities.

	DE Subtype (ADDE/sTBUT)			
	OR (95% CI)	p Value	Adjusted OR (95% CI)	p Value
Hypertension	1.46 (0.82–2.58)	0.20	1.17 (0.64–2.15)	0.61
Insomnia	0.97 (0.51–1.81)	0.92	0.80 (0.41–1.53)	0.49
Depression	1.69 (0.54–5.27)	0.36	1.67 (0.53–5.22)	0.38
	MGD (Yes/No)			
	OR (95% CI)	p Value	Adjusted OR 95% CI)	p Value
Hypertension	2.65 (1.64–4.28)	<0.01	1.33 (0.78–2.27)	0.30
Insomnia	1.94 (1.10–3.42)	0.02	1.21 (0.66–2.21)	0.54
Depression	0.38 (0.09–1.67)	0.20	0.33 (0.07–1.49)	0.15
	FRD (Yes/No)			
	OR (95% CI)	p Value	Adjusted OR (95% CI)	p Value
Hypertension	1.56 (1.00–2.44)	0.05	1.10 (0.68–1.79)	0.70
Insomnia	2.66 (1.57–4.51)	<0.01	2.16 (1.26–3.72)	<0.01
Depression	4.92 (1.85–13.08)	<0.01	4.89 (1.81–13.22)	<0.01

OR, odds ratio; CI, confidence Interval; ADDE, aqueous-deficient dry eye; DE, dry eye; sTBUT, short tear film break up time dry eye; MGD, meibomian gland dysfunction; FRD, friction-related disease.

4. Discussion

In this study, we investigated the relationship between the severity of dry eye disease and systemic comorbidities. Aging is the most clearly documented risk factor for dry eye disease [6], and the elderly tend to be affected by multiple comorbidities. As expected, the average age of subjects in our study was relatively high (62.6 years on average), and approximately half of the patients had systemic comorbidities. Prevalent systemic comorbidities were hypertension, insomnia and depression. We found that patients with dry eye disease and any systemic comorbidity exhibited significantly worse utility, as estimated by HUI-3, than those without. In addition, those with systemic comorbidities had a higher severity of dry eye disease, as demonstrated by objective parameters, such as the TBUT and Schirmer value. These correlations remained statistically significant after adjustment for age. Schein et al. reported that the presence of many systemic comorbidities is strongly associated with reported symptoms of dry eye disease [5], although no association was seen between systemic comorbidity and Schirmer or Rose Bengal test scores. Our findings suggest that the presence of systemic comorbidities may compromise the ocular surface, as well as the QOL of patients with dry eye disease. However, systemic comorbidities include numerous conditions with different pathophysiology, which affect various parts of the body. Our findings are based on a statistical and epidemiological approach and therefore must be re-examined cautiously in further studies.

In this study, we found that patients with dry eye disease and depression showed a significantly shorter TBUT after adjustment for age. Interestingly, those taking antidepressants showed a significantly lower Schirmer value, in addition to a shorter TBUT, after such adjustments. These results suggest that depression and/or anti-depressant use is associated with poor tear film stability, and that antidepressant use may worsen tear secretion in addition to tear stability, which is an indicator of dry eye severity. Previous studies, mostly involving epidemiological questionnaires, have also reported a relationship between depression and dry eye disease [23–26]. In a comparison of depressive and control groups, one case-control study revealed significantly lower Schirmer scores and shorter TBUT, as well as a consistently higher Oxford scores in individuals with depression [27]. Similarly, we demonstrated an association between depression/anti-depressant use and dry eye severity by undertaking objective measurements, although the mechanisms involved in this association remain unknown.

Another interesting finding in our study is that patients with dry eye disease and insomnia showed a significantly shorter TBUT after adjustment for age. Several investigators have recently reported the association of sleep disturbances, like insomnia, and dry eye disease [28–30]. Our results also support such an association. Insomnia is a common problem in the elderly and sedative drugs, including benzodiazepines, are frequently prescribed for this condition in Japan. The mechanism involved in the association between insomnia and dry eye disease may be derived from insomnia itself. Alternatively, the intake of sedative drugs may have some influence. Further studies are needed to clarify this issue.

In addition, we found that FRD was significantly associated with dry eye disease and was a comorbidity with insomnia or depression, even after adjusting for age. The presence of FRD, including conjunctivochalasis and lid wiper epitheliopathy, is a predisposing factor for dry eye disease and its severity. To our knowledge, an association between FRD and depression or insomnia has not yet been reported. We also noted that antidepressant users had decreased tear secretions. Since FRDs are associated with lower tear volume and quality (e.g., secreted mucin), dry eye disease is more likely to be associated with FRD when depression and insomnia are also present than when they are not. Another possible explanation is that anti-depressant and sedative drugs may induce blepharospasm [31,32], as blinking problems induced by drugs may result in the development of FRDs. Although the cause is not known, our study suggests that anti-depressant use may reduce tear secretion and worsen ocular surface conditions.

In this study, we demonstrated that depression and insomnia comorbidity with dry eye disease increased dry eye severity and that, in turn, ocular symptoms may worsen depression/insomnia, thus creating a vicious circle. Therefore, ophthalmologists should be aware of patients' systemic comorbidities in the diagnosis and treatment of dry eye disease. Similarly, psychologists should be aware of patients' eye conditions when considering mental health management. We feel that it is especially important for psychiatrists to take this into account, particularly when prescribing antidepressants, which may aggravate dry eye signs.

Our findings must be considered along with several limitations. First, detailed patient medical information could not be collected regarding the severity of depression, details of medications, duration of systemic comorbidities and duration of oral medicine use. This information is important for establishing the underlying mechanisms of dry eye severity and systemic comorbidities. Dry eye disease is common in patients with depression, especially those of older age who have been experiencing depression and taking antidepressant medication for longer periods. Therefore, future studies should focus on patients with depression and dry eye disease. Second, our study was based on a cross-sectional design; therefore, it is difficult to ascertain whether the observed associations are due to causal effects. Third, we included patients with dry eye disease who had been receiving various treatments. Therefore, there may have been differences in the clinical presentation of these patients.

In conclusion, in the clinical setting ophthalmologists should pay careful attention to the systemic comorbidities of patients with dry eye disease, and especially of older adults who have a higher prevalence of such comorbidities. Comorbidities including depression, insomnia and the use of antidepressants are associated with dry eye disease severity.

Author Contributions: Conceptualization, M.K., M.Y. and Y.H.; data curation, C.S.; formal analysis, Y.H.; funding acquisition, M.Y. and K.S.; investigation, M.K. and C.S.; methodology, M.Y.; project administration, M.Y.; supervision, N.Y. and K.T.; writing—original draft, M.K.; writing—review & editing, M.K., M.Y., C.S., K.S., M.U., Y.H., N.Y. and K.T. All authors have read and agreed to the published version of the manuscript.

Funding: This research was funded by the Japan Dry Eye Society, Tokyo, Japan, and Santen Pharmaceutical Co., Ltd., Osaka, Japan.

Conflicts of Interest: K.S. is an employee of Santen Pharmaceutical Co., Ltd.; M.Y. is a consultant for Otsuka Pharmaceutical Co., Ltd. (Tokyo, Japan) and Johnson & Johnson Vision Care Co. (Paranaque City, Philippines); N.Y. is a speaker's bureau member of Santen Pharmaceutical Co., Ltd. and Otsuka Pharmaceutical Co., Ltd., and is a consultant of Rohto Co., Ltd. (Osaka, Japan) and Alcon Japan Co., Ltd. (Tokyo, Japan), and has patents for ophthalmologic apparatus with Kowa Co., Ltd. (Nagoya, Japan), and is a consultant for Kissei Co., Ltd. (Matsumoto City, Japan) and Rohto Co., Ltd.; K.T. is a consultant, speaker's bureau member, and grant recipient of Santen Pharmaceutical Co., Ltd., as well as a speaker's bureau member and grant recipient of Otsuka Pharmaceutical Co., Ltd. The authors report no other conflicts of interest for this work. This research was conducted by a joint study organization from the Dry Eye Society and Santen Pharmaceutical Co., Ltd. Both organizations contributed to the creation of the documents, including the study protocol; management of the study's progress; both provided information and support to the study sites; disclosed the outcome of the study; and registered and updated the present study in the public registration system.

References

1. Gomes, J.A.P.; Azar, D.T.; Baudouin, C.; Efron, N.; Hirayama, M.; Horwath-Winter, J.; Kim, T.; Mehta, J.S.; Messmer, E.M.; Pepose, J.S.; et al. TFOS DEWS II iatrogenic report. *Ocul. Surf.* **2017**, *15*, 511–538. [CrossRef] [PubMed]
2. Kawashima, M. Systemic Health and Dry Eye. *Investig. Opthalmol. Vis. Sci.* **2018**, *59*, DES138–DES142. [CrossRef] [PubMed]
3. Pinazo-Duran, M.D.; Zanon-Moreno, V.; García-Medina, J.J.; Arévalo, J.F.; Gallego-Pinazo, R.; Nucci, C. Eclectic Ocular Comorbidities and Systemic Diseases with Eye Involvement: A Review. *BioMed Res. Int.* **2016**, 1–10. [CrossRef] [PubMed]
4. Roh, H.C.; Lee, J.K.; Kim, M.; Oh, J.-H.; Chang, M.-W.; Chuck, R.S.; Park, C.Y. Systemic Comorbidities of Dry Eye Syndrome. *Cornea* **2016**, *35*, 1–192. [CrossRef]
5. Schein, O.D.; Muñoz, B.; Tielsch, J.M.; Bandeen-Roche, K.; West, S. Prevalence of dry eye among the elderly. *Am. J. Ophthalmol.* **1997**, *124*, 723–728. [CrossRef]
6. Stapleton, F.; Alves, M.; Bunya, V.Y.; Jalbert, I.; Lekhanont, K.; Malet, F.; Na, K.-S.; Schaumberg, D.; Uchino, M.; Vehof, J.; et al. TFOS DEWS II Epidemiology Report. *Ocul. Surf.* **2017**, *15*, 334–365. [CrossRef]
7. Tan, L.L.; Morgan, P.B.; Cai, Z.Q.; Straughan, R.A. Prevalence of and risk factors for symptomatic dry eye disease in Singapore. *Clin. Exp. Optom.* **2014**, *98*, 45–53. [CrossRef]
8. Dana, R.; Bradley, J.L.; Guerin, A.; Pivneva, I.; Evans, A.M.; Stillman, I. Özer Comorbidities and Prescribed Medications in Patients with or Without Dry Eye Disease: A Population-Based Study. *Am. J. Ophthalmol.* **2019**, *198*, 181–192. [CrossRef]
9. Wang, T.-J.; Wang, I.-J.; Hu, C.-C.; Lin, H.-C. Comorbidities of dry eye disease: A nationwide population-based study. *Acta Ophthalmol.* **2010**, *90*, 663–668. [CrossRef]
10. Kawashima, M.; Yamada, M.; Suwaki, K.; Shigeyasu, C.; Uchino, M.; Hiratsuka, Y.; Yokoi, N.; Tsubota, K. A Clinic-based Survey of Clinical Characteristics and Practice Pattern of Dry Eye in Japan. *Adv. Ther.* **2017**, *34*, 732–743. [CrossRef]
11. Shimazaki, J.; Tsubota, K.; Kinoshita, S. Definition, and diagnosis of dry eye 2006. *Atarashii Ganka* **2007**, *24*, 181–184.
12. Sakane, Y.; Yamaguchi, M.; Yokoi, N.; Uchino, M.; Dogru, M.; Oishi, T.; Ohashi, Y.; Ohashi, Y. Development and Validation of the Dry Eye–Related Quality-of-Life Score Questionnaire. *JAMA Ophthalmol.* **2013**, *131*, 1331–1338. [CrossRef] [PubMed]
13. Horsman, J.; Furlong, W.; Feeny, D.; Torrance, G.W. The Health Utilities Index (HUI®): Concepts, measurement properties and applications. *Heal. Qual. Life Outcomes* **2003**, *1*, 54. [CrossRef] [PubMed]

14. Furlong, W.; Feeny, D.; Torrance, G.W.; Barr, R.D. The Health Utilities Index (HUI) system for assessing health-related quality of life in clinical studies. *Ann. Med.* **2001**, *33*, 375–384. [CrossRef]
15. Lemp, M.A. Report of the National Eye Institute/Industry workshop on Clinical Trials in Dry Eyes. *CLAO J.* **1995**, *21*, 221–232.
16. Van Bijsterveld, O.P. Diagnostic Tests in the Sicca Syndrome. *Arch. Ophthalmol.* **1969**, *82*, 10–14. [CrossRef]
17. Vu, C.H.V.; Kawashima, M.; Yamada, M.; Suwaki, K.; Uchino, M.; Shigeyasu, C.; Hiratsuka, Y.; Yokoi, N.; Tsubota, K. Influence of Meibomian Gland Dysfunction and Friction-Related Disease on the Severity of Dry Eye. *Ophthalmology* **2018**, *125*, 1181–1188. [CrossRef]
18. Bron, A.J.; Benjamin, L.; Snibson, G.R.; Bilaniuk, L.T. Meibomian gland disease. Classification and grading of lid changes. *Eye* **1991**, *5*, 395–411. [CrossRef]
19. Amano, S.; Inoue, K. Clinic-Based Study on Meibomian Gland Dysfunction in Japan. *Investig. Opthalmol. Vis. Sci.* **2017**, *58*, 1283–1287. [CrossRef]
20. Korb, D.R.; Greiner, J.V.; Herman, J.P.; Hebert, E.; Finnemore, V.M.; Exford, J.M.; Glonek, T.; Olson, M.C. Lid-wiper epitheliopathy and dry-eye symptoms in contact lens wearers. *CLAO J.* **2002**, *28*, 211–216.
21. Hirotani, Y.; Yokoi, N.; Komuro, A.; Kinoshita, S. Age-related changes in the mucocutaneous junction and the conjunctivochalasis in the lower lid margins. *Nippon. Ganka Gakkai Zasshi* **2003**, *107*, 363–368. [CrossRef] [PubMed]
22. Korb, D.R.; Herman, J.P.; Greiner, J.V.; Scaffidi, R.C.; Finnemore, V.M.; Exford, J.M.; Blackie, C.A.; Douglass, T. Lid Wiper Epitheliopathy and Dry Eye Symptoms. *Eye Contact Lens Sci. Clin. Pr.* **2005**, *31*, 2–8. [CrossRef] [PubMed]
23. Zheng, Y.; Wu, X.; Lin, X.; Lin, H. The Prevalence of Depression and Depressive Symptoms among Eye Disease Patients: A Systematic Review and Meta-analysis. *Sci. Rep.* **2017**, *7*, 46453. [CrossRef] [PubMed]
24. Labbe, A.; Wang, Y.X.; Jie, Y.; Baudouin, C.; Jonas, J.B.; Xu, L. Dry eye disease, dry eye symptoms and depression: The Beijing Eye Study. *Br. J. Ophthalmol.* **2013**, *97*, 1399–1403. [CrossRef]
25. Kim, K.W.; Han, S.B.; Han, E.R.; Woo, S.J.; Lee, J.J.; Yoon, J.C.; Hyon, J.Y. Association between Depression and Dry Eye Disease in an Elderly Population. *Investig. Opthalmol. Vis. Sci.* **2011**, *52*, 7954–7958. [CrossRef]
26. Wan, K.H.; Chen, L.J.; Young, A.L. Depression and anxiety in dry eye disease: A systematic review and meta-analysis. *Eye* **2016**, *30*, 1558–1567. [CrossRef]
27. Tiskaoglu, N.S.; Yazıcı, A.; Karlıdere, T.; Sari, E.; Oguz, E.Y.; Musaoglu, M.; Aslan, S.; Ermiş, S.S. Dry Eye Disease in Patients with Newly Diagnosed Depressive Disorder. *Curr. Eye Res.* **2016**, *42*, 672–676. [CrossRef]
28. Galor, A.; Seiden, B.; Park, J.J.; Feuer, W.J.; McClellan, A.; Felix, E.R.; Levitt, R.C.; Sarantopoulos, C.D.; Wallace, D.M. The Association of Dry Eye Symptom Severity and Comorbid Insomnia in US Veterans. *Eye Contact Lens Sci. Clin. Pr.* **2018**, *44*, S118–S124. [CrossRef]
29. Hackett, K.; Gotts, Z.M.; Ellis, J.; Deary, V.; Rapley, T.; Ng, W.-F.; Newton, J.L.; Deane, K.H.O. An investigation into the prevalence of sleep disturbances in primary Sjögren's syndrome: A systematic review of the literature. *Rheumatology* **2017**, *56*, 570–580. [CrossRef]
30. Ayaki, M.; Kawashima, M.; Negishi, K.; Tsubota, K. High prevalence of sleep and mood disorders in dry eye patients: Survey of 1,000 eye clinic visitors. *Neuropsychiatr. Dis. Treat.* **2015**, *11*, 889–894. [CrossRef]
31. Wakakura, M.; Tsubouchi, T.; Inouye, J. Etizolam and benzodiazepine induced blepharospasm. *J. Neurol. Neurosurg. Psychiatry* **2004**, *75*, 506–507. [CrossRef] [PubMed]
32. Emoto, Y.; Emoto, H.; Oishi, E.; Hikita, S.; Wakakura, M. Twelve cases of drug-induced blepharospasm improved within 2 months of psychotropic cessation. *Drug Heal. Patient Saf.* **2011**, *3*, 9–14. [CrossRef] [PubMed]

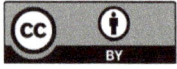

© 2020 by the authors. Licensee MDPI, Basel, Switzerland. This article is an open access article distributed under the terms and conditions of the Creative Commons Attribution (CC BY) license (http://creativecommons.org/licenses/by/4.0/).

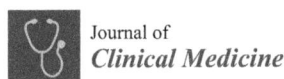

Article

Evaluation of Strip Meniscometry and Association with Clinical and Demographic Variables in a Community Eye Study (in Bangladesh)

Mamunur A.K.M. Rashid [1], Zhang Zhe Thia [2], Calesta Hui Yi Teo [3], Sumaiya Mamun [4], Hon Shing Ong [3,5,6] and Louis Tong [2,3,5,6,*]

1. Ophthalmology, Cornea unit, Al Noor Eye Hospital, 1/9 E, Satmasjid Road, Lalmatia, Dhaka 1207, Bangladesh; mamun3312@gmail.com
2. Yong Loo Lin School of Medicine, National University of Singapore, 10 Medical Drive, Singapore 117597, Singapore; thiazz1995@hotmail.com
3. Ocular Surface Research Group, Singapore Eye Research Institute, The Academia, 20 College Road, Discovery Tower Level 6, Singapore 169856, Singapore; teohuiyicalesta@gmail.com (C.H.Y.T.); honshing@gmail.com (H.S.O.)
4. Nutrition and Epidemiology, Institute of Nutrition & Food Science, University of Dhaka, Dhaka 1000, Bangladesh; sumaiya.mamun@du.ac.bd
5. Corneal and External Eye Disease, Singapore National Eye Centre, 11 Third Hospital Ave, Singapore 168751, Singapore
6. Eye-Academic Clinical Program, Duke-NUS Medical School, 8 College Rd, Singapore 169857, Singapore
* Correspondence: louis.tong.h.t@singhealth.com.sg; Tel.: +65-6227-7255; Fax: +65-6225-2568

Received: 26 August 2020; Accepted: 14 October 2020; Published: 20 October 2020

Abstract: Strip meniscometry (SM) is a relatively new technique for evaluating inferior tear meniscus. We described SM in an epidemiology study and its potential associations with clinical and tear parameters. This cross-sectional study involved 1050 factory garment workers in Gazipur, Bangladesh. The Ocular Surface Disease Index (OSDI) questionnaire and a standard examination for dry eye and meibomian gland dysfunction (MGD), including the five-second SM, were performed by a single ophthalmologist. The participants' ages were 35.56 ± 12.12 years (range 18–59), with 53.8% women. The overall SM was 7.7 ± 3.6 mm, with skewness of 0.126 and kurtosis of 1.84 in frequency distribution. SM values were significantly lower in men than women, and significantly correlated with schirmers (r = 0.71) and tear break up time (TBUT) (r = 0.89). A lower SM value was associated with higher OSDI, lower Schirmer test, increased MG severity and lower TBUT. In multivariable analysis, when adjusted by age, SM values remained associated with schirmers and TBUT, and inversely associated with OSDI. In a separate regression model, higher SM was associated with increasing age, reduced severity of MGD grading, and increased TBUT. To conclude, SM is a rapid clinical test associated with dry eye symptoms and signs, with findings affected by both tear secretion and tear stability.

Keywords: dry eye disease; meibomian gland dysfunction; ocular surface disease; dry eye symptoms; questionnaire; Bangladesh; global health; epidemiology

1. Introduction

Dry Eye Disease (DED), a multifactorial disease of the ocular surface and loss of homeostasis of the tear film, is associated with visual disturbance, symptoms of ocular discomfort, and tear instability [1–3]. Tear film and Ocular Surface Society Dry Eye Workshop (TFOS DEWS) II reported that this disease affects about 5–50% of the population. The large variation is due to a large number of research studies on small geographically homogeneous populations. The epidemiology sub-committee emphasized the need to expand prevalence studies to more geographical regions, and to include different races and ethnicities [4]. Dry eye can have a significant impact in patients' visual function and quality of life, adversely hindering the ability to carry out daily activities, such as reading or driving. This disease of the ocular surface has thus been an increasing public health concern and it poses significant socioeconomic implications [5–9].

Blepharitis and meibomian gland dysfunction (MGD) are major associated factors of DED. MGD is characterized by chronic abnormalities of the meibomian glands, resulting in altered meibum delivery to the tear film, which can result in poor tear film stability or poor breakup times, a type of dry eye classified as evaporative dry eye. On the other hand, dry eye may also be due to aqueous tear deficiency [10,11].

There is scarce data on the epidemiology of dry eye in developing countries within Asia. In developing countries, dry eye has received minimal clinical management and investigative attention compared to other eye diseases. The healthcare burden of dry eye in such countries is essentially unknown [12]. In Indonesia, the age adjusted prevalence of dry eye symptoms is 27.5% (95% CI: 24.8–32.2) [13]. In this report current smoking and pterygium were independent risk factors for the DED [13].

Bangladesh is a country in South Asia located between India and Myanmar, occupying an area of 57,000 square miles, the 8th most populous country in the world. The per capita GDP of Bangladesh is 4992 USD; the country is considered a low income but has the fastest growing real GDP country in the world. As Bangladesh is a populous country of 163 mil, a properly designed epidemiological study will elicit risk factors and knowledge on dry eye that may not be possible in smaller studies elsewhere.

Among the eye diseases in the urban slums of Dhaka, Bangladesh, ocular surface disease forms an important component. A population-based study in Bangladesh found a prevalence of 17.1% for conjunctivitis, 1.4% for blepharitis, 3.2% for DED, and 3.0% for pterygium. This study had limitations in its methodologies of ocular surface diseases assessment. For example, slit-lamp examination was only used in the study for diagnoses and symptoms were not quantified [14]. However, we believe that the reported figures are also underestimated, because the prevalence rates of conditions like dry eye and blepharitis are known to be higher when clinical symptoms are included [14].

Previous studies have shown that strip meniscometry is a rapid clinical test (five seconds per eye) for the assessment of lower meniscal tear volume and may be useful for screening. Unlike tests like Schirmer's I, it does not induce reflex tearing [15,16]. The results of this test have not been reported in a community setting.

In this study, we performed a community-based study of strip meniscometry in a group of garment factory workers in Bangladesh [17], and potential associations with demographic factors and other clinical factors related to tear function.

2. Experimental Section

2.1. Study Design

This was a cross-sectional study conducted in a single garment factory in the town of Gazipur, Bangladesh. Participants had given informed verbal consent. The study obtained approval from the local institutional review board (Bangladesh Medical Research Council BMRC/NREC/2017-2018/1157, approved on 2 August 2018), and only utilized clinically accepted procedures and complied with the Tenets of Declaration of Helsinki for human research.

2.2. Participants

All participants underwent the following clinical procedures on the initial referral visit.

2.3. Study Procedures

2.3.1. Questionnaire

All participants underwent a symptom evaluation using the Ocular Surface Disease Index (OSDI)© questionnaire (Allergan, Inc., Irvine, CA, USA). Briefly, the OSDI questionnaire consisted of 12 questions, each question graded from 0 to 4. The total OSDI scores on the scale of 0 to 100 were then calculated with the OSDI© (Allergan, Inc., Irvine, CA, USA) formula (sum of scores) × 25/(12 questions), with higher scores representing greater symptoms severity [18].

2.3.2. Strip Meniscometry

Strip Meniscometry (SM) Tube (Echo Electricity Co., Ltd., Fukusima, Japan) has been performed as in previous studies [15,16]. Briefly, one end of the strip was held by the investigator against the lower tear meniscus for five seconds, and the length of wetting of the thread read directly from the millimeter markings provided.

2.3.3. Fluorescein Breakup Time (TBUT)

Briefly, a minimally wet (saline) fluorescein strip (Fluorets, Bausch and Lomb, Rochester, NY, USA) was used to instill fluorescein dye. The procedure for this step has been previously described [19,20].

2.3.4. Schirmer's I Test

The Schirmer's I test was done with standard 5 mm wide test strips (Clement Clark®, Essex, UK) with a notch for folding, and without prior anesthesia. The strips were positioned over the inferior temporal half of the lower lid margin in both eyes, and participants' eyes subsequently closed. After 5 min, the extent of tear wetting of the strip was measured to the nearest mm using a ruler [19].

2.3.5. Meibomian Gland Dysfunction Examination

The characteristics of the meibum secreted was evaluated by one ophthalmologist using the right thumb with gentle pressure, under slit-lamp microscopy and graded as follows: 0: clear meibum, 1: colored meibum with normal consistency, 2: viscous meibum, 3: inspissated meibum, and 4: blocked meibomian gland. This was used as a measure of MGD severity.

2.3.6. Slit-Lamp Examination

Other clinical features were examined using a slit lamp biomicroscope. This included scurfing/crusting, subtarsal papillary reaction [19,21], and regularity of the eyelid margin [22]. Corneal sensitivity was also screened using a cotton wisp [23].

2.4. Statistical Analysis

Statistical analysis was performed using StataCorp. 2013. Stata Statistical Software: Release 13.1. College Station, TX: StataCorp LP.

The SM variable was evaluated for its frequency distribution and normality. The univariate association of SM with continuous variables was evaluated by categorizing these variables into binary categories, and the association evaluated with the T-test. Whenever there were more than two categories, analysis of variance was used to determine the statistical significance. Univariate logistic regression was performed between meniscometry category and sex, age, ethnicity, and the six ocular surface signs (tear break up time (TBUT), fluorescein corneal staining, Schirmer's I test, NLMEG, presence of scurf, and inferior fornix papillary grade).

Multivariate logistic regression was performed with meniscometry category as the dependent variable. We performed models using only the clinical signs and demographics of patients, as well as models introducing the predisposing factors of dry eye such as concomitant drugs and medical conditions. We performed logistic regressions with two thresholds for SM as the dependent variable. Statistical significance was based on alpha of 0.05.

3. Results

3.1. Clinical and Characteistics of Participants

In this study, mean age of participants was 35.56 ± 12.12 years (range 18 to 59). 53.8% were women. 64.2% (95%CI: 61.2–67.1) of participants had dry eye defined as OSDI > 12.

3.2. Distribution of Strip Meniscometry Readings

The distribution is bimodal and not normal (Figure 1). The mean readings were 7.7 ± 3.6.

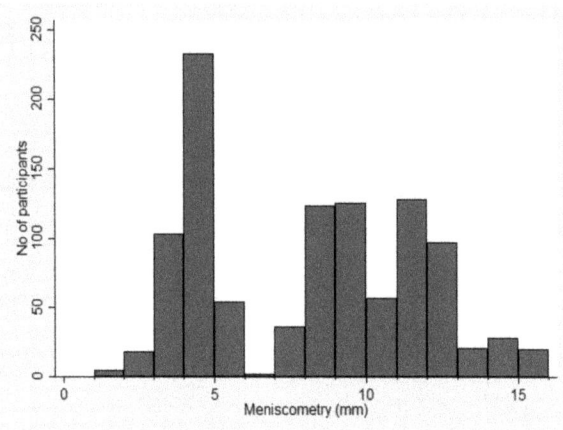

Figure 1. Histogram of strip meniscometry values in factory workers.

3.3. Factors Affecting Strip Meniscometry

The factors associated with SM are shown in (Table 1). When performing a T-test to determine the association between MGD and SM, the three grades of MGD were categorized into two categories for the T-test. The smallest two grades of MGD (MGD Types 0 and 1) are combined into one category, whereas MGD Type 2 was used as the other category.

Table 1. Summary of strip meniscometry readings in this study.

	Participants N (%)	Strip Meniscometry Reading Mean± Standard Deviation (SD) Median (Min, Max)	p Value
Overall	1050 (100%)	7.7 ± 3.6 8 (1, 16)	-
Gender			
Male	485 (46.19%)	7.1 ± 3.8 7 (1, 16)	<0.001
Female	565 (53.81%)	8.1 ± 3.3 9 (2, 16)	
Age			
<30 years	371 (35.33%)	8.4 ± 3.8 10 (2, 16)	<0.001
30–40 years	219 (20.86%)	7.3 ± 3.1 8 (1, 16)	
40–50 years	347 (33.05%)	6.9 ± 3.4 8 (2, 16)	
>50 years	113 (10.76%)	8.1 ± 3.6 9 (2, 14)	

Table 1. Cont.

	Participants N (%)	Strip Meniscometry Reading Mean± Standard Deviation (SD) Median (Min, Max)	p Value
Ocular Surface Disease Index (OSDI)			
Low (<33)	679 (64.67%)	9.7 ± 2.5 10 (3, 16)	<0.001
High (≥33)	371 (35.33%)	3.9 ± 1.4 4 (1, 14)	
Schirmer I test			
Low (<5 mm)	413 (39.33%)	4.0 ± 1.7 4 (1, 14)	<0.001
High (≥5 mm)	637 (60.67%)	10.0 ± 2.3 10 (2, 16)	
Tear Breakup Time (TBUT)			
Low (<5 s)	369 (35.14%)	3.8 ± 1.3 4 (1, 14)	<0.001
High (≥5 s)	681 (64.86%)	9.8 ± 2.5 10 (3, 16)	
Meibomian Gland Dysfunction (MGD) Types			
Type 0	275 (26.19%)	11.2 ± 2.3 11 (3, 16)	<0.001
Type 1	182 (17.33%)	9.8 ± 2.2 10 (4, 16)	
Type 2	593 (56.48%)	5.3 ± 2.4 4 (1, 14)	

Reduced SM readings were associated with increased OSDI (Figure 2A) (r = −0.72, $p < 0.001$), directly correlated with Schirmer (Figure 2B) (r = 0.71, $p < 0.001$), and associated with increased MG severity (Figure 2C) ($p < 0.001$).

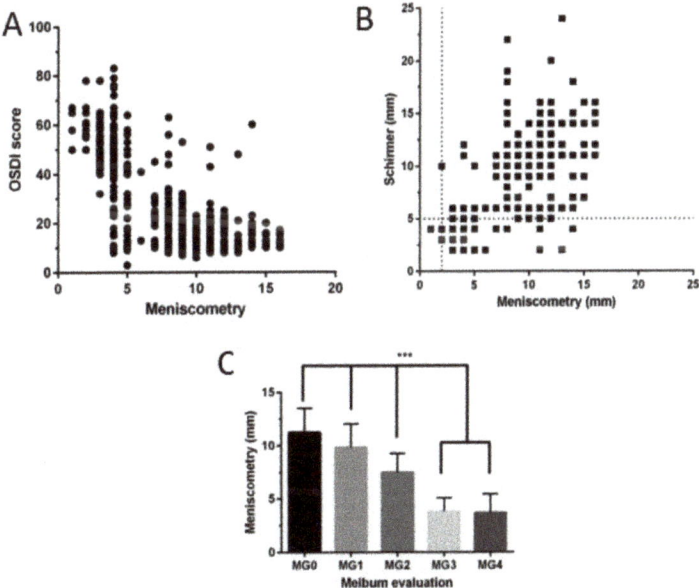

Figure 2. Scatter diagrams showing the relationship between meniscometry and (**A**) Ocular Surface Disease Index (OSDI) scores, (**B**) Schirmer test results. (**C**) Bar graph showing the relationship between meniscometry and meibomian gland dysfunction. MG0: clear meibum, MG1: colored meibum with normal consistency, MG2: viscous meibum, MG3: inspissated meibum, and MG4: blocked meibomian gland. ***: two-tailed p-value for ANOVA and post-hoc tests, $p < 0.001$.

Interestingly, all the 23 subjects with SM < 3 mm had severe dry eye symptoms (OSDI of 33 or more) ($p < 0.001$ on Fischer's exact probability test).

3.4. Multivariate Analysis

We first performed logistic regression with SM categorized as < 7 mm to be low (abnormal), since the mean SM of this study was 7.7 mm. With age, gender, and the clinical parameters as independent variables, we found low values of SM to be significantly associated with higher OSDI and lower Schirmer's readings (Table 2).

Table 2. Multiple logistic regression where dependent variable is the abnormal meniscometry values (< 7 mm)

Parameters	Model 1 Unadjusted Odds Ratio (95% Confidence Interval)	Model 2 [†] Adjusted Odds Ratio (95% Confidence Interval)	Model 3 [††] Adjusted Odds Ratio (95% Confidence Interval)	Model 4 [†††] Adjusted Odds Ratio (95% Confidence Interval)
Age	1.01 (1.00–1.02) *	1.00 (0.99–1.02)	0.97 (0.95–0.99) *	0.97 (0.94–1.00)
Gender	1.85 (1.44–2.38) *	1.83 (1.42–2.35) *	1.67 (1.06–2.63) *	1.09 (0.61–1.94)
OSDI	1.16 (1.15–1.18) *		1.17 (1.15–1.19) *	1.05 (1.02–1.08) *
TBUT	0.43 (0.39–0.47) *			0.87 (0.72–1.05)
Schirmers	0.17 (0.13–0.23) *			0.43 (0.35–0.54) *
MGD	12.15 (8.96–16.48) *			1.42 (0.79–2.57)

[†] Adjusted by Age and Gender; [††] Adjusted by Age, Gender and OSDI; [†††] Adjusted by Age, Gender, ocular surface disease index (OSDI), tear breakup time (TBUT), Schirmers, and meibomian gland dysfunction (MGD); * $p < 0.05$.

However, when we performed logistic regression with SM categorized as <3 mm to be low (abnormal), we found abnormal SM to be significantly associated with higher OSDI and lower TBUT readings after adjustment for the other variables (Model 4 in Table 3). However there were only 23 or 2.19% of participants with SM less than 3 mm, so it may or may not be possible to uncover all the associated factors with this sample size.

Table 3. Multiple logistic regression where dependent variable is the abnormal meniscometry values (< 3 mm).

Parameters	Model 1 Unadjusted Odds Ratio (95% Confidence Interval)	Model 2 [†] Adjusted Odds Ratio (95% Confidence Interval)	Model 3 [††] Adjusted Odds Ratio (95% Confidence Interval)	Model 4 [†††] Adjusted Odds Ratio (95% Confidence Interval)
Age	1.04 (1.00–1.08)	1.03 (1.00–1.08)	1.02 (0.98–1.07)	1.04 (0.99–1.09)
Gender	2.72 (1.11–6.67) *	2.52 (1.02–6.19) *	1.84 (0.70–4.89)	1.37 (0.49–3.82)
OSDI	1.13 (1.09–1.18) *		1.13 (1.08–1.18) *	1.11 (1.06–1.17) *
TBUT	0.41 (0.29–0.60) *			0.48 (0.30–0.77) *
Schirmers	0.59 (0.44–0.78) *			1.33 (0.94–1.86)
MGD grading	4.80 (2.63–8.77) *			1.67 (0.60–4.68)

[†] Adjusted by Age and Gender; [††] Adjusted by Age, Gender and OSDI; [†††] Adjusted by Age, Gender, ocular surface disease index (OSDI), tear breakup time (TBUT), Schirmers, and meibomian gland dysfunction (MGD); * $p < 0.05$.

4. Discussion

The meniscometry readings in this population of garment factory workers in Bangladesh ranged between 1–16 mm, and significantly lower SM readings were found in males, and in participants with higher OSDI, lower TBUT, lower Schirmer's readings, and higher MGD grades.

In the first study performed in a clinic in Japan ($n = 90$), significantly lower SM readings were observed among patients with DED. In addition, the Schirmer's readings, TBUT, mean tear film lipid layer interferometry grade, and vital staining scores were also observed to be lower among patients with DED. With regards to the SM readings, a positive linear correlation exists with the Schirmer's readings as well as the TBUT [16]. In the second study performed in a clinic in Japan ($n = 175$), significantly lower SM readings were observed among patients with DED, with a positive correlation with graticule scale tear meniscus height (TMH) [15].

There were no previous studies of SM in a community setting or study based on the Bangladeshi participants.

In our study (Table 2), lower Schirmer and higher OSDI were associated with abnormal meniscometry values after adjusting for the other clinical variables. This is not surprising since Schirmer's I test, apart from a measure of reflex tear secretion, may also be related to the tear volume in the lower meniscus. With a stricter threshold of SM (Table 3), only lower TBUT and higher OSDI were associated with abnormal SM. This may be related to the pre-existing lower meniscal volume to related to tear stability.

This study involved a large sample in the community within a single occupational group. The use of a uniform protocol by a single ophthalmologist provided an accurate and comprehensive analysis and with a higher confidence of estimates. Since the study did not employ a meibomian gland evaluator, the number of meibomian glands yielding liquid meibum was not documented. The number of subjects with SM less than 3 mm was limited. Another possible limitation is that this study involved only one occupational group. We are not certain why the distribution of SM is bimodal.

5. Conclusions

In conclusion, SM is inexpensive, quick and easy to perform, and may be a suitable tool for epidemiology studies. Although associated with dry eye symptoms, this test is not equivalent to any one of the conventional tests, but still related to some aspect of tear function. It should be explored in other populations.

Author Contributions: Data collection, M.A.K.M.R. and S.M.; methodology, M.A.K.M.R., S.M. and L.T.; conceptualization, L.T.; formal analysis, Z.Z.T., C.H.Y.T. and L.T.; writing—original draft preparation, Z.Z.T., C.H.Y.T. and L.T.; writing—review and editing, Z.Z.T., L.T. and H.S.O.; supervision, L.T.; All authors have read and agreed to the published version of the manuscript.

Funding: This research was funded by National Medical Research Council, grant number NMRC\CSA\017\2017"

Acknowledgments: Funding advisory board or gifts from Santen, Alcon-Novartis, Allergan, B & L, LFAsia, Bioessex, Eye-lens, Dyamed, ZAS Ophthalmic, Bangladesh.

Conflicts of Interest: The authors declare no conflict of interest. The funders had no role in the design of the study; in the collection, analyses, or interpretation of data; in the writing of the manuscript, or in the decision to publish the results.

References

1. Craig, J.P.; Nichols, K.K.; Akpek, E.K.; Caffery, B.; Dua, H.S.; Joo, C.K.; Liu, Z.; Nelson, J.D.; Nichols, J.J.; Tsubota, K.; et al. TFOS DEWS II Definition and Classification Report. *Ocul. Surf.* **2017**, *15*, 276–283. [CrossRef]
2. Wolffsohn, J.S.; Arita, R.; Chalmers, R.; Djalilian, A.; Dogru, M.; Dumbleton, K.; Gupta, P.K.; Karpecki, P.; Lazreg, S.; Pult, H.; et al. TFOS DEWS II Diagnostic Methodology report. *Ocul. Surf.* **2017**, *15*, 539–574. [CrossRef] [PubMed]
3. Craig, J.P.; Nelson, J.D.; Azar, D.T.; Belmonte, C.; Bron, A.J.; Chauhan, S.K.; de Paiva, C.S.; Gomes, J.A.; Hammitt, K.M.; Jones, L.; et al. TFOS DEWS II Report Executive Summary. *Ocul. Surf.* **2017**, *15*, 802–812. [CrossRef]
4. Stapleton, F.; Alves, M.; Bunya, V.Y.; Jalbert, I.; Lekhanont, K.; Malet, F.; Na, K.S.; Schaumberg, D.; Uchino, M.; Vehof, J.; et al. TFOS DEWS II Epidemiology Report. *Ocul. Surf.* **2017**, *15*, 334–365. [CrossRef]
5. Clegg, J.P.; Guest, J.F.; Lehman, A.; Smith, A.F. The annual cost of dry eye syndrome in France, Germany, Italy, Spain, Sweden and the United Kingdom among patients managed by ophthalmologists. *Ophthalmic Epidemiol.* **2006**, *13*, 263–274. [CrossRef] [PubMed]
6. Wlodarczyk, J.; Fairchild, C. United States cost-effectiveness study of two dry eye ophthalmic lubricants. *Ophthalmic Epidemiol.* **2009**, *16*, 22–30. [CrossRef]
7. Sullivan, R.M.; Cermak, J.M.; Papas, A.S.; Dana, M.R.; Sullivan, D.A. Economic and quality of life impact of dry eye symptoms in women with Sjogren's syndrome. *Adv. Exp. Med. Biol.* **2002**, *506*, 1183–1188.

8. Yu, J.; Asche, C.V.; Fairchild, C.J. The economic burden of dry eye disease in the United States: A decision tree analysis. *Cornea* **2011**, *30*, 379–387. [CrossRef]
9. Reddy, P.; Grad, O.; Rajagopalan, K. The economic burden of dry eye: A conceptual framework and preliminary assessment. *Cornea* **2004**, *23*, 751–761. [CrossRef]
10. Chhadva, P.; Goldhardt, R.; Galor, A. Meibomian Gland Disease: The Role of Gland Dysfunction in Dry Eye Disease. *Ophthalmology* **2017**, *124*, S20–S26. [CrossRef] [PubMed]
11. Nichols, K.K.; Foulks, G.N.; Bron, A.J.; Glasgow, B.J.; Dogru, M.; Tsubota, K.; Lemp, M.A.; Sullivan, D.A. The international workshop on meibomian gland dysfunction: Executive summary. *Investig. Ophthalmol. Vis. Sci.* **2011**, *52*, 1922–1929. [CrossRef]
12. Osae, A.E.; Gehlsen, U.; Horstmann, J.; Siebelmann, S.; Stern, M.E.; Kumah, D.B.; Steven, P. Epidemiology of dry eye disease in Africa: The sparse information, gaps and opportunities. *Ocul. Surf.* **2017**, *15*, 159–168. [CrossRef]
13. Lee, A.J.; Lee, J.; Saw, S.M.; Gazzard, G.; Koh, D.; Widjaja, D.; Tan, D.T. Prevalence and risk factors associated with dry eye symptoms: A population based study in Indonesia. *Br. J. Ophthalmol.* **2002**, *86*, 1347–1351. [CrossRef]
14. Sutradhar, I.; Gayen, P.; Hasan, M.; Gupta RDas Roy, T.; Sarker, M. Eye diseases: The neglected health condition among urban slum population of Dhaka, Bangladesh. *BMC Ophthalmol.* **2019**, *19*, 38. [CrossRef]
15. Ibrahim, O.M.A.; Dogru, M.; Ward, S.K.; Matsumoto, Y.; Wakamatsu, T.H.; Ishida, K.; Tsuyama, A.; Kojima, T.; Shimazaki, J.; Tsubota, K. The efficacy, sensitivity, and specificity of strip meniscometry in conjunction with tear function tests in the assessment of tear meniscus. *Investig. Ophthalmol. Vis. Sci.* **2011**, *52*, 2194–2198. [CrossRef]
16. Dogru, M.; Ishida, K.; Matsumoto, Y.; Goto, E.; Ishioka, M.; Kojima, T.; Goto, T.; Saeki, M.; Tsubota, K. Strip meniscometry: A new and simple method of tear meniscus evaluation. *Investig. Ophthalmol. Vis. Sci.* **2006**, *47*, 1895–1901. [CrossRef]
17. Rashid, M.A.K.M.; Teo, C.H.Y.; Mamun, S.; Ong, H.S.; Tong, L. Prevalence and Risk Factors of Severe Dry Eye in Bangladesh-Based Factory Garment Workers. *Diagnostics* **2020**, *10*, 634. [CrossRef]
18. Schiffman, R.M.; Christianson, M.D.; Jacobsen, G.; Hirsch, J.D.; Reis, B.L. Reliability and validity of the Ocular Surface Disease Index. *Arch. Ophthalmol.* **2000**, *118*, 615–621. [CrossRef]
19. Foong, A.W.; Saw, S.M.; Loo, J.L.; Shen, S.; Loon, S.C.; Rosman, M.; Aung, T.; Tan, D.T.; Tai, E.S.; Wong, T.Y. Rationale and methodology for a population-based study of eye diseases in Malay people: The Singapore Malay eye study (SiMES). *Ophthalmic Epidemiol.* **2007**, *14*, 25–35. [CrossRef]
20. Koh, S.; Watanabe, H.; Hosohata, J.; Hori, Y.; Hibino, S.; Nishida, K.; Maeda, N.; Tano, Y. Diagnosing dry eye using a blue-free barrier filter. *Am. J. Ophthalmol.* **2003**, *136*, 513–519. [CrossRef]
21. Peterson, R.C.; Wolffsohn, J.S. Objective grading of the anterior eye. *Optom. Vis. Sci.* **2009**, *86*, 273–278. [CrossRef] [PubMed]
22. Terry, R.L.; Schnider, C.M.; Holden, B.A.; Cornish, R.; Grant, T.; Sweeney, D.; La Hood, D.O.; Back, A.R. CCLRU standards for success of daily and extended wear contact lenses. *Optom. Vis. Sci.* **1993**, *70*, 234–243. [CrossRef] [PubMed]
23. Bruce, A.S. Preliminary Examination. *Contact Lens Pract.* **2018**. [CrossRef]

Publisher's Note: MDPI stays neutral with regard to jurisdictional claims in published maps and institutional affiliations.

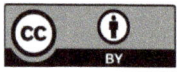

© 2020 by the authors. Licensee MDPI, Basel, Switzerland. This article is an open access article distributed under the terms and conditions of the Creative Commons Attribution (CC BY) license (http://creativecommons.org/licenses/by/4.0/).

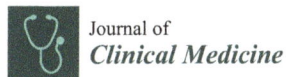

Article

Investigation of Meibomian Gland Function and Dry Eye Disease in Patients with Graves' Ophthalmopathy [†]

Sachiko Inoue [1], Motoko Kawashima [1,*], Reiko Arita [1,2], Ai Kozaki [3] and Kazuo Tsubota [1]

1. Department of Ophthalmology, Keio University School of Medicine, 35 Shinanomachi, Shinjuku-ku, Tokyo 160-8582, Japan; satchin0809@gmail.com (S.I.); ritoh@za2.so-net.ne.jp (R.A.); tsubota@z3.keio.jp (K.T.)
2. Department of Ophthalmology, Itoh Clinic, 626-11 Minaminakano, Minuma-ku, Saitama 337-0042, Japan
3. Olympia Eye Hospital, 2-18-12 Jingumae Shibuya-ku, Tokyo 150-0001, Japan; ai.koz@i.softbank.jp
* Correspondence: motoko-k@a3.keio.jp; Tel.: +81-3-3353-1211
† This paper is an extended version of our paper published in Proceedings of the Japan Cornea Conference 2013, Wakayama, Japan, 14–16 February 2013.

Received: 8 August 2020; Accepted: 28 August 2020; Published: 31 August 2020

Abstract: We prospectively evaluated the relationship between meibomian gland dysfunction (MGD) and Graves' ophthalmopathy (GO) in 19 patients (38 eyes) with subjective dry eye symptoms, compared to 14 age-matched normal participants (14 eyes). Extraocular muscle and lacrimal gland enlargement were evaluated by magnetic resonance imaging (MRI). Ocular surface examinations included fluorescein staining for keratoconjunctival epithelial damage, tear breakup time (TBUT) evaluation, and Schirmer's test. Dry eye symptoms were evaluated with the Dry Eye-related Quality-of-Life Score (DEQS) questionnaire. Lid-margin abnormalities, meibum grade, and meiboscores were assessed using meibography. Clinical activity scores and T2 signal intensity ratios were used to define GO activity. All GO patients had obstructive MGD and 79% exhibited levator muscle enlargement. Ocular surface parameters of TBUT ($p = 0.000$), meibum score ($p = 0.000$), eyelid vasculitis ($p = 0.000$), meiboscore of the upper lid ($p = 0.002$), total meiboscores ($p = 0.001$), and DEQS ($p = 0.000$) significantly differed between GO patients and normal subjects. In addition, GO patients had significantly more abnormalities of the central region of the upper eyelid than normal subjects ($p = 0.000$). Thus, MGD might be related to eye discomfort and deterioration of the ocular surface in GO patients. Inflammation and morphological meibomian gland changes might be characteristic of GO.

Keywords: graves' ophthalmopathy; inflammation; meibomian glands; morphological changes

---

1. Introduction

Graves' ophthalmopathy (GO) is a periocular and orbital inflammatory manifestation that is caused by autoimmune thyroid disease [1]. The pathogenesis of GO involves autoantibodies against thyroid-stimulating hormone (TSH) receptors, which lead to excess production of thyroid hormone. This, in turn, induces an inflammatory response against the periocular and orbital tissues [2–4]. Dry eye disease (DED) is a frequent complaint among patients with GO [2,5], and a high proportion of patients with GO reportedly exhibit dry eye symptoms [5,6]. However, although numerous studies have investigated the pathogenesis of GO, few have offered detailed insight into the association and interaction between GO and DED [2–9]. Moreover, in clinical settings, DED in GO tends to remain neglected.

Regarding the DED mechanism in GO, previous studies have suggested (1) a decrease in tear volume, because the lacrimal gland is one of the target tissues of TSH [2–4], and (2) an increase in palpebral fissure height, leading to accelerated evaporation of tears [10]. Recent studies have suggested that GO pathogenesis is mediated not only by morphological changes but also by immunological causes, including T-cell-mediated inflammation [3] and TSH-receptor expression in the acinar cells of impaired lacrimal glands [2].

Meibomian glands secrete the lipid component of tears, which prevents excessive tear evaporation. Meibomian gland dysfunction (MGD) is considered to be a major cause of evaporative dry eye [11–13]. However, few reports have investigated the relationship between GO and the ocular surface, including both MGD and DED. Therefore, here we investigated the relationship between GO and MGD in patients with GO and dry eye symptoms, using detailed GO information obtained using various modalities, such as magnetic resonance imaging (MRI).

2. Experimental Section

2.1. Patients

This study was a prospective, clinic-based, descriptive study and adhered to the guidelines of the Declaration of Helsinki (as amended in 2013). The study protocol was approved by the institutional review board of the Keio University School of Medicine (No. 20120210). All patients received a full explanation of the study procedures and written informed consent was obtained from each subject prior to enrolment. To ensure privacy, all records were identified by an anonymous subject identification number.

All GO patients were referred to our clinic from Olympia Eye Hospital, Tokyo, Japan. They were diagnosed with GO in accordance with previously described criteria [14]. Additionally, the patients underwent diagnostic imaging by MRI at the hospital. The patients with subjective dry eye symptoms—such as dry eye sensation, foreign body sensation, and photophobia—had been referred to the Keio University Hospital MGD clinic consecutively. Normal participants without GO were also included in this study as controls. All patients underwent a general ophthalmic examination and slit-lamp biomicroscopy. Furthermore, they underwent a more detailed examination of MGD and the ocular surface.

2.2. Ocular Surface Examination

Two investigators with experience of investigation of the ocular surface (M.K. and S.I.) evaluated the tear breakup time (TBUT) as well as keratoconjunctival epithelial damage, on the basis of fluorescein staining scores (0–9) of the cornea and conjunctiva, as described previously [15]. For these tests, 2 μL of preservative-free 0.5% fluorescein dye was instilled into each eye using a micropipette, to avoid altering the tear dynamics. Then, conjunctival rose bengal staining was performed to detect superior limbic keratoconjunctivitis (SLK) and lid wiper syndrome. Finally, Schirmer's test was performed without topical anesthesia.

2.3. Criteria for Dry Eye Diagnosis

A dry eye diagnosis was made according to the latest Japanese dry eye diagnostic criteria (2016) [16]. Briefly, the presence of dry eye symptoms and the presence of qualitative disturbance of the tear film (TBUT ≤ 5 s) both had to be present for a diagnosis of dry eye [16].

2.4. Criteria for Diagnosis of Meibomian Gland Dysfunction

Obstructive MGD was diagnosed when an eye tested positive for all 3 of the following criteria: (1) symptoms of MGD, such as dry eye sensation, burning sensation, foreign body sensation; (2) abnormal findings around the orifices of the glands, and (3) findings indicating meibomian gland orifice obstruction. The presence of any two or more of these findings was defined as a lid margin abnormality in this study. An eye was judged positive for abnormal findings around the orifices when at least 1 of 3 findings, i.e., irregular lid margin, vascular engorgement, or anterior/posterior displacement of the mucocutaneous junction, was recognized. Vascular engorgement was defined as the presence of moderate or severe telangiectasia or redness. An eye was judged positive for orifice obstruction when both findings indicative of meibomian gland orifice obstruction, i.e., decreased meibomian secretion, and plugging, pouting, and ridging were recognized [17]. Meibomian secretion (meibum) was graded as follows: grade 0, clear meibum, easily expressed; grade 1, cloudy meibum, expressed with mild pressure; grade 2, cloudy meibum, expressed with more than moderate pressure; and grade 3, no meibum expression, even with hard pressure [18]. Morphological changes in the meibomian glands were observed using a non-contact mobile meibography system (Japan Focus Corporation, Tokyo, Japan) and graded accordingly [19]. Partial or complete meibomian gland loss was scored using the following grades for each eyelid, as previously described: grade 0, no meibomian gland loss; grade 1, area of meibomian gland loss < 1/3 of the total meibomian gland area; grade 2, area of meibomian gland loss between 1/3 and 2/3 of the total area; and grade 3, area of meibomian gland loss > 2/3 of the total area. Meiboscores (0–6) were summed to obtain a score from 0 through 6 for each eye [20]. The central region was also defined as the middle 1/3 part of the lid width.

2.5. Examination for Graves' Ophthalmopathy

Proptosis (protrusion > 15 mm) was measured using a Hertel exophthalmometer (Handaya, Tokyo, Japan). Lid retraction was defined as a palpebral fissure height > 7 mm [14] and exposure of the upper sclera. In the MRI investigation, levator muscle enlargement was determined in a sagittal section. Swelling of the lacrimal gland and extraocular muscle enlargement was determined in a coronal section. Muscles that were clearly thicker than the optic nerve were determined to be enlarged. GO activity was defined based on clinical activity score (CAS) [21] and T2 signal intensity ratios (T2SIR) [22]. Each patient was assigned a CAS after examination by an ophthalmologist. This score is based on 4 well-known classic signs of inflammation, i.e., pain, redness, swelling, and impaired function, and consists of scores for 10 items. Each sign judged as present is scored 1 point, and each sign has the same weight. The active phase of GO was defined by CAS ≥ 4 points. The T2SIR was defined by the ratio of signal strengths of extraocular muscles and the ipsilateral temporal muscle on T2-weighted images.

The severity of GO was classified using Olympia Eye Hospital diagnostic criteria. The classification of mild GO was as follows: palpebral fissure height was 7–10 mm, lid swelling was mild (eyelids mildly swollen with fluid), the conjunctiva showed chemosis, injection, or congestion; the range of proptosis was 15–18 mm, the extra-ocular muscles exhibited no or intermittent diplopia. Additionally, no optic nerve, retina, or corneal findings were exhibited.

The classification of moderate GO was as follows: palpebral fissure height was 10–12 mm; lid swelling was moderate (eyelid skin showed obvious swelling but the tissue was not tense); the conjunctiva showed SLK; the range of proptosis was 18–21 mm; the extra-ocular muscle showed disorder, as exhibited by diplopia of the peripheral field-of-view; and the cornea showed infiltration due to lagophthalmos that affected the entire cornea. Additionally, no optic nerve or retina findings were exhibited.

Severe GO was classified as severe if the following were present: palpebral fissure height was 12 mm or more, lid swelling was severe (the upper eyelid skin-fold was ballooned out, filled with fluid, and the skin was taught), the conjunctiva showed upper scleral vessel engorgement, the range of proptosis was 21 mm or more, the extra-ocular muscle disorder extended to diplopia of the 1st eye position, the cornea shows infiltration due to lagophthalmos, affecting the entire cornea. Additionally, no optic nerve or retina findings were present.

Furthermore, the most severe form of GO was classified when, in addition to the findings of severe GO, corneal perforation, ulcer, or optic neuropathy were present. If even one of these findings was present, the condition was regarded as the most severe GO.

2.6. Assessment of Subjective Symptoms, Self-Reported via a Questionnaire

A validated dry eye symptom questionnaire, the Dry Eye-related Quality-of-Life Score (DEQS) questionnaire, was administered. The DEQS questionnaire was recently developed in Japan and its internal consistency, test-retest reliability, discriminant validity, and responsiveness to change have all been validated previously [23]. It comprises 15 questions; 6 questions assess ocular symptoms and 9 assess the effect of DED on the quality of life. The 6 questions related to ocular symptoms query respondents on the presence and severity of foreign body sensations, dry eye sensations, pain or soreness, ocular fatigue, eyelid heaviness, and eye redness. The frequency of symptoms is scored from 0 (none) to 4 (highest frequency), and the severity of symptoms is scored from 1 (low) to 4 (high) [23]. The summary scale score ranges from 0 (best) to 100 (worst).

2.7. Statistical Analysis

Data were analyzed using the Statistical Package for the Social Sciences version 26.0 (IBM Corp., Armonk, NY, USA) and Excel® version 14.1.0 (Microsoft®, Redmond, WA, USA). The t-test was used for continuous variables, the Mann–Whitney U-test for ordinal variables and chi-squared test for nominal variables. Statistical significance was indicated at $p < 0.05$.

3. Results

In total, 36 patients were included in this study; 19 were patients with GO and 14 were normal participants. Table 1 shows the characteristics of the 19 GO patients, among whom 1 (2 eyes) had active GO, 18 had hyperthyroidism, and 1 had hypothyroidism. The mean duration of GO was 52.9 ± 21.5 months (Table 1). The mean age of all patients was 44.1 ± 7.9 years (range, 27–56 years). The mean age of GO patients was 44.0 ± 10.0 years (range, 27–56 years) and that of control participants was 44.6 ± 7.6 years (range, 27–56 years). There were no statistically significant differences between GO patients and normal patients ($p = 0.4$). The GO patients comprised of 17 women and 2 men whereas normal participants were all women (Table 2).

Table 1. Clinical characteristics and ophthalmologic parameter of the 19 patients with Graves' ophthalmopathy.

Parameter	Patients with GO ($n = 19$)
Clinical parameters	
Duration of GO, months	52.9 ± 21.5
Active GO, n (CAS ≥ 4)	1
Smokers, n (%)	8 (42.1)
Thyroid function	
Hyperthyroidism, n	18
Hypothyroidism, n	1
Euthyroidism, n	0
Ophthalmologic parameter	
Severity of GO, mild n, (%)	10/19 (52.6)
Moderate n (%)	9/19 (47.4)
Proptosis (>15 mm) n, mm, (%)	38/38, 18.8 ± 1.8, (100)
Eyelid retraction, n (%)	4/38 (10.5)
Palpebral fissure height (>7 mm) n, mm, (%)	33/38, 9.0 ± 2.0 (91.7)
Eyelid swelling, n (%)	22/38 (57.9)
Engorgement of the levator muscle, n (%)	30/38 (78.9)
Engorgement of the extra ocular muscle, n (%)	17/38 (44.7)
Swelling of the lacrimal gland, n (%)	28/38 (73.7)

GO: Graves' ophthalmopathy, CAS: clinical activity score.

Table 2. Clinical parameters of ophthalmic evaluations.

Parameter	Patients with GO (n = 19)	Normal Participants (n = 14)	p Value
Mean age, years (mean ± SD)	44.0 ± 10.0	44.6 ± 2.2	$p = 0.6$
Male, n	2	0	$p = 0.4$
Ocular surface examination			
Lid margin abnormalities, n	19		
Vasculitis, n	19	2	$p = 0.000$
Fluorescein score	0.6 ± 0.8	0.3 ± 0.5	$p = 0.4$
TBUT, s	4.7 ± 3.2	7.1 ± 1.6	$p = 0.000$
SLK, n	0	0	-
Schirmer's test, mm	10.5 ± 8.8	9.2 ± 3.5	$p = 0.5$
Meibum score	1.6 ± 0.5	0.3 ± 0.5	$p = 0.000$
Meibography			
Meiboscores			
Upper lid	1.0 ± 0.6	0.3 ± 0.5	$p = 0.002$
Lower lid	0.9 ± 0.6	0.4 ± 0.5	$p = 0.07$
Total meiboscores	1.9 ± 1.1	0.7 ± 0.8	$p = 0.001$
Abnormalities of central part, n	12	0	$p = 0.000$
DEQS	35.2 ± 28.3	4.3 ± 1.3	$p = 0.000$

TBUT = tear breakup time; SLK = superior limbic keratoconjunctivitis; DEQS = Dry Eye-related Quality-of-Life Score, GO: Graves' ophthalmopathy. All values are expressed as mean ± standard deviation (SD). p-value, vs. normal participants.

3.1. Ocular Surface Examination

In ocular surface investigations, the right eye was selected in GO patients, and their 19 eyes were compared to the 14 eyes of normal participants. Overall, 32 of 38 eyes (84.2%) of patients with GO were diagnosed with DED. Notably, all patients exhibited obstructive MGD. Objective ocular surface parameters are summarized in Table 2. TBUT was significantly shorter in patients with GO than that in normal participants ($p = 0.000$; Table 2). Vasculitis, meibum score, and DEQS were significantly higher in patients with GO than those in normal participants ($p = 0.000$, $p = 0.000$, $p = 0.000$ respectively; Table 2). Upper eyelid meiboscore and total meiboscore (upper and lower eyelid) were significantly higher in patients with GO than in normal participants ($p = 0.002$, $p = 0.001$ respectively; Table 2). Furthermore, abnormalities of the central part of the upper eyelid were significantly more common in patients with GO than in normal participants ($p = 0.000$; Table 2). The fluorescein staining score, Schirmer's test findings, and meiboscore of the lower lid were not significantly different between the two groups. There were no patients with SLK (Table 2; Figures 1 and 2).

3.2. Examination for Graves' Ophthalmopathy

Proptosis was observed in 38 of 38 eyes (100%); the mean proptosis value was 18.8 ± 1.8 mm. The mean palpebral fissure height was 9.0 ± 2.0 mm; of the 38 eyes, 33 (91.7%) exhibited palpebral fissure height > 7 mm. Twenty of 38 eyes (52.6%) exhibited thickening of the eyelids (eyelid swelling). Engorgement of the levator muscle on MR images was seen in 30 of 38 eyes (78.9%) (Figure 1; Figure 2). Engorgement of the extra-ocular muscles on MR images was seen in 17 of 38 eyes (44.7%). Lacrimal gland swelling was observed in 28 of 38 eyes (73.7%), and eyelid retraction was observed in 4 of 38 (10.5%) eyelids (Table 1). In terms of severity of GO, 10 patients were classified as having mild and 9 patients were classified as having moderate disease (Table 1). Only 1 patient was in the acute phase (Table 1).

Detailed data of the ocular surface parameters and GO parameters of the patients are presented in Table 3.

3.3. Representative Cases

3.3.1. Case 1

A 53-year-old woman presented with GO, (disease duration of 60 months), in the inactive phase at presentation. The DEQS score was 25. The patient exhibited eyelid swelling, as well as exophthalmos (19 mm and 18 mm in the right and left eyes, respectively; Figure 1). There was no obvious eyelid retraction; the palpebral fissure height of the right and left eyes was relatively normal and mild (7 mm and 8 mm, respectively). The patient complained of dry eye symptoms, and the TBUT in both eyes was 6 s. In both eyes, the corneo-conjunctival staining score was 1, and the Schirmer's test value was 2 mm. The eyelid margins exhibited plugging (upper lid margin), displacement of the mucocutaneous junction, vascular engorgement (upper and lower lid margins), and inflammation (eyelid and ocular conjunctiva) (Figure 1d). The meibum grade was 1. On the basis of these findings, the patient was diagnosed with MGD. Meibography findings indicated meibomian gland dropout in the upper and lower eyelids of the right eye and the central region of the upper eyelid of the left eye (Figure 1b,c,e,f). Levator muscle swelling in the upper eyelids and lacrimal gland swelling were observed in MR images (Figure 1g–i). The CAS score was 0.

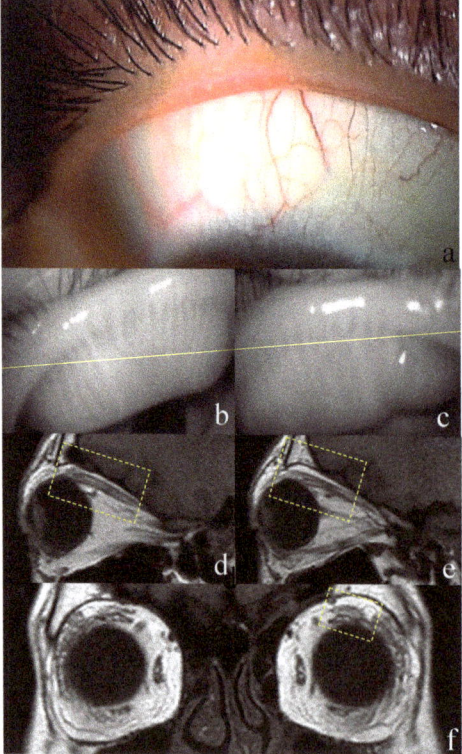

Figure 1. Representative case of a 53-year-old woman with Graves' ophthalmopathy. The patient presented with vascular engorgement, lid-margin inflammation, and plugging of the lid margin (**a**). The meibomian glands at the central region of the eyelids exhibit abnormal findings, particularly in the upper eyelid (**b**,**c**). Magnetic resonance imaging findings show enlargement of the levator muscle and lacrimal gland (**d**–**f**).

3.3.2. Case 2

A 56-year-old woman presented with GO (disease duration of 96 months), in the inactive phase at presentation. The DEQS score was 8.3. Initially, the patient exhibited swelling, chronic inflammation, and pigmentation of the eyelids. Exophthalmos was observed in both eyes (17 mm and 16 mm in the right and left eyes, respectively; Figure 2a). In the follow-up evaluation (current status), no lid retraction was observed, and the palpebral fissure height of both eyes was mild (8 mm, both eyes). The patient complained of dry eye symptoms at presentation, and the TBUT in the right and left eyes was 3 s and 5 s, respectively. The corneo-conjunctival score in both eyes was 0. Schirmer's test values in the right and left eyes were 4 mm and 13 mm, respectively. Evaluation of eyelid margins revealed plugging and vascular engorgement (upper and lower eyelid margins) as well as inflammation (palpebral and ocular conjunctiva) (Figure 2d). Meibum grades in the right and left eyes were 2 and 1, respectively. On the basis of these findings, the patient was diagnosed with DED and MGD. Meibography findings revealed meibomian gland dropout in the upper and lower eyelids of both eyes; both eyes exhibited a meiboscore of 3 (Figure 2b,c,e,f). Levator muscle swelling in the upper eyelid, as well as swelling of the superior, medial, and inferior rectus muscles and lacrimal glands, were observed on MR images (Figure 1g–i). The CAS score was 1.

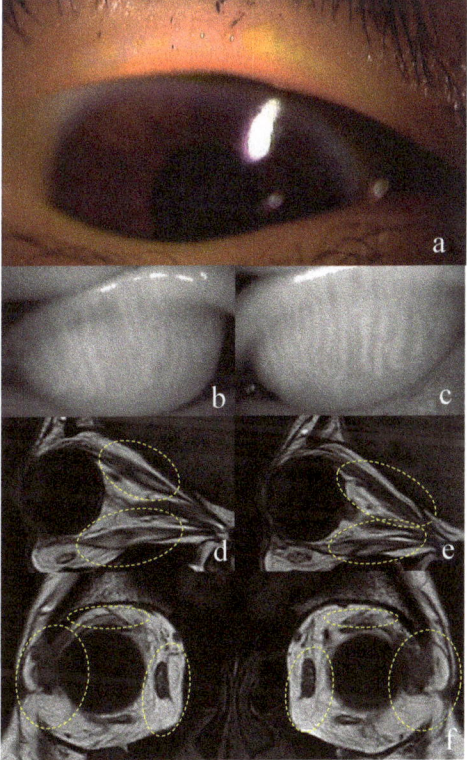

Figure 2. Representative case of a 56-year-old woman with Graves' ophthalmopathy. The patient presented with lid-margin inflammation (**a**). The meibomian glands in the central region of the upper eyelid exhibit abnormal findings (**b,c**). Magnetic resonance imaging findings show (**d,e**) levator muscle and superior and inferior rectus muscle enlargement, as well as (**f**) medial rectus muscle enlargement and swelling of the lacrimal glands.

Table 3. Ocular surface parameters and Graves' ophthalmopathy (GO) severity.

			Fluorescein		Lid margin Vasculitis		Schirmer's Test (mm)	Meibum Grade	Meiboscore			Abnormalities Central Part		DEQS	CAS	GO Severity	Disease Duration	Proptosis	Palpebral Fissure	Engorgement			Swelling	
	Age	Sex	Eye	Score	TBUT (s)	Upper Lid	Lower Lid			Upper Lid	Lower Lid	Total	Upper Lid	Lower Lid							Levator Muscle	Extra-Ocular Muscles	Lacrimal Gland	Eyelid Swelling	Lid Retraction
1	53	F	R	1	6	1	1	2	1	2	2	4	1	0	25	0	2	60	19	7	1	0	1	1	0
2			L	1	6	1	1	2	1	2	0	2	1	0					18	8	1	0	1	1	0
2	56	F	R	2	6	1	1	23	2	1	0	1	1	0	55	5	2	53	19	8	1	0	1	1	0
			L	2	4	1	1	13	2	2	0	0	1	0					18	10	1	1	1	0	0
3	41	F	R	3	4	0	0	9	2	0	0	0	0	0	60	2	1	58	18	8	1	0	1	0	0
			L	0	4	0	0	9	2	0	0	0	0	0					17	9	1	1	1	0	0
4	38	F	R	0	4	1	1	9	1	2	1	3	0	0	55	0	2	60	20	8	1	0	1	1	0
			L	0	3	1	1	6	2	2	1	3	0	0					21	9	1	0	1	1	0
5	47	F	R	1	3	1	1	4	1	0	1	1	1	1	56.7	0	1	24	16	10	1	0	1	1	0
			L	0	2	1	1	0	2	2	0	3	0	0					16	9	1	0	1	1	0
6	38	F	R	0	3	1	1	4	1	1	1	2	0	0	11.6	2	2	60	19	8	1	0	1	1	0
			L	0	4	1	1	19	1	1	0	1	1	0					22	12	1	0	1	1	1
7	42	F	R	0	2	1	1	17	1	1	2	3	1	0	16.6	0	1	24	18	8	0	0	0	0	0
			L	0	2	1	1	2	1	1	0	1	1	1					18	10	0	0	1	1	1
8	28	F	R	0	2	1	0	0	1	2	0	2	1	0	26.7	2	2	48	20	11	1	1	1	1	1
			L	1	0	1	1	3	1	1	1	3	1	1					18	11	1	0	1	1	1
9	45	F	R	0	4	1	0	0	2	2	0	2	1	0	23.3	0	1	60	19	10	1	1	0	1	0
			L	0	4	1	1	1	2	1	1	2	0	0					18	9	1	0	0	1	0
10	39	F	R	2	8	1	1	11	2	2	0	2	0	0	30	1	2	7	18	10	1	1	1	1	0
			L	2	5	1	1	12	2	1	1	2	1	0					19	11	1	0	1	1	0
11	44	F	R	1	4	1	1	6	2	1	1	2	1	0	20	1	1	65	18	6	0	0	0	1	0
			L	0	5	1	0	11	2	1	0	1	1	0					19	8	0	0	0	1	0
12	39	M	R	0	5	1	1	17	1	2	1	3	1	1	21.7	1	1	75	18	9	1	1	1	0	0
			L	0	5	1	1	11	1	1	1	2	1	0					18	9	1	1	1	0	0
13	67	F	R	0	5	1	1	14	2	2	1	3	1	0	35.7	0	1	72	18	8	1	0	1	1	0
			L	0	5	1	1	12	2	1	1	2	0	0					17	7	1	0	1	1	0
14	29	F	R	0	5	1	1	20	1	0	0	0	1	0	3.3	1	1	24	18	9	1	1	1	1	0
			L	0	3	1	1	14	1	1	1	2	1	0					19	9	1	1	1	1	0
15	48	M	R	0	3	1	1	14	2	1	1	2	1	0	58.9	2	2	64	23	9	1	1	1	1	0
			L	0	3	1	1	15	2	2	2	4	0	0					21	12	1	1	0	1	0
16	27	F	R	0	5	1	1	12	2	2	3	4	1	0	10	1	2	48	22	12	1	1	1	1	1
			L	1		1	1	22	2	1	3	4	0	0					23	12	1	1	1	1	0
17	56	F	R	1	3	1	1	3	2	1	2	3	0	0	8.3	1	2	55	18	8	1	1	1	1	0
			L	0	2	1	1	3	2	1	1	2	0	0					20	8	1	1	1	1	1
18	38	F	R	1	6	1	1	35	1	1	1	2	0	0	91.7	1	1	8	16	6	1	1	1	1	1
			L	0	7	1	1	35	2	1	1	2	0	0					17	7	1	1	1	1	1
19	52	F	R	0	3	1	1	4	1	2	1	3	1	0	58.9	0	1	96	17	8	1	0	0	1	1
			L	0	5	1	1	13	2	1	2	3	1	0					16	8	1	0	0	1	0

TBUT: tear breakup time, DEQS: Dry eye-Related Quality-of-Life Score, F: female, M: male, R: right, L: left.

4. Discussion

This study investigated the relationship between ocular surface parameters, including MGD and DED, and GO in patients with dry eye symptoms. A high percentage (84.2%) of the patients were diagnosed with DED. More surprisingly, all patients in this study exhibited obstructive MGD; this proportion was higher than the proportion of patients with DED. Our findings revealed that patients presented with clinical features of vascular engorgement and inflammation of eyelid margins, levator muscle thickening, and in some patients, meibomian gland changes in the central region of the eyelids, based on meibography. TBUT, vasculitis, DEQS, and meiboscores (upper lid and total score) were significantly worse in GO patients than those in the normal controls. Recently, Kim et al. reported that patients with GO exhibited morphological changes in the meibomian glands, which correlated with proptosis and palpebral fissure height [24]. The authors considered that lack of blinking by proptosis and palpebral fissure height in patients with GO was caused by decreased excretion of meibum and gave rise to obstructive MGD. The patients in this study had high meibum grades, which were similar to those previously reported in 60-year-old patients with MGD [25,26]. Recent studies reported that oxidative stress is associated with GO [27,28]. According to another study, oxidative stress resulted in changes in the meibomian glands and meibum composition [29]. In this study, most patients exhibited proptosis and increased palpebral fissure height. Based on previous studies and the results of the present study, we speculated that MGD and deterioration of meibum were caused by morphological changes related to GO and oxidative stress. The meiboscores of patients with GO were significantly higher than that of normal participants in this study, and those previously reported [24]. Furthermore, we found that patients with GO exhibited meibomian gland changes in the central region of the eyelids, particularly of the upper lid, which has not been reported previously. In a previous study of contact-lens users [30], meibography findings revealed negative changes. Hence, the authors concluded that this condition was correlated to the duration of use and chronic irritation caused by the contact-lenses. Most patients (nearly 80%) in the study exhibited levator muscle enlargement. This position might correspond to the superior levator muscles and also SLK. SLK is often observed in patients with GO and is caused by abnormal friction and ocular surface inflammation [31,32]. In a previous study, SLK had a stronger correlation with lid retraction and extra-ocular muscle enlargement in GO patients than in individuals without GO [31,33]. Although, none of our patients exhibited SLK and eyelid retraction, because most patients were in the inactive phase of GO. These results suggest that levator muscle condition may affect the upper central meibomian gland morphology. However, considering the results of our own and previous reports, patients with meibography changes in the center of the eyelids might have inflammation and friction. Furthermore, they may have SLK and lid retraction during the active phase of GO. Hence, we speculated that friction and inflammation may be caused by GO; prolonged duration of GO might lead to changes in the center of the eyelids that are noted by meibography. We also hypothesized that these findings would be a characteristic meibography sign in some GO patients with dry eye symptoms. As in previous studies, TBUT in this study was lower than normal participants. [3,7,8,24]. Proptosis and increased palpebral fissure height have been reported as causes of ocular surface damage in patients with GO [2,4]. In particular, increased palpebral fissure height has been reported to be the most influential factor for tear evaporation [10,34,35]. In our study, most patients exhibited proptosis and increased palpebral fissure height; therefore, we speculated that these anatomical factors were among the reasons for the relatively short TBUT. Furthermore, excessive tear evaporation has been proposed as a cause of hyperosmolarity [35,36].

Tear hyperosmolarity stimulates the production of proinflammatory cytokines at the ocular surface [35,36]. These inflammatory responses are known to be related to T-lymphocytes. It has been reported that GO is caused by T-lymphocyte-mediated stimulation of orbital cells [2,4]. Expression of TSH receptors in GO patients has also been demonstrated, and the lacrimal gland is known as the target organ for TSH [2]. Previously, computed tomography findings have revealed swollen lacrimal glands in patients with GO [37]. In this study, MRI findings showed lacrimal gland swelling, and our patients' Schirmer's test values were lower than those reported in previous studies [7,33]. The rate of vascular engorgement of the lid margin in this study was 97.3%, although, a previous study showed that the rate of this phenomenon in normal controls in women of the same age range was only 14% [20]. We also recognized inflammatory signs around the eyes. Since GO is caused by inflammation and immune-related mechanisms, GO is likely to result in MGD and DED.

This study had a few limitations. First, this was a pilot study and, therefore, the sample size was small; however, we will be conducting a similar study with a larger sample size in the future and include additional comparisons such as those of the active and inactive phases of GO. Second, some selection bias might have occurred, although we included consecutive patients with GO. Inclusion of patients with GO at different stages of activity (active/chronic) and different disease durations might have helped to define the details of the relationship between GO and MGD more specifically, thereby helping to elucidate the point of occurrence of MGD in GO eyes. In addition, in further studies, quantitative markers, such as those reflecting ocular surface oxidative stress and inflammation, should be studied in patients with GO. Furthermore, we would like to investigate the pathophysiological mechanisms and inflammatory pathways (e.g., T-lymphocyte-related pathways and oxidative stress-related pathways) related to MGD in GO patients, using experimental models.

5. Conclusions

In summary, we found strong associations between dry eye symptoms in GO patients and ocular surface parameters, including MGD and DED. These were characterized by meibomian gland dropout at the center of the eyelids, as well as eyelid margin vascular engorgement and inflammation. Inflammation and morphological changes of meibomian glands might be characteristic findings in patients with GO. Although further investigations are required to elucidate the mechanism underlying the association between the ocular surface state, including MGD and DED, and GO, the present findings indicate the possibility that MGD may be involved in causing eye discomfort in patients with GO.

Author Contributions: Conceptualization, M.K. and R.A.; formal analysis, S.I.; investigation, M.K. and S.I.; writing—original draft preparation, S.I.; writing—review and editing, M.K., R.A., A.K. and K.T.; visualization, M.K.; supervision, A.K., K.T.; project administration, M.K. All authors have read and agreed to the published version of the manuscript.

Funding: This research received no external funding.

Conflicts of Interest: R.A. holds the patent of the non-invasive meibography system (JP Patent Registration No. 5281846, US Patent Publication No. 2011-0273550A1, EP Patent Publication No. 2189108A1). R.A. is a consultant for Japan Focus Corporation. No conflicting relationship exists for the other authors.

References

1. Bothun, E.D.; Scheurer, R.A.; Harrison, A.R.; Lee, M.S. Update on thyroid eye disease and management. *Clin. Ophthalmol.* **2009**, *3*, 543–551. [PubMed]
2. Bahn, R.S.; Dutton, C.M.; Natt, N.; Joba, W.; Spitzweg, C.; Heufelder, A.E. Thyrotropin receptor expression in Graves' orbital adipose/connective tissues: Potential autoantigen in Graves' ophthalmopathy. *J. Clin. Endocrinol. Metab.* **1998**, *83*, 998–1002. [CrossRef] [PubMed]
3. Lehmann, G.M.; Feldon, S.E.; Smith, T.J.; Phipps, R.P. Immune mechanisms in thyroid eye disease. *Thyroid* **2008**, *18*, 959–965. [CrossRef]
4. Eckstein, A.K.; Finkenrath, A.; Heiligenhaus, A.; Renzing-Köhler, K.; Esser, J.; Krüger, C.; Quadbeck, B.; Steuhl, K.P.; Gieseler, R.K. Dry eye syndrome in thyroid-associated ophthalmopathy: Lacrimal expression of TSH receptor suggests involvement of TSHR-specific autoantibodies. *Acta Ophthalmol. Scand.* **2004**, *82*, 291–297. [CrossRef] [PubMed]
5. Gürdal, C.; Saraç, O.; Genç, I.; Kırımlıoğlu, H.; Takmaz, T.; Can, I. Ocular surface and dry eye in Graves' disease. *Curr. Eye Res.* **2011**, *36*, 8–13. [CrossRef] [PubMed]
6. Coulter, I.; Frewin, S.; Krassas, G.E.; Perros, P. Psychological implications of Graves' orbitopathy. *Eur. J. Endocrinol.* **2007**, *157*, 127–131. [CrossRef]
7. Selter, J.H.; Gire, A.I.; Sikder, S. The relationship between Graves' ophthalmopathy and dry eye syndrome. *Clin. Ophthalmol.* **2014**, *9*, 57–62.

8. Villani, E.; Viola, F.; Sala, R.; Salvi, M.; Mapelli, C.; Currò, N.; Vannucchi, G.; Beck-Peccoz, P.; Ratiglia, R. Corneal involvement in Graves' orbitopathy: An in vivo confocal study. *Investig. Ophthalmol. Vis. Sci.* **2010**, *51*, 4574–4578. [CrossRef]
9. Rocha, E.M.; Mantelli, F.; Nominato, L.F.; Bonini, S. Hormones and dry eye syndrome: An update on what we do and don't know. *Curr. Opin. Ophthalmol.* **2013**, *24*, 348–355. [CrossRef]
10. Brasil, M.V.; Brasil, O.F.; Vieira, R.P.; Vaisman, M.; do Amaral Filho, O.M. Tear film analysis and its relation with palpebral fissure height and exophthalmos in Graves' ophthalmopathy. *Arq. Bras. Oftalmol.* **2005**, *68*, 615–618. [CrossRef]
11. Lemp, M.A. Report of the National Eye Institute/Industry workshop on clinical trials in dry eyes. *Clao. J.* **1995**, *21*, 221–232. [PubMed]
12. Mathers, W.D. Ocular evaporation in meibomian gland dysfunction and dry eye. *Ophthalmology* **1993**, *100*, 347–351. [CrossRef]
13. Shimazaki, J.; Sakata, M.; Tsubota, K. Ocular surface changes and discomfort in patients with meibomian gland dysfunction. *Arch. Ophthalmol.* **1995**, *113*, 1266–1270. [CrossRef]
14. Kozaki, A.; Inoue, R.; Komoto, N.; Maeda, T.; Inoue, Y.; Inoue, T.; Ayaki, M. Proptosis in dysthyroid ophthalmopathy: A case series of 10,931 Japanese cases. *Optom. Vis. Sci.* **2010**, *87*, 200–204. [CrossRef] [PubMed]
15. Uchino, Y.; Uchino, M.; Dogru, M.; Ward, S.; Yokoi, N.; Tsubota, K. Changes in dry eye diagnostic status following implementation of revised Japanese dry eye diagnostic criteria. *Jpn. J. Ophthalmol.* **2014**, *56*, 8–13. [CrossRef] [PubMed]
16. Tsubota, K.; Yokoi, N.; Shimazaki, J.; Watanabe, H.; Dogru, M.; Yamada, M.; Kinoshita, S.; Kim, H.M.; Tchah, H.W.; Hyon, J.Y.; et al. Asia Dry Eye Society. New perspectives on dry-eye definition and diagnosis: A consensus report by the Asia Dry eye Society. *Ocul. Surf.* **2017**, *15*, 65–76. [CrossRef]
17. Meibomian Gland Dysfunction Working Group. Definition and diagnostic criteria for meibomian gland dysfunction. *Atarashii Ganka.* **2010**, *27*, 627–631.
18. Shimazaki, J.; Goto, E.; Ono, M.; Shimmura, S.; Tsubota, K. Meibomian gland dysfunction in patients with Sjögren syndrome. *Ophthalmology* **1998**, *105*, 1485–1488. [CrossRef]
19. Arita, R.; Itoh, K.; Maeda, S.; Maeda, K.; Amano, S. A newly developed noninvasive and mobile pen-shaped meibography system. *Cornea* **2013**, *32*, 242–247. [CrossRef]
20. Arita, R.; Itoh, K.; Inoue, K.; Amano, S. Noncontact infrared meibography to document age-related changes of the meibomian glands in a normal population. *Ophthalmology* **2008**, *115*, 911–915. [CrossRef]
21. Mourits, M.P.; Prummel, M.F.; Wiersinga, M.; Koornneef, L. Clinical activity score as a guide in the management of patients with Graves' ophthalmopathy. *Clin. Endocrinol.* **1997**, *47*, 9–14. [CrossRef]
22. Tortora, F.; Cirillo, M.; Ferrara, M.; Belfiore, M.P.; Carella, C.; Caranci, F.; Cirillo, S. Disease activity in Graves' ophthalmopathy: Diagnosis with orbital MR imaging and correlation with clinical score. *Neuroradiol. J.* **2013**, *26*, 555–564. [CrossRef]
23. Sakane, Y.; Yamaguchi, M.; Yokoi, N.; Uchino, M.; Dogru, M.; Oishi, T.; Ohashi, Y.; Ohashi, Y. Development and validation of the Dry-eye-Related Quality-of-Life Score questionnaire. *JAMA Ophthalmol.* **2013**, *131*, 1331–1338. [CrossRef]
24. Kim, Y.S.; Kwak, A.Y.; Lee, S.Y.; Yoon, J.S.; Jang, S.Y. Meibomian gland dysfunction in Graves' orbitopathy. *Can. J. Ophthalmol.* **2015**, *50*, 278–282. [CrossRef]
25. Arita, R.; Morishige, N.; Koh, S.; Shirakawa, R.; Kawashima, M.; Sakimoto, T.; Suzuki, T.; Tsubota, K. Increased tear fluid production as a compensatory response to meibomian gland loss: A multicenter cross-sectional study. *Ophthalmology* **2015**, *122*, 925–933. [CrossRef]
26. Arita, R.; Minoura, I.; Morishige, N.; Shirakawa, R.; Fukuoka, S.; Asai, K.; Goto, T.; Imanaka, T.; Nakamura, M. Development of definitive and reliable grading scales for meibomian gland dysfunction. *Am. J. Ophthalmol.* **2016**, *169*, 125–137. [CrossRef]
27. Tsai, C.C.; Wu, S.B.; Cheng, C.Y.; Kao, S.C.; Kau, H.C.; Lee, S.M.; Wei, Y.H. Increased response to oxidative stress challenge in Graves' ophthalmopathy orbital fibroblasts. *Mol. Vis.* **2011**, *17*, 2782–2788.
28. Zarković, M. The role of oxidative stress on the pathogenesis of graves' disease. *J. Thyroid Res.* **2012**, *2012*, 302537. [CrossRef]
29. Ibrahim, O.M.; Dogru, M.; Matsumoto, Y.; Igarashi, A.; Kojima, T.; Wakamatsu, T.H.; Inaba, T.; Shimizu, T.; Shimazaki, J.; Tsubota, K. Oxidative stress induced age dependent meibomian gland dysfunction in Cu, Zn-superoxide dismutase-1 (Sod1) knockout mice. *PLoS ONE* **2014**, *9*, e99328. [CrossRef]

30. Arita, R.; Itoh, K.; Inoue, K.; Kuchiba, A.; Yamaguchi, T.; Amano, S. Contact lens wear is associated with decrease of meibomian glands. *Ophthalmology* **2009**, *116*, 379–384. [CrossRef]
31. Kabat, A.G. Lacrimal occlusion therapy for the treatment of superior limbic keratoconjunctivitis. *Optom. Vis. Sci.* **1998**, *75*, 714–718. [CrossRef]
32. Takahashi, Y.; Ichinose, A.; Kakizaki, H. Topical rebamipide treatment for superior limbic keratoconjunctivitis in patients with thyroid eye disease. *Am. J. Ophthalmol.* **2014**, *157*, 807–812. [CrossRef]
33. Murakami, Y.; Kanamoto, T.; Tuboi, T.; Maeda, T.; Inoue, Y. Evaluation of extraocular muscle enlargement in dysthyroid ophthalmopathy. *Jpn. J. Ophthalmol.* **2001**, *45*, 622–627. [CrossRef]
34. Iskeleli, G.; Karakoc, Y.; Abdula, A. Tear film osmolarity in patients with thyroid ophthalmopathy. *Jpn. J. Ophthalmol.* **2008**, *52*, 323–326. [CrossRef]
35. Gilbard, J.P.; Farris, R.L. Ocular surface drying and tear film osmolarity in thyroid eye disease. *Acta Ophthalmol.* **1983**, *61*, 108–116. [CrossRef]
36. Achtsidis, V.; Tentolouris, N.; Theodoropoulou, S.; Panagiotidis, D.; Vaikoussis, E.; Saldana, M.; Gouws, P.; Theodossiadis, P.G. Dry eye in Graves' ophthalmopathy: Correlation with corneal hypoesthesia. *Eur. J. Ophthalmol.* **2013**, *23*, 473–479. [CrossRef]
37. Harris, M.A.; Realini, T.; Hogg, J.P.; Sivak-Callcott, J.A. CT dimensions of the lacrimal gland in Graves orbitopathy. *Ophthal. Plast. Reconstr. Surg.* **2012**, *28*, 69–72. [CrossRef]

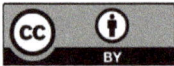

© 2020 by the authors. Licensee MDPI, Basel, Switzerland. This article is an open access article distributed under the terms and conditions of the Creative Commons Attribution (CC BY) license (http://creativecommons.org/licenses/by/4.0/).

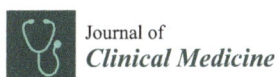

Article

Proposed Algorithm for Management of Meibomian Gland Dysfunction Based on Noninvasive Meibography

Reiko Arita [1,2,*], Shima Fukuoka [2,3] and Motoko Kawashima [2,4]

1. Department of Ophthalmology, Itoh Clinic, 626-11 Minami-Nakano, Minumaku, Saitama 337-0042, Japan
2. Lid and Meibomian Gland Working Group (LIME), Tokyo 112-0006, Japan; fshima3271@gmail.com (S.F.); motoko326@gmail.com (M.K.)
3. Omiya Hamada Eye Clinic, 1-169-1, Sakuragicho, Omiyaku, Saitama 330-0854, Japan
4. Department of Ophthalmology, Keio University, 35 Shinanomachi, Shinjuku-ku, Tokyo 160-8582, Japan
* Correspondence: ritoh@za2.so-net.ne.jp; Tel.: +81-48-686-5588

Received: 15 November 2020; Accepted: 24 December 2020; Published: 27 December 2020

Abstract: Although the pathophysiology of meibomian gland dysfunction (MGD) remains incompletely understood, many treatment options have recently become available. According to an international workshop report, treatment selection for MGD should be based on a comprehensive stage classification dependent on ocular symptoms, lid margin abnormalities, meibum grade, and ocular surface staining. However, it is often difficult to evaluate all parameters required for such classification in routine clinical practice. We have now retrospectively evaluated therapeutic efficacy in MGD patients who received five types of treatment in the clinic setting: (1) meibocare (application of a warm compress and practice of lid hygiene), (2) meibum expression plus meibocare, (3) azithromycin eyedrops plus meibocare, (4) thermal pulsation therapy plus meibocare, or (5) intense pulsed light (IPL) therapy plus meibocare. Patients in each treatment group were classified into three subsets according to the meiboscore determined by noncontact meibography at baseline. Eyes in the IPL group showed improvement even if the meiboscore was high (5 or 6), whereas meibocare tended to be effective only if the meiboscore was low (1 or 2). The meiboscore may thus serve to guide selection of the most appropriate treatment in MGD patients. Prospective studies are warranted to confirm these outcomes.

Keywords: meibomian gland; meibography; meiboscore; meibomian gland dysfunction

1. Introduction

Meibomian gland dysfunction (MGD) is the leading cause of dry eye [1] and has a prevalence that varies widely from 3.5% to 70% according to age, sex, and ethnicity [2]. A population-based study (Hirado-Takushima study) performed on Takushima island in Japan found the prevalence of MGD to be 32.3% [3]. A survey of cataract surgery patients found that 63% of such individuals showed signs of MGD, and MGD was found to adversely affect visual acuity and patient satisfaction after such surgery [4]. According to the European Society of Cataract and Refractive Surgeons (ESCRS) and American Society of Cataract and Refractive Surgery (ASCRS) guidelines for cataract surgery, MGD should be diagnosed and treated before such surgery [5].

MGD is a chronic condition of the meibomian glands that is characterized by terminal duct obstruction or qualitative or quantitative changes in glandular secretion (meibum) [6]. In the obstructive form of MGD, hyperkeratinization of the ductal epithelium results in a reduced availability of meibum to coat the aqueous layer of the tear film [7]. This meibum deficiency thus gives rise to increased tear evaporation and consequent tear hyperosmolarity [8].

MGD is diagnosed on the basis of subjective symptoms, lid margin abnormalities, the condition of the gland orifices, and meibum grade [9]. Approaches such as conventional meibography and confocal microscopy for observation of the morphology of meibomian glands as well as tear interferometry for evaluation of gland function are also available [9], but they are not widely adopted in the clinic. Noncontact meibography is a recently developed noninvasive method that allows relatively rapid imaging of meibomian glands [10] with high reproducibility and which yields images convincing to patients of the need for treatment [11]. It is now widely adopted in clinical practice for evaluation of meibomian gland–related diseases.

Treatment options for MGD have increased greatly—in particular, with the recent advent of nonpharmaceutical treatments [12]—since the International Workshop on Meibomian Gland Dysfunction in 2011 [8]. Selection of a treatment for MGD is currently based on the stage classification proposed at the 2011 workshop [13]. Such stage classification is itself based on a comprehensive evaluation of subjective symptoms, lid margin abnormalities (plugging, vascularity), meibum grade, and degree of ocular surface staining [13]. However, it is often difficult to select a treatment method according to this complicated classification in the clinic. Moreover, it is unclear at what stage nonpharmaceutical treatment options, such as intraductal probing [14], thermal pulsation therapy [15], and intense pulsed light [16], should be performed.

We have therefore now conducted a retrospective examination of the characteristics of MGD patients who visited Itoh Clinic and received one of five types of treatment. The efficacy of each treatment was reevaluated from the viewpoint of noninvasive meibography grading (meiboscore) at baseline [10].

2. Experimental Section

This retrospective randomized study was conducted at Itoh Clinic in Saitama, Japan, adhered to the tenets of the Declaration of Helsinki, and was approved by the Institutional Review Board of the Faculty of Medicine at Itoh Clinic (approval code: IRIN201302-05). Written informed consent was obtained from all participants.

2.1. Patients and Treatment

Patients with MGD who attended Itoh Clinic between April 2014 and September 2020 were eligible for enrollment. One clinician (R.A.) who is an expert on MGD diagnosed the condition and enrolled MGD patients. The patients were consecutively enrolled in the study, with their baseline characteristics being found not to differ significantly among the treatment groups. Inclusion criteria were as follows: (1) an age of at least 20 years; (2) a diagnosis of MGD according to Japanese diagnostic criteria [17] including ocular symptoms, plugged gland orifices, vascularity and irregularity of lid margins, and decreased meibum quality and quantity (Shimazaki grading) [18]. Exclusion criteria comprised active ocular infection, ocular inflammatory disease, or aqueous-deficient dry eye (Schirmer test value of ≤5 mm). All enrolled patients performed meibocare, defined as warming of eyelids and the practice of lid hygiene twice a day. Five types of therapy were conducted during the study period: (1) meibocare alone for 3 months (years 2014–2016), (2) four sessions of meibum expression with an Arita meibomian gland compressor (Katena) 3 weeks apart together with meibocare over 3 months (MGX group) (years 2015–2016), (3) instillation of azithromycin eyedrops, Azimychin, Senju) for 2 weeks together with meibocare (AZM group) (years 2019–2020), (4) one session of treatment with a LipiFlow thermal pulsation system (Johnson & Johnson) together with meibocare for 1 month (years 2015–2017), and (5) four sessions of treatment with intense pulsed light (M22, Lumenis) 3 weeks apart together with meibocare over 3 months (IPL group) (years 2016–2019). All patients were allowed to apply artificial tears four times a day. All patients were examined before and 1 month after the end of the treatment period.

2.2. Clinical Examinations

Ocular symptoms were assessed with the Standardized Patient Evaluation of Eye Dryness (SPEED) questionnaire [19]. The thickness of the lipid layer of the tear film (LLT) was measured with a LipiView interferometer (Johnson & Johnson). Lid margin abnormalities [20]—including plugging (scale of 0–3) and vascularity (scale of 0–3)—as well as the fluorescein-based breakup time of the tear film (FBUT), corneal-conjunctival fluorescein staining (fluo) score (scale of 0–9) [21], and grade of meibum expressed with digital pressure (scale of 0–3) [18] were evaluated by slitlamp microscopy. The meiboscore (0–3 for each eyelid), which reflects the extent of meibomian gland loss, was determined with a noncontact meibography system (Topcon) [10], and the meiboscore for both eyelids was summed (total of 0–6) (Figure 1) [10]. The volume of tear fluid was measured by Schirmer's test performed without the administration of anesthetic [22]. Eyes were categorized as showing an improvement (that is, treatment was effective) if the SPEED score had decreased by ≥4 points [23] and meibum grade had decreased by ≥1 point after treatment compared with before treatment. Data for this study were obtained from the right eye of each subject unless the right eye was excluded, in which case data from the left eye were used.

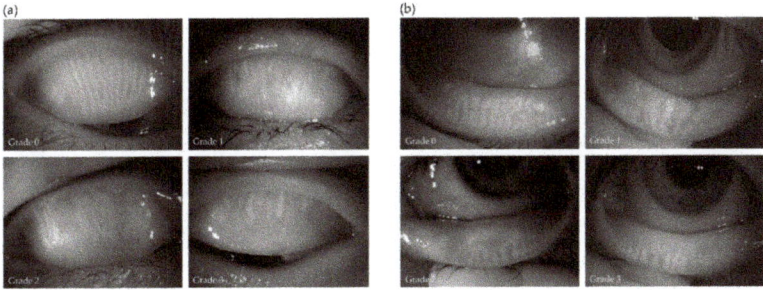

Figure 1. Representative images obtained by noncontact meibography from upper (**a**) and lower (**b**) eyelids with a meiboscore of 0 to 3. The lost area of meibomian glands was graded as 0 for no loss (upper left panels), 1 for a lost area of less than one-third (upper right panels), 2 for a lost area of between one-third and two-thirds (lower left panels), or 3 for a lost area of more than two-thirds (lower right panels).

2.3. Statistical Analysis

Data were found to be nonnormally distributed with the Shapiro-Wilk test ($p < 0.05$), and nonparametric testing was therefore applied. Baseline variables were compared among the treatment groups with Dunn's multiple-comparison test. The Wilcoxon signed-rank test was used to compare variables between baseline and after treatment. The outcome variables of the study were the SPEED score and meibum grade before and after treatment. We performed a statistical power analysis for both the SPEED score and meibum grade. For the SPEED score, the mean difference between before after treatment was 5.3, with a corresponding SD of 4.5; for meibum grade, the mean difference was 1.1 with an SD of 1.0. These changes were calculated from the results of all 165 eyes in the current study. The average number of eyes in each group was 33. The power ($1 - \beta$) was 0.91 and 0.86 at the level of $\alpha = 0.05$ for the SPEED score and meibum grade, respectively, and the sample size was sufficient. Statistical analysis was performed with JMP Pro version 15 software (SAS). Statistical tests were two sided, and a p value of <0.05 was considered statistically significant.

3. Results

3.1. Patient Characteristics

A total of 165 patients was enrolled in this study. The characteristics of the study subjects before and after treatment are presented in Table 1. None of the measured parameters at baseline differed significantly among the five treatment groups (Table 2).

Table 1. Characteristics of the study subjects with meibomian gland dysfunction before and after treatment in the meibocare, meibomian gland expression (MGX), azithromycin eyedrop (AZM), LipiFlow, and intense pulsed light (IPL) groups.

Characteristic	Pre- or Posttreatment	Meibocare (n = 30 Eyes)	MGX (n = 30 Eyes)	AZM (n = 38 Eyes)	LipiFlow (n = 30 Eyes)	IPL (n = 37 Eyes)
Sex (male/female)		17/13	16/14	20/18	16/14	22/15
Age (years)		59.1 ± 18.7	58.9 ± 15	60.2 ± 16	62.9 ± 14.2	60.5 ± 18
Duration of dry eye (years)		4.4 ± 2.5	4.2 ± 2.3	4.4 ± 2.2	4.3 ± 3.5	4.3 ± 2.3
SPEED score (0–28)	Pre	12.2 ± 3.9	12.5 ± 4.2	12.6 ± 4	11.3 ± 3	13.4 ± 3.2
	Post	9.0 ± 3.6	8.9 ± 4.9	6.2 ± 4.5	8.7 ± 4.2	3.7 ± 2.8
	p value	<0.001 **	<0.001 **	<0.001 **	<0.001 **	<0.001 **
LLT (nm)	Pre	54.8 ± 19.6	53.4 ± 11.6	57.9 ± 20.5	59.8 ± 17.9	56.2 ± 23.7
	Post	53.0 ± 18.3	59.3 ± 14.8	61.7 ± 19.2	65.2 ± 27.8	65.4 ± 22.5
	p value	0.11	0.031 *	0.36	0.015 *	0.10
Plugging (0–3)	Pre	2.1 ± 0.8	2.1 ± 0.8	2.0 ± 0.6	2.0 ± 0.8	2.3 ± 0.9
	Post	1.9 ± 0.9	1.6 ± 0.9	0.9 ± 0.8	1.4 ± 0.9	0.2 ± 0.4
	p value	0.057	<0.001 **	<0.001 **	<0.001 **	<0.001 **
Vascularity (0–3)	Pre	1.3 ± 0.5	1.4 ± 0.9	1.6 ± 0.6	1.7 ± 1.0	1.4 ± 0.7
	Post	1.3 ± 0.4	1.4 ± 0.9	0.6 ± 0.6	1.4 ± 1.0	0.2 ± 0.4
	p value	0.33	1	0.006 *	<0.001 **	<0.001 **
FBUT (s)	Pre	3.1 ± 1.2	3.0 ± 1.1	3.2 ± 1.0	3.3 ± 0.7	3.1 ± 1.2
	Post	3.4 ± 1.3	3.9 ± 0.6	5.8 ± 2.8	3.1 ± 1.7	6.7 ± 2.4
	p value	0.030 *	<0.001 **	0.37	<0.001 **	<0.001 **
Fluo score (0–9)	Pre	0.8 ± 0.6	0.8 ± 0.8	1.0 ± 1.2	0.9 ± 0.6	1.0 ± 1.1
	Post	0.6 ± 0.6	0.5 ± 0.7	0.4 ± 1.0	0.8 ± 0.6	0.1 ± 0.3
	p value	0.006 *	0.001 **	0.043 *	<0.001 **	<0.001 **
Meibum grade (0–3)	Pre	2.3 ± 0.5	2.4 ± 0.5	2.3 ± 0.4	2.3 ± 0.4	2.6 ± 0.5
	Post	1.8 ± 0.9	1.6 ± 0.9	1.2 ± 0.8	1.7 ± 1.0	0.1 ± 0.4
	p value	<0.001 **	<0.001 **	<0.001 **	<0.001 **	<0.001 **
Meiboscore (0–6)	Pre	3.8 ± 1.7	3.8 ± 1.7	3.8 ± 1.6	3.8 ± 1.8	3.9 ± 1.5
Schirmer test value (mm)	Pre	10.9 ± 4.2	12.4 ± 9.1	10.6 ± 5.8	9.7 ± 5.6	11.0 ± 6.7
	Post	10.3 ± 4.3	12.0 ± 9	8.5 ± 4.6	9.0 ± 7.3	10.6 ± 6.9
	p value	0.056	0.169	0.16	0.11	0.003 *

Data are means ± SD. p values for comparisons between pre- and posttreatment were determined with the Wilcoxon signed-rank test (* $p < 0.05$, ** $p < 0.001$). SPEED, Standardized Patient Evaluation of Eye Dryness; LLT, lipid layer thickness of the tear film; FBUT, tear film breakup time with fluorescein; fluo, fluorescein staining.

Table 2. Comparison of the baseline characteristics of the study subjects with meibomian gland dysfunction in the meibocare, meibomian gland expression (MGX), azithromycin eyedrop (AZM), LipiFlow, and intense pulsed light (IPL) groups.

Characteristic				*p* Value		
Age	Treatment	Meibocare	MGX	AZM	LipiFlow	
	MGX	1				
	AZM	1	1			
	LipiFlow	1	1	1		
	IPL	1	1	1	1	
Duration of dry eye	Treatment	Meibocare	MGX	AZM	LipiFlow	
	MGX	1				
	AZM	1	1			
	LipiFlow	1	1	1		
	IPL	1	1	1	1	
SPEED score	Treatment	Meibocare	MGX	AZM	LipiFlow	
	MGX	1				
	AZM	1	1			
	LipiFlow	1	1	1		
	IPL	0.62	1	1	0.098	
LLT	Treatment	Meibocare	MGX	AZM	LipiFlow	
	MGX	1				
	AZM	1	1			
	LipiFlow	1	1	1		
	IPL	1	1	1	1	
Plugging	Treatment	Meibocare	MGX	AZM	LipiFlow	
	MGX	1				
	AZM	1	1			
	LipiFlow	1	1	1		
	IPL	1	1	0.50	0.99	
Vascularity	Treatment	Meibocare	MGX	AZM	LipiFlow	
	MGX	1				
	AZM	0.68	1			
	LipiFlow	0.44	1	1		
	IPL	1	1	1	1	
FBUT	Treatment	Meibocare	MGX	AZM	LipiFlow	
	MGX	1				
	AZM	1	1			
	LipiFlow	1	1	1		
	IPL	1	1	1	1	
Fluo score	Treatment	Meibocare	MGX	AZM	LipiFlow	
	MGX	1				
	AZM	1	1			
	LipiFlow	1	1	1		
	IPL	1	1	1	1	

Table 2. Cont.

Characteristic			p Value		
Meibum grade	Treatment	Meibocare	MGX	AZM	LipiFlow
	MGX	1			
	AZM	1	1		
	LipiFlow	1	1	1	
	IPL	0.24	0.90	0.062	0.11
Meiboscore	Treatment	Meibocare	MGX	AZM	LipiFlow
	MGX	1			
	AZM	1	1		
	LipiFlow	1	1	1	
	IPL	1	1	1	1
Schirmer test value	Treatment	Meibocare	MGX	AZM	LipiFlow
	MGX	1			
	AZM	1	1		
	LipiFlow	0.83	1	1	
	IPL	1	1	1	1

p values were determined with Dunn's multiple-comparison test. SPEED, Standardized Patient Evaluation of Eye Dryness; LLT, lipid layer thickness of the tear film; FBUT, tear film breakup time with fluorescein; fluo, fluorescein staining.

Previous therapies for the enrolled patients are shown in Table 3, with most individuals having been prescribed eyedrops including hyaluronic acid eyedrops, preservative-free artificial tears, diquafosol eyedrops, topical steroid eyedrops, and rebamipide eyedrops. About half of the patients had performed meibocare or undergone meibomian gland expression. None of them had previously received azithromycin eyedrops, LipiFlow treatment, or intense pulsed light therapy.

Table 3. Previous therapies for the study patients with meibomian gland dysfunction in the meibocare, meibomian gland expression (MGX), azithromycin eyedrop (AZM), LipiFlow, and intense pulsed light (IPL) groups.

Therapy	No. (%) of Patients				
	Meibocare ($n = 30$)	MGX ($n = 30$)	AZM ($n = 38$)	LipiFlow ($n = 30$)	IPL ($n = 37$)
Hyaluronic acid eyedrops	17 (56.7%)	20 (66.7%)	25 (65.8%)	25 (83.3%)	30 (81.1%)
Preservative-free artificial tears	15 (50.0%)	18 (60.0%)	15 (39.5%)	10 (33.3%)	14 (37.8%)
Diquafosol eyedrops	5 (16.7%)	7 (23.3%)	10 (26.3%)	15 (50.0%)	20 (54.1%)
Topical steroid eyedrops	8 (26.7%)	6 (20.0%)	10 (26.3%)	9 (30.0%)	10 (27.0%)
Rebamipide eyedrops	3 (10.0%)	5 (16.7%)	6 (15.8%)	8 (26.7%)	10 (27.0%)
Meibocare	-	12 (40.0%)	16 (42.1%)	15 (50.0%)	20 (54.1%)
Meibomian gland expression	12 (40.0%)	-	15 (39.4%)	15 (50.0%)	15 (40.5%)
Azithromycin eyedrops	0 (0.0%)	0 (0.0%)	-	0 (0.0%)	0 (0.0%)
LipiFlow	0 (0.0%)	0 (0.0%)	0 (0.0%)	-	0 (0.0%)
Intense pulsed light	0 (0.0%)	0 (0.0%)	0 (0.0%)	0 (0.0%)	-

3.2. Treatment Efficacy

The SPEED score was significantly reduced at 1 month after the end of the treatment period for all treatment groups (Table 1). LLT was significantly increased in the MGX group and the LipiFlow group. Plugging was significantly improved in all groups with the exception of the meibocare group. Vascularity was significantly improved in the AZM group, the LipiFlow group, and the IPL group. FBUT was significantly prolonged in all groups with the exception of the AZM group and the LipiFlow group. The fluo score was significantly decreased in all groups. Meibum grade was significantly improved in all groups.

3.3. Treatment Efficacy According to the Meiboscore

Eyes in each treatment group were graded on the basis of the meiboscore (1 or 2, mild gland loss; 3 or 4, moderate gland loss; 5 or 6, severe gland loss) at baseline (Figure 1). Eyes were also categorized as showing improvement (treatment was effective) if the SPEED score decreased by ≥4 points and meibum grade decreased by ≥1 point compared with the values before treatment. In the meibocare group, 100% of patients with mild gland loss showed improvement (Table 4). However, none of those with moderate or severe gland loss showed improvement. In the MGX group, 88% of patients with mild gland loss improved, compared with 55% of those with moderate gland loss and none of those with severe gland loss. In the AZM group, 92% of patients with mild gland loss and 100% of those with moderate gland loss improved, whereas none of those with severe gland loss did so. In the LipiFlow group, 75%, 10%, and 0% of patients with mild, moderate, or severe gland loss, respectively, showed improvement. Finally, in the IPL group, all patients with mild to severe gland loss improved.

Table 4. Improvement of eyes with meibomian gland dysfunction after treatment in the meibocare, meibomian gland expression (MGX), azithromycin eyedrop (AZM), LipiFlow, and intense pulsed light (IPL) groups according to the meiboscore at baseline.

Meiboscore	Meibocare Improved/Total	MGX Improved/Total	AZM Improved/Total	LipiFlow Improved/Total	IPL Improved/Total
1 or 2	8/8 (100%)	7/8 (88%)	11/12 (92%)	6/8 (75%)	10/10 (100%)
3 or 4	0/11 (0%)	6/11 (55%)	13/13 (100%)	1/10 (10%)	14/14 (100%)
5 or 6	0/11 (0%)	0/11 (0%)	0/13 (0%)	0/12 (0%)	13/13 (100%)

Eyes were categorized as showing improvement if the SPEED score decreased by ≥4 points and meibum grade decreased by ≥1 point compared with the values before treatment.

4. Discussion

Diagnosis of MGD is largely made on the basis of the combination of subjective symptoms and the findings of slitlamp microscopy [9], but the guidelines for treatment selection according to disease severity are not clear. Given that more than half of MGD patients have no symptoms [20] and it is difficult to estimate the disease duration [20], existing guidelines are insufficient for accurate determination of MGD severity. We have now performed a retrospective assessment of the efficacy of five different types of treatment based on the meiboscore for MGD patients who attended Itoh Clinic. Our findings suggest that some treatment options can be selected according to the extent of disruption of meibomian gland morphology apparent in images obtained by noncontact meibography.

Meibography has been improved substantially since its introduction by Tapie in 1977 [24], but it was originally invasive and was not widely applied clinically. The development of noninvasive meibography based on infrared light [10] made it possible to observe meibomian glands of patients in general clinical practice, and it has served as a basis for many clinical studies [11,25]. It has thus not only revealed changes in meibomian gland morphology associated with various ocular surface diseases and provided insight into disease pathophysiology [25], but also highlighted the importance of diagnosis and treatment of MGD in many types of ophthalmology patients, including those treated with antiglaucoma eyedrops [26,27] or undergoing cataract surgery [4], as well as children and adolescents [28,29]. The specificity and sensitivity for MGD diagnosis based on the morphology of meibomian glands are high at 85% and 96.7%, respectively [30]. Meibography images convince patients of the need for treatment and are useful for obtaining informed consent in clinical studies. However, it is difficult to finely quantify meibomian gland area in such images, and they are not suitable for monitoring because gland area is not readily recovered by treatment. Tests of meibomian gland function such as meibum grading are relatively subjective. Tear interferometry is quantitative, but the findings are readily influenced by conditions such as humidity, room and body temperature, and eye makeup. On the other hand, meibography is objective and highly reproducible and can accurately diagnose MGD [31] and evaluate disease status [31,32]. Assessment of both gland morphology and function would be the ideal way to evaluate the efficacy of MGD treatment in the future. Given the retrospective nature of the present study, however, the efficacy of MGD treatment was evaluated by one expert clinician according to the meiboscore in order to minimize potential bias.

The five types of treatment performed at Itoh Clinic during the study period are administered (prescribed) for MGD in Japan. Given that the times the various treatments were launched in Japan differ, the times they were performed also differed. Patients were consecutively enrolled in the study, and there was no significant difference in baseline characteristics among the treatment groups. All five treatment types significantly improved subjective symptoms and objective tear parameters compared with baseline. However, our analysis of treatment efficacy according to the meiboscore at baseline revealed that meibocare tended to be effective only for eyes at the mild stage of MGD and that intense pulsed light was effective at all stages and was the only effective treatment for eyes at the severe stage of the disease characterized by many gland dropouts. The efficacies of meibomian gland expression and the LipiFlow device tended to be similar, consistent with the results of a previous study suggesting that LipiFlow is not effective in eyes with many gland dropouts [33]. We defined improvement of eyes with MGD as a decrease in the SPEED score of ≥4 points and a decrease in meibum grade of ≥1 point in our study. Our results do not imply that intense pulsed light induced regeneration of meibomian glands, however. The efficacy of intense pulsed light may depend on an anti-inflammatory action as well as on melting of meibum, and it may therefore be more effective for severe MGD associated with many gland dropouts than is the LipiFlow device, whose efficacy is thought to rely on meibum melting and gland massage. In addition, the standard protocol for intense pulsed light therapy applied in the present study consists of four sessions at 3-week intervals, whereas the standard protocol for LipiFlow is a single application. This difference might have affected the results of our study. Moreover, MGD patients treated with the LipiFlow device showed a significant improvement in symptoms and most signs.

In the present study, we summed the meiboscores for the upper and lower eyelids [10]. It remains controversial, however, whether the meiboscore should be evaluated for the upper eyelid alone, the lower eyelid alone, or both eyelids [34]. Changes apparent in the upper and lower eyelids are not always similar, and it is important to determine the reserve capacity of both upper and lower meibomian glands from the viewpoint of the oil reservoir for coating the entire ocular surface. With regard to assessment of the severity of MGD and selection of a treatment method, it would be desirable to make a comprehensive judgment based on the sum of the meiboscores of the upper and lower meibomian glands.

Tear film breakup time was measured with fluorescein in this study, which began before publication of the TFOS DEWS II report [35] that recommended the use of noninvasive measures of tear film stability. The invasiveness of the procedure in the present study was minimized by gently applying the fluorescein-stained paper to the conjunctival sac and asking the patient to blink twice.

Limitations of the present study include its retrospective nature, with the result that there was no washout period for previous treatments prior to the selected treatment. All patients also received meibocare in addition to the selected specific treatment option. In addition, the treatment periods and applications were set according to the treatment protocols and so differed among the patient groups. It should be considered in the future whether these differences can be minimized.

In conclusion, our results suggest that the most appropriate treatment can be selected for each MGD patient on the basis of the meiboscore. When meibomian gland loss is early and mild or moderate, several treatment options are available. When meibomian gland loss is severe, intense pulsed light treatment is recommended. Meibography may thus predict the effectiveness of future treatment and thereby inform selection of the best treatment option for each patient, especially for individuals with many gland dropouts. Future prospective studies are needed to confirm the outcomes of the present study.

Author Contributions: Conceptualization, R.A.; formal analysis, S.F.; investigation, R.A.; writing—original draft preparation, R.A.; writing—review and editing, S.F. and M.K.; supervision, R.A.; project administration, R.A. All authors have read and agreed to the published version of the manuscript.

Funding: This research received no external funding.

Institutional Review Board Statement: The study was conducted according to the guidelines of the Declaration of Helsinki, and approved by the Institutional Review Board of Itoh Clinic (approval code: IRIN201302-05, date of approval: 25 February 2013).

Informed Consent Statement: Informed consent was obtained from all subjects involved in the study.

Data Availability Statement: The data presented in this study are available on request from the corresponding author.

Conflicts of Interest: R.A. has the patent of the non-invasive meibography system (JP Patent Registration No. 5281846, US Patent Publication No.2011-0273550A1, EP Patent Publication No. 2189108A1). R.A. is a consultant for Inami Co., KOWA company and TOPCON Japan. No conflicting relationship exists for the other authors.

References

1. Lemp, M.A.; Crews, L.A.; Bron, A.J.; Foulks, G.N.; Sullivan, B.D. Distribution of aqueous-deficient and evaporative dry eye in a clinic-based patient cohort: A retrospective study. *Cornea* **2012**, *31*, 472–478. [CrossRef] [PubMed]
2. Schaumberg, D.A.; Nichols, J.J.; Papas, E.B.; Tong, L.; Uchino, M.; Nichols, K.K. The international workshop on meibomian gland dysfunction: Report of the subcommittee on the epidemiology of, and associated risk factors for, MGD. *Investig. Ophthalmol. Vis. Sci.* **2011**, *52*, 1994–2005. [CrossRef] [PubMed]
3. Arita, R.; Mizoguchi, T.; Kawashima, M.; Fukuoka, S.; Koh, S.; Shirakawa, R.; Suzuki, T.; Morishige, N. Meibomian Gland Dysfunction and Dry Eye are Similar, but Different based on a Population-Based Study (Hirado-Takushima Study) in Japan. *Am. J. Ophthalmol.* **2019**, *207*, 410–418. [CrossRef] [PubMed]
4. Cochener, B.; Cassan, A.; Omiel, L. Prevalence of meibomian gland dysfunction at the time of cataract surgery. *J. Cataract. Refract. Surg.* **2018**, *44*, 144–148. [CrossRef] [PubMed]
5. Starr, C.E.; Gupta, P.K.; Farid, M.; Beckman, K.A.; Chan, C.C.; Yeu, E.; Gomes, J.A.P.; Ayers, B.D.; Berdahl, J.P.; Holland, E.J.; et al. An algorithm for the preoperative diagnosis and treatment of ocular surface disorders. *J. Cataract. Refract. Surg.* **2019**, *45*, 669–684. [CrossRef]
6. Nelson, J.D.; Shimazaki, J.; Benitez-del-Castillo, J.M.; Craig, J.P.; McCulley, J.P.; Den, S.; Foulks, G.N. The international workshop on meibomian gland dysfunction: Report of the definition and classification subcommittee. *Investig. Ophthalmol. Vis. Sci.* **2011**, *52*, 1930–1937. [CrossRef]
7. Knop, E.; Knop, N.; Millar, T.; Obata, H.; Sullivan, D.A. The international workshop on meibomian gland dysfunction: Report of the subcommittee on anatomy, physiology, and pathophysiology of the meibomian gland. *Investig. Ophthalmol. Vis. Sci.* **2011**, *52*, 1938–1978. [CrossRef]

8. Nichols, K.K.; Foulks, G.N.; Bron, A.J.; Glasgow, B.J.; Dogru, M.; Tsubota, K.; Lemp, M.A.; Sullivan, D.A. The international workshop on meibomian gland dysfunction: Executive summary. *Investig. Ophthalmol. Vis. Sci.* **2011**, *52*, 1922–1929. [CrossRef]
9. Tomlinson, A.; Bron, A.J.; Korb, D.R.; Amano, S.; Paugh, J.R.; Pearce, E.I.; Yee, R.; Yokoi, N.; Arita, R.; Dogru, M. The international workshop on meibomian gland dysfunction: Report of the diagnosis subcommittee. *Investig. Ophthalmol. Vis. Sci.* **2011**, *52*, 2006–2049. [CrossRef]
10. Arita, R.; Itoh, K.; Inoue, K.; Amano, S. Noncontact infrared meibography to document age-related changes of the meibomian glands in a normal population. *Ophthalmology* **2008**, *115*, 911–915. [CrossRef]
11. Fineide, F.; Arita, R.; Utheim, T.P. The role of meibography in ocular surface diagnostics: A review. *Ocul. Surf* **2020**, in press. [CrossRef] [PubMed]
12. Arita, R.; Fukuoka, S. Non-pharmaceutical treatment options for meibomian gland dysfunction. *Clin. Exp. Optom.* **2020**, *103*, 742–755. [CrossRef] [PubMed]
13. Geerling, G.; Tauber, J.; Baudouin, C.; Goto, E.; Matsumoto, Y.; O'Brien, T.; Rolando, M.; Tsubota, K.; Nichols, K.K. The international workshop on meibomian gland dysfunction: Report of the subcommittee on management and treatment of meibomian gland dysfunction. *Investig. Ophthalmol. Vis. Sci.* **2011**, *52*, 2050–2064. [CrossRef] [PubMed]
14. Maskin, S.L. Intraductal meibomian gland probing relieves symptoms of obstructive meibomian gland dysfunction. *Cornea* **2010**, *29*, 1145–1152. [CrossRef]
15. Greiner, J.V. A single LipiFlow(R) Thermal Pulsation System treatment improves meibomian gland function and reduces dry eye symptoms for 9 months. *Curr. Eye Res.* **2012**, *37*, 272–278. [CrossRef]
16. Toyos, R.; McGill, W.; Briscoe, D. Intense pulsed light treatment for dry eye disease due to meibomian gland dysfunction; a 3-year retrospective study. *Photomed. Laser Surg.* **2015**, *33*, 41–46. [CrossRef]
17. Amano, S.; Arita, R.; Kinoshita, S.; Japanese Dry Eye Society MGD Working Group. Definition and diagnostic criteria for meibomian gland dysfunction. *Atarashii Ganka (J. Eye).* **2010**, *27*, 627–631.
18. Shimazaki, J.; Sakata, M.; Tsubota, K. Ocular surface changes and discomfort in patients with meibomian gland dysfunction. *Arch. Ophthalmol.* **1995**, *113*, 1266–1270. [CrossRef]
19. Finis, D.; Pischel, N.; Konig, C.; Hayajneh, J.; Borrelli, M.; Schrader, S.; Geerling, G. Comparison of the OSDI and SPEED questionnaires for the evaluation of dry eye disease in clinical routine. *Ophthalmologe* **2014**, *111*, 1050–1056. [CrossRef]
20. Arita, R.; Minoura, I.; Morishige, N.; Shirakawa, R.; Fukuoka, S.; Asai, K.; Goto, T.; Imanaka, T.; Nakamura, M. Development of Definitive and Reliable Grading Scales for Meibomian Gland Dysfunction. *Am. J. Ophthalmol.* **2016**, *169*, 125–137. [CrossRef]
21. van Bijsterveld, O.P. Diagnostic tests in the Sicca syndrome. *Arch. Ophthalmol.* **1969**, *82*, 10–14. [CrossRef] [PubMed]
22. Schirmer, O. Studiun zur Physiologie und Pathologie der Tranenabsonderung und Tranenabfuhr. *Albrecht Graefes Arch. Ophthalmol.* **1903**, *56*, 197–291. [CrossRef]
23. Asiedu, K.; Kyei, S.; Mensah, S.N.; Ocansey, S.; Abu, L.S.; Kyere, E.A. Ocular Surface Disease Index (OSDI) Versus the Standard Patient Evaluation of Eye Dryness (SPEED): A Study of a Nonclinical Sample. *Cornea* **2016**, *35*, 175–180. [CrossRef] [PubMed]
24. Tapie, R. Biomicroscopical study of Meibomian glands. *Ann. Ocul.* **1977**, *210*, 637–648.
25. Arita, R. Meibography: A Japanese Perspective. *Investig. Ophthalmol. Vis. Sci.* **2018**, *59*, DES48–DES55. [CrossRef] [PubMed]
26. Arita, R.; Itoh, K.; Maeda, S.; Maeda, K.; Furuta, A.; Tomidokoro, A.; Aihara, M.; Amano, S. Effects of long-term topical anti-glaucoma medications on meibomian glands. *Graefe's Arch. Clin. Exp. Ophthalmol.* **2012**, *250*, 1181–1185. [CrossRef]
27. Uzunosmanoglu, E.; Mocan, M.C.; Kocabeyoglu, S.; Karakaya, J.; Irkec, M. Meibomian Gland Dysfunction in Patients Receiving Long-Term Glaucoma Medications. *Cornea* **2016**, *35*, 1112–1116. [CrossRef]
28. Mizoguchi, T.; Arita, R.; Fukuoka, S.; Morishige, N. Morphology and function of meibomian glands and other tear film parameters in junior high school students. *Cornea* **2017**, *36*, 922–926. [CrossRef]

29. Gupta, P.K.; Stevens, M.N.; Kashyap, N.; Priestley, Y. Prevalence of meibomian gland atrophy in a pediatric population. *Cornea* **2018**, *37*, 426–430. [CrossRef]
30. Adil, M.Y.; Xiao, J.; Olafsson, J.; Chen, X.; Lagali, N.S.; Raeder, S.; Utheim, O.A.; Dartt, D.A.; Utheim, T.P. Meibomian gland morphology is a sensitive early indicator of meibomian gland dysfunction. *Am. J. Ophthalmol.* **2019**, *200*, 16–25. [CrossRef]
31. Xiao, J.; Adil, M.Y.; Olafsson, J.; Chen, X.; Utheim, O.A.; Raeder, S.; Lagali, N.S.; Dartt, D.A.; Utheim, T.P. Diagnostic test efficacy of meibomian gland morphology and function. *Sci. Rep.* **2019**, *9*, 17345. [CrossRef] [PubMed]
32. Xiao, J.; Adil, M.Y.; Chen, X.; Utheim, O.A.; Raeder, S.; Tonseth, K.A.; Lagali, N.S.; Dartt, D.A.; Utheim, T.P. Functional and morphological evaluation of meibomian glands in the assessment of meibomian gland dysfunction subtype and severity. *Am. J. Ophthalmol.* **2020**, *209*, 160–167. [CrossRef] [PubMed]
33. Greiner, J.V. Long-term (3 year) effects of a single thermal pulsation system treatment on meibomian gland function and dry eye symptoms. *Eye Contact Lens.* **2016**, *42*, 99–107. [CrossRef] [PubMed]
34. Eom, Y.; Choi, K.E.; Kang, S.Y.; Lee, H.K.; Kim, H.M.; Song, J.S. Comparison of meibomian gland loss and expressed meibum grade between the upper and lower eyelids in patients with obstructive meibomian gland dysfunction. *Cornea* **2014**, *33*, 448–452. [CrossRef]
35. Wolffsohn, J.S.; Arita, R.; Chalmers, R.; Djalilian, A.; Dogru, M.; Dumbleton, K.; Gupta, P.K.; Karpecki, P.; Lazreg, S.; Pult, H.; et al. TFOS DEWS II diagnostic methodology report. *Ocul. Surf.* **2017**, *15*, 539–574. [CrossRef]

Publisher's Note: MDPI stays neutral with regard to jurisdictional claims in published maps and institutional affiliations.

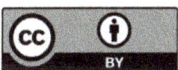

© 2020 by the authors. Licensee MDPI, Basel, Switzerland. This article is an open access article distributed under the terms and conditions of the Creative Commons Attribution (CC BY) license (http://creativecommons.org/licenses/by/4.0/).

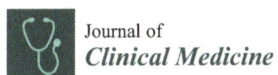

Article

Relation of Dietary Fatty Acids and Vitamin D to the Prevalence of Meibomian Gland Dysfunction in Japanese Adults: The Hirado–Takushima Study

Shima Fukuoka [1,2,3], Reiko Arita [1,4,*], Takanori Mizoguchi [1,5], Motoko Kawashima [1,6], Shizuka Koh [1,7], Rika Shirakawa [1,3], Takashi Suzuki [1,8], Satoshi Sasaki [9] and Naoyuki Morishige [1,10]

1. Lid and Meibomian Gland Working Group (LIME), 626-11 Minami-Nakano, Minumaku, Saitama 337-0042, Japan; fshima3271@gmail.com (S.F.); t-mizo@siren.ocn.ne.jp (T.M.); motoko326@gmail.com (M.K.); cizciz@gmail.com (S.K.); rikadream@hotmail.com (R.S.); takashisuzuki58@gmail.com (T.S.); morishig@corneajp.com (N.M.)
2. Omiya Hamada Eye Clinic, 1-169-1 Sakuragicho, Omiyaku, Saitama 330-0854, Japan
3. Department of Ophthalmology, The University of Tokyo, 7-3-1 Hongo, Bunkyoku, Tokyo 113-8655, Japan
4. Department of Ophthalmology, Itoh Clinic, 626-11 Minami-Nakano, Minumaku, Saitama 337-0042, Japan
5. Mizoguchi Eye Clinic, 6-13 Tawaramachi, Sasebo, Nagasaki 857-0016, Japan
6. Department of Ophthalmology, Keio University, 35 Shinanomachi, Shinjukuku, Tokyo 160-8582, Japan
7. Department of Ophthalmology, Osaka University, 2-15 Yamadaoka, Suita 565-0871, Japan
8. Department of Ophthalmology, Toho University Omori Medical Center, 6-11-1 Omorinishi, Otaku, Tokyo 143-8541, Japan
9. Department of Social and Preventive Epidemiology, School of Public Health, The University of Tokyo, 7-3-1 Hongo, Bunkyoku, Tokyo 113-0033, Japan; stssasak@m.u-tokyo.ac.jp
10. Division of Cornea and Ocular Surface, Ohshima Eye Hospital 11-8 Kamigofukumachi, Hakataku, Fukuoka 812-0036, Japan
* Correspondence: ritoh@za2.so-net.ne.jp; Tel.: +81-48-686-5588

Received: 1 December 2020; Accepted: 14 January 2021; Published: 18 January 2021

Abstract: Intervention studies have shown that n-3 polyunsaturated fatty acid (PUFA) supplementation is effective for the treatment of meibomian gland dysfunction (MGD). Ointment containing an analog of vitamin D has also been found to improve symptoms and signs of MGD. We have now evaluated the relation of MGD prevalence to dietary intake of fatty acids (FAs) and vitamin D among a Japanese population. Subjects comprised 300 adults aged 20 to 92 years residing on Takushima Island. MGD was diagnosed on the basis of subjective symptoms, lid margin abnormalities, and meibomian gland obstruction. Dietary FA and vitamin D intake was estimated with a brief-type self-administered diet history questionnaire. MGD prevalence was 35.3%. Multivariate adjusted odds ratios (95% confidence intervals) between extreme quintiles of intake for MGD prevalence were 0.40 (0.16–0.97) for total fat, 0.40 (0.17–0.97) for saturated FAs, 0.40 (0.17–0.97) for oleic acid, 0.52 (0.23–1.18) for n-3 PUFAs, 0.63 (0.27–1.49) for n-6 PUFAs, 1.32 (0.59–2.95) for the n-6/n-3 PUFA ratio, and 0.38 (0.17–0.87) for vitamin D. Total fat, saturated FA, oleic acid, and vitamin D intake may thus be negatively associated with MGD prevalence in the Japanese.

Keywords: fatty acids; vitamin D; meibomian gland dysfunction; brief-type self-administered diet history questionnaire; Japanese

1. Introduction

The ocular surface is covered and protected by the tear film comprised of lipid, aqueous, and mucin layers. Meibomian glands are sebaceous glands in the eyelids and secrete meibum, which is composed of >600 types of lipid [1], most of which are unsaturated wax esters and derived from oleic acid [2]. Meibum forms the lipid layer of the tear film, which plays an important role in the stabilization of the tear film [3,4] and prevents excessive evaporation of tear fluid [5]. Meibomian gland dysfunction (MGD) is defined by the International Workshop on Meibomian Gland Dysfunction as "a chronic, diffuse abnormality of the meibomian glands that is commonly characterized by terminal duct obstruction or qualitative or quantitative changes in glandular secretion" [6]. MGD is thus associated with tear film instability as a result of deficiency of the lipid layer. MGD is also a major cause of dry eye disease—in particular, of evaporative dry eye [6–8]. Population-based studies have revealed prevalence rates for MGD ranging from 38% to 68% among individuals over the age of 40 years [9]. We previously found that the prevalence of symptomatic MGD was 32.9% among Japanese individuals aged 6 years or older and 44.5% among those aged 40 years or older in a population-based study (Hirado-Takushima study) [10].

Therapies for MGD aim to improve the quality and quantity of meibum, to stabilize the tear film, to reduce inflammation, and to ameliorate subjective symptoms. Dietary supplementation with n-3 polyunsaturated fatty acids (PUFAs) is recommended both by the International Workshop on Meibomian Gland Dysfunction [11] and by the International Dry Eye Workshop [12]. Given that the human body is not able to synthesize n-3 or n-6 PUFAs, these essential fatty acids must be obtained from the diet. Several randomized, double-masked trials found that n-3 PUFA supplementation improved subjective symptoms [13–15], tear film stability [13–15], lid margin telangiectasia [13,14], as well as meibum quality [13,15] and expressibility [14,15] in individuals with MGD. A cross-sectional study also reported that dietary intake of n-3 PUFAs was negatively related and that the n-6/n-3 PUFA ratio was positively related to the prevalence of dry eye in women [16]. However, another cross-sectional study found that neither dietary intake of n-3 or n-6 PUFAs nor the n-6/n-3 PUFA ratio was associated with dry eye in postmenopausal women [17]. This latter study did detect a negative relation between dietary intake of n-3 and n-6 PUFAs and the prevalence of MGD [17].

Topical application of an analog of the active form of vitamin D3 was shown to ameliorate ocular symptoms and objective signs of MGD compared with baseline [18]. Oral vitamin D supplementation was also found to improve meibomian gland expressibility in MGD patients with vitamin D deficiency [19]. As far as we are aware, however, no observational study has previously examined the relationship between dietary intake of vitamin D and MGD.

Given the paucity of evidence regarding the relation between diet and MGD, we have now performed a cross-sectional study to investigate the relation of dietary consumption of specific types of fatty acids and vitamin D to the prevalence of MGD among adult Japanese in the Hirado-Takushima study.

2. Experimental Section

2.1. Study Design and Subjects

The present study is based on the Hirado-Takushima study, a population-based cross-sectional study that investigated the prevalence and risk factors of MGD and dry eye in Japan [10]. The subjects of this cross-sectional study were adult residents of Takushima Island, Hirado, Nagasaki, Japan, and the study adhered to the tenets of the Declaration of Helsinki and was approved by the Institutional Review Board of Itoh Clinic and registered in the University Hospital Medical Information Network database (UMIN000028310). Written informed consent was obtained from all participants before inclusion in the study. The dietary and lifestyle assessments of the study subjects were based on questionnaires conducted in August 2017. The ocular assessments were performed in November 2017. A total of 338 adult residents (119 men, 219 women) was recruited to the study. A set of three self-administered questionnaires was completed by the participants at home. Responses to the questionnaires were checked once by a physician who did not participate in the ocular examinations. If any missing or erroneous responses to questions considered essential for the analysis were detected, the subject was asked to complete or correct those responses. Exclusion criteria for the present study included pregnancy ($n = 0$) or nursing ($n = 8$) for women, an extremely low (<500 kcal/day, $n = 2$) or high (>4000 kcal/day, $n = 0$) reported energy intake, missing data for ophthalmologic measurements included in multivariate analysis ($n = 27$), and missing answers to the diet history questionnaire ($n = 1$). The final analysis was thus performed for 300 residents (109 men, 191 women) aged 20 to 92 years.

2.2. Dietary Assessment

Dietary habits during the preceding month were assessed with a brief-type self-administered diet history questionnaire (BDHQ) that was designed to assess the habitual dietary intake of Japanese adults and had been previously validated [20,21]. Details of the structure of the questionnaire, its method for calculation of dietary intake, and its validity for commonly studied food and nutrient intake have been described previously [20,21]. Participants were asked about the frequency of intake for food and nonalcoholic beverage items, daily intake of rice and miso soup, frequency and amount of alcoholic beverage consumption, and usual cooking methods. The BDHQ allows estimation of the daily intake of 58 food items, energy, and specific nutrients, including fats and vitamins, on the basis of the Standard Tables of Food Composition in Japan [22]. It is a four-page fixed-portion questionnaire. To facilitate reading and completion of the BDHQ, the present study adopted a large-print version that increased the printed size to 10 pages but which contained no other changes to the structure or content for participants aged >55 years. Fish and shellfish, meat, eggs, and dairy products were included in animal food. Cereals, pulses, potatoes, confectionaries, fruits, vegetables, and seasonings and spices were included in plant food. Dietary supplements were not included in the calculation of nutrient or fatty acid intake because of the lack of a reliable composition table for dietary supplements in Japan. Supplement use was queried in the BDHQ and treated as a confounding factor. The percentage contribution of each food group to total fat or vitamin D intake was calculated by dividing daily fat or vitamin D intake from each food group by total daily consumption of fat or vitamin D.

2.3. Assessment of Subjective Symptoms and Other Variables

Subjective ocular symptoms related to dry eye were assessed with the Dry Eye-Related Quality-of-Life Score (DEQS) [23]. The subjects reported their birth date, body weight, and height in the BDHQ. Body mass index (BMI) was calculated by dividing self-reported body weight (kg) by the square of self-reported height (m^2). A questionnaire on lifestyle also elicited information on occupation, history of ocular surgery, eyedrop use, contact lens wear, history of chronic systemic disease, history of dyslipidemia, taking of lipid-lowering agents, smoking and alcohol habits, and taking of supplements. Details were described previously [10].

2.4. Ocular Examinations

The ocular surface of both eyes was assessed according to standardized protocols by a team of seven ophthalmologists with expertise in dry eye and MGD (members of the Lid and Meibomian Gland Working Group) [10]. Participants were diagnosed with MGD [24] on the basis of (1) the presence of any chronic ocular symptom [23]; (2) the detection of more than one lid margin abnormality among vascularity, displacement of the mucocutaneous junction, and irregularity; and (3) obstruction of meibomian glands as revealed by the detection of plugging and reduced meibum expression in response to moderate digital pressure [25] in at least one eye. The ophthalmologists performing the examinations remained masked to the responses to the BDHQ throughout the assessment.

2.5. Statistical Analysis

All dietary variables were adjusted for energy by the residual method with the use of a linear regression model. The data were found to be non-normally distributed with the Shapiro–Wilk test ($p < 0.05$), and nonparametric testing was thus performed. The characteristics of the subjects with or without MGD were compared with the Mann–Whitney U test for continuous variables or Fisher's exact test for categorical variables.

The intake of specific nutrients adjusted by the residual method was categorized at quintile points on the basis of the distribution for all study subjects. The odds ratio (OR) and its 95% confidence interval (CI) for fat, fatty acids, the n-6/n-3 PUFA ratio, and vitamin D with regard to MGD were calculated by different logistic regression models after adjustment for potential confounding factors: age, sex, BMI, energy intake, occupation, history of ocular surgery, eyedrop use, contact lens wear, history of chronic systemic disease, history of dyslipidemia, taking of lipid-lowering agents, current smoking, alcohol habit, and taking of supplements, with the lowest quintile as the reference. The initial logistic regression model was a crude model (that is, an unadjusted model), to which covariates were added with a forward selection method. In a second multivariate model (Model 1), age (years, continuous) and sex (male or female) were used as potential confounding factors. The final multivariate model (Model 2) included age (years, continuous), sex (male or female), BMI (kg/m^2, continuous), history of chronic systemic disease (yes or no), and alcohol consumption (yes or no) as potential confounding factors. Other variables—energy intake (kcal/day, continuous), occupation (fisherman, farmer, local government official, or other), history of ocular surgery (yes or no), eyedrop use (yes or no), contact lens wear (yes or no), history of dyslipidemia (yes or no), taking of lipid-lowering agents (yes or no), current smoking (yes or no), and taking of supplements (yes or no)—were not included in Models 1 and 2 because they had no influence on the relationship between dietary variables and MGD ($p > 0.10$).

Data are presented as means ± standard deviations. Statistical analysis was performed with JMP Pro version 14 software (SAS, Cary, NC, USA), all statistical tests were two sided, and a p value of <0.05 was considered statistically significant.

3. Results

3.1. Subsection

Table 1 shows the distribution of selected variables among all subjects as well as in the non-MGD and MGD groups. A total of 106 subjects (35.3%) was diagnosed with MGD. Mean age of the study population was 61.7 ± 15.6 years, and mean BMI was 23.9 ± 3.5 kg/m^2. Compared with the non-MGD group, the MGD group was significantly older ($p < 0.001$) and included a larger proportion of men ($p = 0.006$). BMI did not differ significantly between the two groups ($p = 0.99$). A higher proportion of subjects with MGD had a history of chronic systemic disease ($p < 0.001$). No significant differences between the two groups were apparent for history of dyslipidemia ($p = 0.39$), taking of lipid-lowering agents ($p = 1.0$), or taking of dietary supplements ($p = 0.89$).

3.2. Daily Intake of Fatty Acids and Vitamin D in Subjects with or Without MGD

Table 2 shows the daily intake of specific dietary components in all subjects as well as in those of the non-MGD or MGD groups, with p values for comparisons between the latter two groups being determined with the Mann–Whitney U test. Mean intake of total fat, animal fat, or plant fat for all subjects was 50.7 ± 11.7, 23.3 ± 8.3, and 27.4 ± 7.2 g/day, respectively. The mean intake of fatty acids was 13.7 ± 4.0 g/day for saturated fatty acids (SFAs), 18.1 ± 4.5 g/day for monounsaturated fatty acids (MUFAs), 12.3 ± 2.9 g/day for PUFAs, 2.6 ± 1.0 g/day for n-3 PUFAs, and 9.7 ± 2.4 g/day for n-6 PUFAs. Mean intake of the MUFA oleic acid was 16.4 ± 4.1 g/day, whereas that of the n-3 PUFAs eicosapentaenoic acid (EPA) and docosahexaenoic acid (DHA) was 0.33 ± 0.27 and 0.55 ± 0.40 g/day, respectively. Mean intake of vitamin D was 15.4 ± 11.9 μg/day. Intake of total fat and animal fat was significantly lower in the MGD group than in the non-MGD group (p = 0.007 and 0.002, respectively). There was no significant difference in plant fat intake between the two groups (p = 0.60). Intake of SFAs, MUFAs, PUFAs, and n-3 PUFAs was also significantly lower in the MGD group than in the non-MGD group (p = 0.015, 0.005, 0.039, and 0.017, respectively), as was intake of oleic acid and EPA (p = 0.007 and 0.044, respectively). There was no significant difference in n-6 PUFA intake or in the n-6/n-3 PUFA ratio between the two groups (p = 0.10 and 0.40, respectively). Vitamin D intake in the MGD group was significantly lower than that in the non-MGD group (p = 0.039). The main contributors to total fat intake in the study population were cooking oil (20%), meat (15%), fish and shellfish (12%), and dairy products (11%), whereas those to vitamin D intake were fish and shellfish (92%) and eggs (4%) (Table 3).

Table 1. Characteristics of adult subjects with or without meibomian gland dysfunction (MGD) in the Hirado–Takushima study.

Characteristic	Total (n = 300)	Non-MGD (n = 194)	MGD (n = 106)	p
Age (years)	61.7 ± 15.6	57.9 ± 15.7	68.2 ± 12.8	<0.001 **
Male sex, n (%)	109 (36.3)	59 (30.4)	50 (47.2)	0.006 [†]
Body height (cm)	158.2 ± 8.2	158.5 ± 8.1	157.7 ± 8.3	0.51
Body weight (kg)	60.2 ± 11.6	69.5 ± 12.2	59.5 ± 10.5	0.72
Body mass index (kg/m^2)	23.9 ± 3.5	24.0 ± 3.5	23.8 ± 3.4	0.99
Occupation, n (%)				
Fisherman	38 (12.7)	27 (13.9)	11 (10.4)	
Farmer	28 (9.3)	8 (4.1)	5 (4.7)	0.52
Local government official	13 (4.3)	15 (7.7)	13 (12.3)	
Other	221 (73.7)	144 (74.2)	77 (72.6)	
History of ocular surgery, n (%)	51 (17.0)	27 (13.9)	24 (22.6)	0.076
Eyedrop use, n (%)	131 (43.7)	81 (41.8)	50 (47.2)	0.40
Contact lens wear, n (%)	15 (5.0)	13 (6.7)	2 (1.9)	0.095
History of chronic systemic disease, n (%)	171 (57.0)	93 (47.9)	78 (73.6)	<0.001 [††]
History of dyslipidemia, n (%)	13 (4.3)	7 (3.6)	6 (5.7)	0.39
Taking lipid-lowering agents, n (%)	3 (1.0)	2 (1.0)	1 (0.9)	1.0
Current smoking, n (%)	26 (8.7)	19 (9.8)	7 (6.6)	0.40
Alcohol drinking, n (%)	254 (84.7)	165 (85.1)	89 (84.0)	0.87
Dietary supplement use, n (%)	77 (25.7)	49 (25.3)	28 (26.4)	0.89

Data are means ± standard deviations or n (%), as indicated. p values for comparisons between the non-MGD and MGD groups were determined with the Mann–Whitney U test (age, body height, body weight, and body mass index; ** p < 0.001) or Fisher's exact test (other characteristics; [†] p < 0.05, [††] p < 0.001).

Table 2. Daily intake of dietary components in adult subjects with or without meibomian gland dysfunction (MGD) in the Hirado–Takushima study.

Dietary Component	Total (n = 300)	Non-MGD (n = 194)	MGD (n = 106)	p
Energy intake (kcal/day)	1782.9 ± 564.3	1744.6 ± 550.4	1853.0 ± 585.0	0.057
Total fat (g/day)	50.7 ± 11.7	52.1 ± 11.1	48.0 ± 12.4	0.007 *
Animal fat (g/day)	23.3 ± 8.3	24.5 ± 8.3	21.0 ± 8.0	0.002 *
Plant fat (g/day)	27.4 ± 7.2	27.6 ± 6.9	27.0 ± 7.9	0.60
Saturated fatty acids (g/day)	13.7 ± 4.0	14.2 ± 4.0	12.8 ± 3.9	0.015 *
Monounsaturated fatty acids (g/day)	18.1 ± 4.5	18.7 ± 4.2	17.1 ± 4.7	0.005 *
Oleic acid (g/day)	16.4 ± 4.1	16.9 ± 3.9	15.5 ± 4.3	0.007 *
Polyunsaturated fatty acids (g/day)	12.3 ± 2.9	12.6 ± 2.8	11.8 ± 3.1	0.039 *
n-3 Polyunsaturated fatty acids (g/day)	2.6 ± 1.0	2.7 ± 1.0	2.5 ± 0.9	0.017 *
α-Linolenic acid (g/day)	1.5 ± 0.4	1.6 ± 0.4	1.5 ± 0.5	0.10
Eicosapentaenoic acid (g/day)	0.33 ± 0.27	0.35 ± 0.30	0.30 ± 0.22	0.044 *
Docosahexaenoic acid (g/day)	0.55 ± 0.40	0.58 ± 0.44	0.50 ± 0.33	0.051
n-6 Polyunsaturated fatty acids (g/day)	9.7 ± 2.4	9.8 ± 2.3	9.3 ± 2.5	0.10
Linoleic acid (g/day)	9.4 ± 2.3	9.5 ± 2.2	9.1 ± 2.5	0.11
Arachidonic acid (g/day)	0.16 ± 0.05	0.17 ± 0.05	0.16 ± 0.06	0.17
n-6/n-3 Polyunsaturated fatty acid ratio	4.1 ± 1.3	4.0 ± 1.2	4.0 ± 1.6	0.40
Cholesterol (mg/day)	377.3 ± 132.6	381.8 ± 126.6	369.0 ± 143.1	0.49
Vitamin D (µg/day)	15.4 ± 11.9	16.4 ± 13.0	13.6 ± 9.6	0.039 *

Data are means ± standard deviations. Nutrient intake was adjusted for energy according to the residual method. p values for comparisons between the non-MGD and MGD groups were determined with the Mann–Whitney U test (* p < 0.05).

Table 3. Contribution of each food group to total fat and vitamin D estimated by a brief-type diet history questionnaire in adult subjects of the Hirado–Takushima study.

Food Group	Total Fat (%)	Vitamin D (%)
Cooking oil	20.2 ± 9.1	0.0 ± 0.0
Animal food		
Meat	15.4 ± 10.9	0.4 ± 4.7
Fish and shellfish	11.8 ± 10.1	92.4 ± 55.4
Dairy products	10.8 ± 8.7	0.7 ± 11.2
Eggs	7.4 ± 5.0	3.8 ± 34.8
Plant food		
Seasonings and spices	10.3 ± 7.6	0.3 ± 1.9
Confectionaries	8.9 ± 9.6	0.6 ± 13.7
Cereals	7.5 ± 4.3	0.2 ± 1.9
Pulses	6.7 ± 4.1	0.0 ± 0.0
Vegetables	0.8 ± 0.5	1.5 ± 5.1
Fruits	0.2 ± 0.3	0.0 ± 0.0
Potatoes	0.1 ± 0.1	0.0 ± 0.0

Data are mean ± standard deviations.

3.3. Multivariate Adjusted ORs for Fatty Acid and Vitamin D Intake with Regard to MGD

The ORs and 95% CIs for the prevalence of MGD according to dietary intake of specific types of fatty acids and vitamin D are shown in Table 4 and Figure 1. Intake of SFAs was inversely associated with the prevalence of MGD after adjustment for sex and age (p for trend = 0.026, Model 1), and this association was maintained after further multivariate adjustment (p for trend = 0.020, Model 2). The multivariate adjusted ORs and 95% CIs for MGD prevalence in the first, second, third, fourth, and fifth quintiles of SFA intake were 1.00 (reference), 0.34 (0.15– 0.78), 0.44 (0.19–1.02), 0.94 (0.42–2.13), and 0.40 (0.17–0.97), respectively, in Model 2. Intake of n-3 PUFAs was also inversely associated with MGD after adjustment for sex and age (p for trend = 0.049, Model 1), but this association was not maintained after further multivariate adjustment (p for trend = 0.077, Model 2) and none of the multivariate adjusted ORs for the second to fifth quintiles differed significantly relative to the first quintile. The multivariate adjusted ORs and 95% CIs for the fifth quintile compared with the first quintile in Model 2 were 0.40 (0.16–0.97) for total fat, 0.40 (0.17–0.97) for oleic acid, and 0.38 (0.17–0.87) for vitamin D. For EPA, the multivariate adjusted OR (and 95% CI) for the fourth quintile compared with the first quintile in Model 2 was 0.41 (0.17–0.97), but that in the fifth quintile compared with the first quintile was 0.68 (0.31–1.50). Whereas intake of animal fat, MUFAs, or PUFAs was significantly lower in the MGD group than in the non-MGD group by the Mann–Whitney U test (Table 2), none of these dietary components was significantly related to the prevalence of MGD in either Model 1 or 2 of the multivariate analysis (Table 4). There was no significant difference in intake of plant fat, α-linolenic acid, DHA, n-6 PUFAs, linoleic acid, arachidonic acid, or cholesterol or in the n-6/n-3 PUFA ratio between the MGD and non-MGD groups by the Mann–Whitney U test (Table 2), and there was no significant relationship between these parameters and the prevalence of MGD in Model 1 or 2 of the multivariate analysis (Table 4).

Table 4. Multivariate adjusted odds ratios (ORs) and 95% confidence intervals (CIs) for the prevalence of meibomian gland dysfunction (MGD) by quintile (Q) of intake of specific fats and vitamin D among adult subjects in the Hirado–Takushima study.

Dietary Component			Q1 (Lowest) n = 60	Q2 (n = 60)	Q3 (n = 60)	Q4 (n = 60)	Q5 (Highest) n = 60	p for Trend
Total fat								
	Intake	(g/day)	≤41.5	41.5–47.7	47.9–53.9	54.1–61.7	≥61.7	
	MGD	(%)	48.3	31.7	41.7	33.3	21.7	
	Model 1	OR (95% CI)	1.00	0.61 (0.28–1.34)	1.07 (0.49–2.34)	0.94 (0.42–2.13)	0.46 (0.20–1.07)	0.20
	Model 2	OR (95% CI)	1.00	0.60 (0.27–1.35)	1.02 (0.46–2.26)	0.86 (0.37–1.97)	0.40 (0.16–0.97)	0.16
Animal fat								
	Intake	(g/day)	≤16.9	16.9–21.0	21.2–25.0	25.1–29.8	≥29.8	
	MGD	(%)	46.7	40.0	36.7	30.0	23.3	
	Model 1	OR (95% CI)	1.00	0.92 (0.42–2.00)	0.76 (0.35–1.66)	0.87 (0.38–1.97)	0.59 (0.25–1.36)	0.75
	Model 2	OR (95% CI)	1.00	0.93 (0.42–2.06)	0.69 (0.31–1.53)	0.75 (0.32–1.76)	0.55 (0.23–1.32)	0.66
Plant fat								
	Intake	(g/day)	≤21.5	21.9–25.8	25.9–28.7	28.9–33.0	≥33.1	
	MGD	(%)	41.7	35.0	36.7	23.3	40.0	
	Model 1	OR (95% CI)	1.00	0.87 (0.39–1.93)	1.10 (0.49–2.46)	0.64 (0.27–1.49)	1.09 (0.50–2.39)	0.70
	Model 2	OR (95% CI)	1.00	0.79 (0.35–1.79)	0.99 (0.43–2.28)	0.54 (0.22–1.30)	0.95 (0.42–2.16)	0.58
Saturated fatty acids								
	Intake	(g/day)	≤10.2	10.2–12.6	12.6–14.5	14.5–16.7	≥16.8	
	MGD	(%)	53.3	26.7	31.7	41.7	23.3	
	Model 1	OR (95% CI)	1.00	0.34 (0.15–0.77)	0.55 (0.25–1.21)	1.04 (0.47–2.28)	0.46 (0.20–1.09)	0.026 *
	Model 2	OR (95% CI)	1.00	0.34 (0.15–0.78)	0.44 (0.19–1.02)	0.94 (0.42–2.13)	0.40 (0.17–0.97)	0.020 *
Monounsaturated fatty acids								
	Intake	(g/day)	≤14.4	14.5–17.1	17.1–19.5	19.5–22.1	≥22.1	
	MGD	(%)	46.7	30.0	50.0	23.3	26.7	
	Model 1	OR (95% CI)	1.00	0.57 (0.25–1.27)	1.33 (0.62–2.88)	0.62 (0.27–1.46)	0.58 (0.25–1.30)	0.13
	Model 2	OR (95% CI)	1.00	0.55 (0.24–1.25)	1.27 (0.58–2.80)	0.58 (0.24–1.38)	0.50 (0.21–1.17)	0.094
Oleic acid								
	Intake	(g/day)	≤13.3	13.4–15.2	15.3–17.6	17.6–19.9	≥19.9	
	MGD	(%)	48.3	30.0	46.7	28.3	23.3	
	Model 1	OR (95% CI)	1.00	0.50 (0.22–1.11)	1.14 (0.53–2.49)	0.74 (0.33–1.69)	0.46 (0.20–1.07)	0.10
	Model 2	OR (95% CI)	1.00	0.54 (0.24–1.21)	1.08 (0.49–2.39)	0.68 (0.29–1.58)	0.40 (0.17–0.97)	0.11
Polyunsaturated fatty acids								
	Intake	(g/day)	≤9.9	10.0–11.5	11.5–13.1	13.2–14.7	≥14.7	
	MGD	(%)	45.0	35.0	40.0	31.7	25.0	
	Model 1	OR (95% CI)	1.00	0.82 (0.37–1.82)	1.20 (0.54–2.64)	0.93 (0.41–2.12)	0.51 (0.22–1.15)	0.31
	Model 2	OR (95% CI)	1.00	0.79 (0.35–1.78)	1.16 (0.51–2.62)	0.83 (0.36–1.93)	0.46 (0.19–1.07)	0.25
n-3 Polyunsaturated fatty acids								
	Intake	(g/day)	≤1.9	1.9–2.4	2.4–2.7	2.7–3.1	≥3.2	
	MGD	(%)	45.0	48.3	23.3	31.7	28.3	
	Model 1	OR (95% CI)	1.00	1.33 (0.60–2.94)	0.45 (0.19–1.05)	0.66 (0.29–1.48)	0.53 (0.24–1.18)	0.049 *
	Model 2	OR (95% CI)	1.00	1.29 (0.57–2.89)	0.47 (0.20–1.12)	0.64 (0.28–1.47)	0.52 (0.23–1.18)	0.077
α-Linolenic acid								
	Intake	(g/day)	≤1.2	1.2–1.4	1.4–1.6	1.6–1.9	≥1.9	
	MGD	(%)	45.0	33.3	36.7	31.7	30.0	
	Model 1	OR (95% CI)	1.00	0.71 (0.32–1.57)	1.01 (0.45–2.23)	0.75 (0.34–1.68)	0.67 (0.30–1.50)	0.77
	Model 2	OR (95% CI)	1.00	0.75 (0.34–1.67)	0.96 (0.42–2.18)	0.68 (0.30–1.55)	0.62 (0.27–1.43)	0.74

Table 4. Cont.

Dietary Component			Q1 (Lowest) n = 60	Q2 (n = 60)	Q3 (n = 60)	Q4 (n = 60)	Q5 (Highest) n = 60	p for Trend
Eicosapentaenoic acid								
	Intake	(g/day)	≤0.15	0.15–0.26	0.26–0.34	0.34–0.47	≥0.47	
	MGD	(%)	45.0	40.0	35.0	21.7	35.0	
	Model 1	OR (95% CI)	1.00	0.87 (0.39–1.91)	0.90 (0.40–2.02)	0.40 (0.17–0.94)	0.63 (0.29–1.36)	0.20
	Model 2	OR (95% CI)	1.00	0.84 (0.37–1.87)	0.93 (0.41–2.12)	0.41 (0.17–0.97)	0.68 (0.31–1.50)	0.24
Docosahexaenoic acid								
	Intake	(g/day)	≤0.28	0.28–0.44	0.44–0.57	0.57–0.75	≥0.76	
	MGD	(%)	43.3	46.7	23.3	31.7	31.7	
	Model 1	OR (95% CI)	1.00	1.18 (0.54–2.58)	0.55 (0.24–1.30)	0.70 (0.31–1.56)	0.57 (0.26–1.26)	0.24
	Model 2	OR (95% CI)	1.00	1.20 (0.54–2.66)	0.58 (0.24–1.38)	0.74 (0.33–1.67)	0.61 (0.28–1.37)	0.34
n-6 Polyunsaturated fatty acids								
	Intake	(g/day)	≤7.7	7.7–9.2	9.2–10.2	10.2–11.5	≥11.5	
	MGD	(%)	43.3	33.3	40.0	31.7	28.3	
	Model 1	OR (95% CI)	1.00	0.79 (0.36–1.76)	1.22 (0.55–2.71)	1.54 (0.70–3.41)	0.97 (0.43–2.02)	0.74
	Model 2	OR (95% CI)	1.00	0.71 (0.31–1.62)	1.16 (0.51–2.63)	0.82 (0.35–1.92)	0.63 (0.27–1.49)	0.61
Linoleic acid								
	Intake	(g/day)	≤7.4	7.5–8.9	8.9–9.9	9.9–11.1	≥11.2	
	MGD	(%)	43.3	31.7	41.7	31.7	28.3	
	Model 1	OR (95% CI)	1.00	0.72 (0.32–1.62)	1.31 (0.59–2.90)	1.00 (0.44–2.28)	0.74 (0.32–1.68)	0.57
	Model 2	OR (95% CI)	1.00	0.66 (0.29–1.50)	1.25 (0.56–2.83)	0.83 (0.35–1.94)	0.63 (0.27–1.49)	0.44
Arachidonic acid								
	Intake	(g/day)	≤0.12	0.12–0.15	0.15–0.17	0.17–0.20	≥0.20	
	MGD	(%)	45.0	38.3	21.7	36.7	35.0	
	Model 1	OR (95% CI)	1.00	0.87 (0.40–1.91)	0.42 (0.18–0.99)	0.95 (0.43–2.11)	0.78 (0.35–1.69)	0.27
	Model 2	OR (95% CI)	1.00	0.94 (0.42–2.09)	0.44 (0.18–1.03)	0.46 (0.20–1.10)	1.00 (0.44–2.25)	0.26
n-6/n-3 Polyunsaturated fatty acid ratio								
	Ratio	(%)	≤3.2	3.2–3.6	3.6–4.0	4.0–4.7	≥4.7	
	MGD		36.7	31.7	28.3	38.3	41.7	
	Model 1	OR (95% CI)	1.00	0.89 (0.40–1.99)	0.97 (0.43–2.21)	1.44 (0.65–3.21)	1.53 (0.70–3.34)	0.58
	Model 2	OR (95% CI)	1.00	0.86 (0.38–1.95)	0.93 (0.40–2.17)	1.36 (0.60–3.07)	1.32 (0.59–2.95)	0.75
Cholesterol								
	Intake	(mg/day)	≤270.6	270.8–330.7	331.2–395.0	399.1–479.8	≥480.6	
	MGD	(%)	40.0	35.0	26.7	40.0	35.0	
	Model 1	OR (95% CI)	1.00	1.04 (0.47–2.33)	0.63 (0.27–1.45)	1.41 (0.63–3.14)	0.73 (0.33–1.63)	0.33
	Model 2	OR (95% CI)	1.00	1.07 (0.47–2.44)	0.60 (0.25–1.41)	1.36 (0.60–3.11)	0.70 (0.31–1.58)	0.30
Vitamin D								
	Intake	(μg/day)	≤7.6	7.6–11.7	11.7–14.9	15.0–22.3	≥22.6	
	MGD	(%)	46.7	35.0	38.3	28.3	28.3	
	Model 1	OR (95% CI)	1.00	0.55 (0.24–1.23)	0.98 (0.44–2.20)	0.55 (0.24–1.24)	0.38 (0.17–0.86)	0.087
	Model 2	OR (95% CI)	1.00	0.56 (0.25–1.27)	1.00 (0.44–2.27)	0.51 (0.22–1.19)	0.38 (0.17–0.87)	0.081

Nutrient intake was adjusted for energy by the residual method. Model 1: adjusted for age (years, continuous) and sex (male or female). Model 2: adjusted for age (years, continuous), sex (male or female), body mass index (kg/m^2, continuous), history of chronic systemic disease (yes or no), and alcohol drinking (yes or no). * $p < 0.05$.

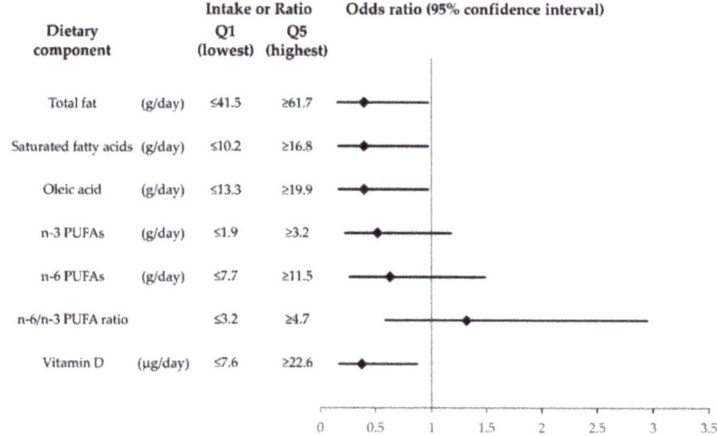

Figure 1. Multivariate adjusted odds ratios and 95% confidence intervals for the prevalence of meibomian gland dysfunction according to extreme quintiles (Q1 and Q5) of intake of specific fats and vitamin D among adult subjects in the Hirado–Takushima study. Nutrient intake was adjusted for energy by the residual method. The results are for Model 2, with adjustment for age (years, continuous), sex (male or female), body mass index (kg/m2, continuous), history of chronic systemic disease (yes or no), and alcohol drinking (yes or no). PUFA, polyunsaturated fatty acid.

4. Discussion

Our cross-sectional study investigated the relation of dietary intake of fatty acids and vitamin D to the prevalence of MGD. The results revealed that SFA intake was inversely associated with MGD prevalence (p for trend = 0.020, Model 2) among adult residents of Takushima Island, and that the highest quintiles for dietary intake of total fat, SFAs, oleic acid, and vitamin D were significantly associated with a lower prevalence of MGD compared with the first quintiles (Model 2). There was no significant association between either the intake of n-3 PUFAs, n-6 PUFAs, or cholesterol or the n-6/n-3 PUFA ratio and the prevalence of MGD by multivariate logistic regression analysis.

Diet and oral supplementation are different things. In our study, multivariate logistic regression analysis revealed that there was no significant association between intake of n-3 PUFAs or n-6 PUFAs or the n-6/n-3 PUFA ratio and the prevalence of MGD. A previous cross-sectional study found that the prevalence of MGD was 21.9% in 319 postmenopausal women and that high n-3 PUFA intake (OR and 95% CI, 0.22 and 0.06–0.78) and moderate n-6 PUFA intake (0.37 and 0.15–0.91) were significantly associated with a lower prevalence of MGD [17]. In this previous study, however, only postmenopausal women 50 years of age and older were recruited and the diagnosis of MGD was based only on reduced meibum expressibility with digital pressure for the 10 central meibomian glands of the lower eyelids [26]. In our study, we recruited both men and women at least 20 years of age and diagnosed MGD on the basis of subjective symptoms, lid margin abnormalities, and obstruction of meibomian glands [24]. In the MGD group of the previous study [17], the mean daily intake of n-3 PUFAs (1.87 g/day) was lower, that of n-6 PUFAs (15.24 g/day) was higher, and the mean n-6/n-3 PUFA ratio (8.35) was higher compared with the corresponding values for the MGD group of our study (2.5 g/day, 9.3 g/day, and 4.0, respectively). Another previous cross-sectional study of the Mediterranean diet found that the daily intake of n-3 PUFAs was not significantly associated with tear film breakup time as measured with fluorescein (OR and 95% CI, 0.87 and 0.38–2.01), with meibum quality (1.06 and 0.48–2.39), or with plugging of the inferior eyelid margin (0.91

and 0.37–2.20) in 247 men aged 55 to 95 years [27]. Although meibomian gland parameters were assessed and dry eye was diagnosed in this previous study, the diagnosis of MGD was not made [27]. The typical Western diet is heavy on red and processed meats, poultry, and full-fat dairy products, and it tends to be low in n-3 PUFAs, to be high in n-6 PUFAs, and to have a high n-6/n-3 PUFA ratio of between 15 and 25 [28,29]. In contrast, the Mediterranean-style diet is characterized by a high intake of non-refined cereals, fruits, vegetables, legumes, olive oil, fish, and potatoes and a low intake of SFAs [30,31], with a low n-6/n-3 PUFA ratio of ~4 [13]. The traditional Japanese diet is characterized by a high intake of fish and plant foods and a low intake of refined carbohydrates and meat [32]. The participants of our study had a relatively high n-3 PUFA intake, low n-6 PUFA intake, and low n-6/n-3 PUFA ratio. An inverse relationship between n-3 PUFA intake and the prevalence of MGD, and the lack of an association between the n-6/n-3 PUFA ratio and MGD prevalence, might therefore be apparent only when consumption of n-3 PUFAs is low.

There have been only three observational studies that have assessed the relation of dietary intake of fatty acids to the prevalence of dry eye. A cross-sectional study with a large cohort of female health professionals (the Women's Health Study) showed an association between lower dietary intake of n-3 PUFAs and a higher n-6/n-3 PUFA ratio and a higher prevalence of dry eye [16]. There was no association between n-6 PUFA intake and dry eye prevalence. Dry eye in this study was defined on the basis of asking participants whether they had been clinically diagnosed with dry eye syndrome [16], and MGD was not assessed. Two other cross-sectional studies found that dietary intake of n-3 PUFAs was not associated with the prevalence of dry eye disease [17,27]. An interventional study showed that consumption of a Mediterranean diet for 6 months was associated with amelioration of subjective symptoms of dry eye, an increase in both the fluorescein breakup time of the tear film (FBUT) and Schirmer's test value, and reduced fluorescein staining of the ocular surface [30]. There is a consensus that dry eye and MGD are similar and overlapping diseases. We previously showed that the ocular symptoms of MGD and dry eye are similar, but that the pathogenesis and risk factors of the two conditions differ [10]. The results of research on dry eye thus need to be considered separately from those of studies on MGD. The Hirado–Takushima study was designed to focus on dry eye and MGD, and we therefore believe that the current study is equipped to specifically reveal the relation between diet and MGD prevalence.

Several randomized, controlled studies have investigated the efficacy of n-3 PUFA supplements for MGD [13–15,33]. A prospective, randomized, double-masked trial found that n-3 PUFA supplementation with EPA at 1050 mg/day and DHA at 127.5 mg/day together with the practice of lid hygiene and administration of preservative-free artificial tears for 3 months improved subjective symptoms, FBUT, lid margin inflammation, and meibomian gland expression compared with baseline [14]. The placebo (sunflower oil) together with lid hygiene and preservative-free artificial tears ameliorated subjective symptoms but did not change other objective parameters [14]. A prospective, randomized, placebo-controlled, masked trial showed that dietary supplementation with EPA at 720 mg/day and DHA at 480 mg/day for 12 weeks improved contrast sensitivity under photopic and mesopic testing conditions, subjective symptoms, FBUT, the fluorescein staining score, meibum expressibility, and meibum quality in patients with moderate MGD compared with the placebo group treated with vitamin E at 400 mg/day [15]. Another such trial showed that dietary supplementation with EPA at 1680 mg/day and DHA at 560 mg/day for 12 weeks improved subjective symptoms, tear osmolarity, and FBUT compared with the placebo group treated with linoleic acid (safflower oil) at 3136 mg/day [34]. Yet another trial showed that dietary supplementation with n-3 PUFAs at 3 g/day for 12 months improved subjective symptoms, FBUT, lid margin telangiectasia, meibum quality, meibomian gland blockage, and the number of visible ducts of meibomian glands compared with baseline in patients with blepharitis and obstructive MGD [13]. On the other hand, the placebo (olive oil) improved FBUT, meibum quality, meibomian gland stenosis, and the number of visible ducts of meibomian glands. The changes in FBUT and meibum quality did not differ significantly between the n-3 PUFA and placebo groups [13]. A prospective, randomized, multicenter clinical trial (Dry Eye Assessment and Management, or DREAM, trial) recently failed to detect a superior improvement in subjective symptoms and objective parameters of dry eye in individuals receiving n-3 PUFAs at 3 g/day (EPA at 2 g/day and DHA at 1 g/day) compared with those receiving placebo (olive oil at 5 g/day) [35]. There were no significant differences in the corneal and conjunctival staining score, FBUT, or Schirmer's test value between the n-3 PUFA supplement group and the placebo group [35]. Parameters related to meibomian glands were not assessed in this previous study. In our study, the multivariate adjusted OR and 95% CI for MGD prevalence and the highest quintile of oleic acid intake compared with the lowest quintile were 0.40 and 0.17 to 0.97 in Model 2. This result suggests the possibility that oleic acid intake may protect against the development of MGD. Gas chromatography revealed that the major components of olive oil were oleic acid (C18:1cis, n-9) at 66.4%, palmitic acid (C16:0) at 16.5%, and linoleic acid (C18:2cis, n-6) at 16.4%, whereas those of sunflower oil were linoleic acid at 62.2% and oleic acid at 28.0% [36]. Oleic acid has been shown to be a major constituent of meibum [2,37,38] and to protect against oxidative stress [39]. The use of olive oil containing oleic acid as a placebo might thus have influenced the results of previous studies of the relation between n-3 PUFA supplementation and MGD or dry eye [13,35]. The average dietary intake of n-3 PUFAs was 2.6 ± 1.0 g/day for all subjects of our study, with values of 1.5 ± 0.4 and 4.0 ± 1.0 g/day for those in the lowest and highest quintiles, respectively. The participants of our study thus had an n-3 PUFA intake similar to that for patients of previous interventional studies with n-3 PUFA supplements. It is possible that we did not detect a protective effect of n-3 PUFAs on MGD in our study as a result of the relatively high intake even in the lowest intake group.

Both n-3 PUFAs and n-6 PUFAs are essential fatty acids and have been shown to play an important role in regulation of inflammatory and immune responses. The metabolic pathways for n-3 and n-6 PUFAs share enzymes with the inflammation-related metabolism of arachidonic acid. Whereas n-3 PUFAs are thought to be anti-inflammatory, n-6 PUFAs are thought to inhibit this function of n-3 PUFAs in a competitive manner [12,13,29]. The role of inflammation in MGD is not clearly understood [40], but n-3 PUFA intake may reduce the inflammatory state of the eyelid margin.

The balanced composition of meibum is important for maintenance of the stability of the tear film [38,41]. The oleic acid content of meibum was shown to be higher in patients with meibomian seborrhea than in those with meibomianitis or in healthy individuals [41]. Fatty acids in meibum of MGD patients were found to include a higher proportion of branched-chain fatty acids and a lower proportion of SFAs, especially of palmitic (C16) and stearic (C18) acids, compared with those in healthy meibum [38]. Supplementation with n-3 PUFAs increased n-3 fatty acid levels and reduced the n-6/n-3 fatty acid ratio in both plasma [13] and red blood cells [13,35] compared with placebo. A randomized, controlled-feeding, double-blind, crossover study reported that a diet containing oil with a high level of oleic acid lowered circulating concentrations of total cholesterol, low-density-lipoprotein cholesterol, apolipoprotein B, and non-high-density-lipoprotein cholesterol compared with a diet containing a Western-type control oil with a low level of oleic acid [42]. Previous studies have revealed an association between dyslipidemia and MGD [10,43–47]. In the current study, no difference in the history of dyslipidemia ($p = 0.39$) or in the taking of lipid-lowering agents ($p = 1.0$) was apparent between the non-MGD and MGD groups. In our previous report of the Hirado–Takushima study, however, we found that the use of lipid-lowering agents was significantly and independently associated with MGD (OR and 95% CI of 3.22 and 1.05–9.87) by multivariate logistic regression analysis [10]. Exposure to n-3 and n-6 PUFAs for up to 7 days in vitro was found to increase the quantity of intracellular small secretory lipid vesicles and the cellular content of triglycerides in human meibomian gland epithelial cells [48]. Dietary intake of n-3 PUFAs and other unsaturated fatty acids was also found to be associated with a significant change in the lipid profile of meibum in 18 women with Sjögren's syndrome [49]. Dietary fatty acid intake and its balance may thus affect not only the composition of lipids in blood but also that of meibum.

We found that the multivariate adjusted OR (and 95% CI) for the prevalence of MGD and the fifth quintiles of total fat or SFAs in Model 2 was 0.40 (0.16–0.97) and 0.40 (0.17–0.97), respectively, suggesting that a high intake of total fat and SFAs might protect against MGD. As far as we are aware, the relation between total fat or SFA intake and MGD has not previously been examined. Dietary guidelines recommend that SFA intake be limited to <10% of energy intake or be as low as possible in order to reduce ischemic heart disease and stroke [50,51]. Recent meta-analyses, however, found that SFAs were not associated with cardiovascular disease [52,53], coronary heart disease [52], ischemic stroke [52], type 2 diabetes [52], or breast cancer [54]. Another meta-analysis showed that odd-chain SFAs reduced the risk of type 2 diabetes, whereas even- and very long-chain SFAs increased it [55]. Total fat was also not associated with cardiovascular disease [53] or breast cancer [54] in previous meta-analyses. The human body is made up of nutrients from the diet. The quantity and quality of lipids secreted from meibomian glands is altered in MGD [7]. Although the role of fatty acid intake and its balance in MGD is not clearly understood, excessive, insufficient, or unbalanced intake of dietary fatty acids may induce MGD. Further research is needed to clarify the role of dietary fatty acid intake in MGD.

Serum levels of 25-hydroxyvitamin D have been associated with dry eye [27,56,57]. There has been no previous study of the relation between dietary intake or serum levels of vitamin D and MGD. In our present study, the highest quintile of vitamin D intake was associated with a low prevalence of MGD. A previous case study reported that oral vitamin D supplementation ameliorated persistent symptoms in a 40-year-old patient with ocular pain, bilateral MGD, evaporative dry eye, and vitamin D deficiency [58]. A single-arm clinical study of 40 patients with vitamin D deficiency found that oral vitamin D supplementation for 8 weeks improved meibomian gland expressibility, eyelid margin condition, Schirmer's test value, FBUT, and subjective symptoms compared with baseline [19]. Eight-week topical application of an analog of the active form of vitamin D3 was also found to be associated with improved ocular symptoms, plugging and vascularity of lid margins, FBUT, corneal fluorescein staining, meibum grade, and meibomian gland area in patients with obstructive MGD [18]. Recent studies have provided a new insight into the physiological role of vitamin D in extra skeletal tissues [59]. Hyperkeratinization is thought to be a major cause of obstructive MGD [40,60], and the active form of vitamin D3 was found to inhibit the proliferation of keratinocytes and to promote their differentiation [61–64]. Vitamin D and the vitamin D receptor are also implicated in the control of inflammation and immunity [59,65], as well as in that of lipid metabolism [66]. Vitamin D deficiency has been found to be related to dyslipidemia [67,68]. Meibum is composed of many types of lipid. Dietary vitamin D intake might thus be expected to be associated with MGD. Further studies focusing on the relation between vitamin D and MGD may help to elucidate the pathogenesis of MGD and develop new treatment strategies for this condition.

The present study has several limitations. First, many of the male subjects work as fishermen but fish away from the island. Our results thus cannot be readily extended to the general Japanese population. Epidemiological studies in urban areas may yield different results. We would like to do another population-based cross-sectional study in an urban area of Japan and compare the results with the present study in the future. Second, the BDHQ is a self-reported diet history questionnaire. We excluded subjects reporting low or high energy intake, and we used energy-adjusted values of dietary component intake, to minimize the effect of writing errors. Third, we were unable to include the intake of dietary supplements in calculating intake of fatty acids and vitamin D, given that reliable data for composition of dietary supplements were not available in Japan. We included dietary supplement use (yes or no) as a confounder. Fourth, although we attempted to adjust for a wide range of potential confounding variables, we were unable to rule out residual ones. Fifth, we did not perform blood tests. Sixth, we did not assess the impact of sedentary behavior and physical activity. And finally, the study has a cross-sectional design, precluding assessment of causal effects of fatty acid or vitamin D intake on the prevalence of MGD.

5. Conclusions

We have performed a population-based study to assess the relationship between dietary intake of fatty acids and vitamin D and the prevalence of MGD among residents of Takushima Island, Japan. Our results suggest that high intake of total fat, SFAs, oleic acid, and vitamin D may be inversely associated with the prevalence of MGD in Japanese individuals. No significant association was detected between the prevalence of MGD and either dietary intake of n-3 PUFAs or n-6 PUFAs or the n-6/n-3 PUFA ratio by multivariate logistic regression analysis. Further epidemiological studies are warranted to clarify dietary strategies for prevention of MGD.

Author Contributions: Conceptualization, R.A. and S.F.; formal analysis, S.F.; investigation, R.A., S.F., T.M., M.K., S.K., R.S., T.S., and N.M.; writing—original draft preparation, S.F.; writing—review and editing, R.A., and N.M.; supervision, N.M.; project administration, R.A.; software, S.S.; All authors have read and agreed to the published version of the manuscript.

Funding: This research received no external funding. It was financially supported by the Lid and Meibomian Gland Working Group.

Institutional Review Board Statement: The study was conducted according to the guidelines of the Declaration of Helsinki and approved by the Institutional Review Board of Itoh Clinic (protocol code: IRIN201707-04, date of approval: 10th July 2017).

Informed Consent Statement: Informed consent was obtained from all subjects involved in the study.

Data Availability Statement: The data presented in this study are available on request from the corresponding author.

Conflicts of Interest: R.A. holds patents of a noninvasive meibography system (JP patent registration no. 5281846, U.S. patent publication no. 2011-0273550A1, and EP patent publication no. 2189108A1) and is a consultant for Inami Co., Kowa Co., and Topcon Japan. The remaining authors declare no conflict of interest.

References

1. Lam, S.M.; Tong, L.; Duan, X.; Petznick, A.; Wenk, M.R.; Shui, G. Extensive characterization of human tear fluid collected using different techniques unravels the presence of novel lipid amphiphiles. *J. Lipid Res.* **2014**, *55*, 289–298. [CrossRef] [PubMed]
2. Butovich, I.A.; Arciniega, J.C.; Lu, H.; Molai, M. Evaluation and quantitation of intact wax esters of human meibum by gas-liquid chromatography-ion trap mass spectrometry. *Investig. Ophthalmol. Vis. Sci.* **2012**, *53*, 3766–3781. [CrossRef] [PubMed]
3. Rosenfeld, L.; Fuller, G.G. Consequences of interfacial viscoelasticity on thin film stability. *Langmuir* **2012**, *28*, 14238–14244. [CrossRef] [PubMed]
4. Georgiev, G.A.; Yokoi, N.; Ivanova, S.; Tonchev, V.; Nencheva, Y.; Krastev, R. Surface relaxations as a tool to distinguish the dynamic interfacial properties of films formed by normal and diseased meibomian lipids. *Soft Matter* **2014**, *10*, 5579–5588. [CrossRef]
5. Tomlinson, A.; Doane, M.G.; McFadyen, A. Inputs and outputs of the lacrimal system: Review of production and evaporative loss. *Ocul. Surf.* **2009**, *7*, 186–198. [CrossRef]
6. Nelson, J.D.; Shimazaki, J.; Benitez-Del-Castillo, J.M.; Craig, J.P.; McCulley, J.P.; Den, S.; Foulks, G.N. The international workshop on meibomian gland dysfunction: Report of the definition and classification subcommittee. *Investig. Ophthalmol. Vis. Sci.* **2011**, *52*, 1930–1937. [CrossRef] [PubMed]
7. Nichols, K.K.; Foulks, G.N.; Bron, A.J.; Glasgow, B.J.; Dogru, M.; Tsubota, K.; Lemp, M.A.; Sullivan, D.A. The international workshop on meibomian gland dysfunction: Executive summary. *Investig. Ophthalmol. Vis. Sci.* **2011**, *52*, 1922–1929. [CrossRef] [PubMed]

8. Lemp, M.A. Report of the national eye institute/industry workshop on clinical trials in dry eyes. *CLAO J.* **1995**, *21*, 221–232.
9. Stapleton, F.; Alves, M.; Bunya, V.Y.; Jalbert, I.; Lekhanont, K.; Malet, F.; Fiona, S.; Schaumberg, D.; Uchino, M.; Vehof, J.; et al. TFOS DEWS II epidemiology report. *Ocul. Surf.* **2017**, *15*, 334–365. [CrossRef]
10. Arita, R.; Mizoguchi, T.; Kawashima, M.; Fukuoka, S.; Koh, S.; Shirakawa, R.; Suzuki, T.; Morishige, N. Meibomian gland dysfunction and dry eye are similar but different based on a population-based study: The hirado-takushima study in Japan. *Am. J. Ophthalmol.* **2019**, *207*, 410–418. [CrossRef]
11. Geerling, G.; Tauber, J.; Baudouin, C.; Goto, E.; Matsumoto, Y.; O'Brien, T.; Rolando, M.; Tsubota, K.; Nichols, K.K. The international workshop on meibomian gland dysfunction: Report of the subcommittee on management and treatment of mei-bomian gland dysfunction. *Investig. Ophthalmol. Vis. Sci.* **2011**, *52*, 2050–2064. [CrossRef] [PubMed]
12. Jones, L.; Downie, L.E.; Korb, D.; Benitez-Del-Castillo, J.M.; Dana, R.; Deng, S.X.; Dong, P.N.; Geerling, G.; Hida, R.Y.; Liu, Y.; et al. TFOS DEWS II management and therapy report. *Ocul. Surf.* **2017**, *15*, 575–628. [CrossRef] [PubMed]
13. Macsai, M.S. The Role of omega-3 dietary supplementation in blepharitis and meibomian gland dysfunction (an AOS thesis). *Trans. Am. Ophthalmol. Soc.* **2008**, *106*, 336–356. [PubMed]
14. Oleñik, A.; Jiménez-Alfaro, I.; Alejandre-Alba, N.; Mahillo-Fernández, I. A randomized, double-masked study to evaluate the effect of omega-3 fatty acids supplementation in meibomian gland dysfunction. *Clin. Interv. Aging* **2013**, *8*, 1133–1138. [CrossRef] [PubMed]
15. Malhotra, C.; Singh, S.; Chakma, P.; Jain, A.K. Effect of oral omega-3 Fatty Acid supplementation on contrast sensitivity in patients with moderate meibomian gland dysfunction: A prospective placebo-controlled study. *Cornea* **2015**, *34*, 637–643. [CrossRef] [PubMed]
16. Miljanović, B.; Trivedi, K.A.; Dana, M.R.; Gilbard, J.P.; Buring, J.E.; Schaumberg, D.A. Relation between dietary n−3 and n−6 fatty acids and clinically diagnosed dry eye syndrome in women. *Am. J. Clin. Nutr.* **2005**, *82*, 887–893. [CrossRef]
17. Ziemanski, J.F.; Wolters, L.R.; Jones-Jordan, L.; Nichols, J.J.; Nichols, K.K. Relation between dietary essential fatty acid intake and dry eye disease and meibomian gland dysfunction in postmenopausal women. *Am. J. Ophthalmol.* **2018**, *189*, 29–40. [CrossRef]
18. Arita, R.; Kawashima, M.; Ito, M.; Tsubota, K. Clinical safety and efficacy of vitamin D3 analog ointment for treatment of obstructive meibomian gland dysfunction. *BMC Ophthalmol.* **2017**, *17*, 1–6. [CrossRef]
19. Karaca, E.E.; Kemer, Ö.E.; Özek, D.; Berker, D.; Imga, N.N. Clinical outcomes of ocular surface in patients treated with vitamin D oral replacement. *Arq. Bras. Oftalmol.* **2020**, *83*, 312–317. [CrossRef]
20. Kobayashi, S.; Murakami, K.; Sasaki, S.; Okubo, H.; Hirota, N.; Notsu, A.; Fukui, M.; Date, C. Comparison of relative validity of food group intakes estimated by comprehensive and brief-type self-administered diet history questionnaires against 16 d dietary records in Japanese adults. *Public Health Nutr.* **2011**, *14*, 1200–1211. [CrossRef]
21. Kobayashi, S.; Honda, S.; Murakami, K.; Sasaki, S.; Okubo, H.; Hirota, N.; Notsu, A.; Fukui, M.; Date, C. Both comprehensive and brief self-administered diet history questionnaires satisfactorily rank nutrient intakes in japanese adults. *J. Epidemiol.* **2012**, *22*, 151–159. [CrossRef] [PubMed]
22. Science and Technology Agency. *Standard Tables of Food Composition in Japan 2015*; 7th Revised Rersion; Ministry of Education, Culture, Sports, Science and Technology: Tokyo, Japan, 2015.
23. Sakane, Y.; Yamaguchi, M.; Yokoi, N.; Uchino, M.; Dogru, M.; Oishi, T.; Ohashi, Y.; Ohashi, Y. Development and validation of the dry eye–related quality-of-life score questionnaire. *JAMA Ophthalmol.* **2013**, *131*, 1331–1338. [CrossRef] [PubMed]
24. Amano, S.; Arita, R.; Kinoshita, S.; Yokoi, N.; Sotozono, C.; Komuro, A.; Suzuki, T.; Shimazaki, J. Definition and diagnostic criteria for meibomian gland dysfunction. *Atarashii Ganka* **2010**, *27*, 627–631.
25. Shimazaki, J.; Sakata, M.; Tsubota, K. Ocular surface changes and discomfort in patients with meibomian gland dysfunction. *Arch. Ophthalmol.* **1995**, *113*, 1266–1270. [CrossRef]

26. Tomlinson, A.; Bron, A.J.; Korb, D.R.; Amano, S.; Paugh, J.R.; Pearce, E.I.; Yee, R.; Yokoi, N.; Arita, R.; Dogru, M. The international workshop on meibomian gland dysfunction: Report of the diagnosis subcommittee. *Investig. Ophthalmol. Vis. Sci.* **2011**, *52*, 2006–2049. [CrossRef]
27. Galor, A.; Gardener, H.; Pouyeh, B.; Feuer, W.; Florez, H. Effect of a mediterranean dietary pattern and vitamin d levels on dry eye syndrome. *Cornea* **2014**, *33*, 437–441. [CrossRef]
28. Simopoulos, A.P. The Mediterranean Diets: What is so special about the diet of Greece? The scientific evidence. *J. Nutr.* **2001**, *131*, 3065S–3073S. [CrossRef]
29. James, M.J.; Gibson, R.A.; Cleland, L.G. Dietary polyunsaturated fatty acids and inflammatory mediator production. *Am. J. Clin. Nutr.* **2000**, *71*, 343s–348s. [CrossRef]
30. Molina-Leyva, I.; Molina-Leyva, A.; Riquelme-Gallego, B.; Cano-Ibáñez, N.; García-Molina, L.; Bueno-Cavanillas, A. Effectiveness of mediterranean diet implementation in dry eye parameters: A study of PREDIMED-PLUS trial. *Nutrients* **2020**, *12*, 1289. [CrossRef]
31. Panagiotakos, D.; Pitsavos, C.; Arvaniti, F.; Stefanadis, C. Adherence to the Mediterranean food pattern predicts the prevalence of hypertension, hypercholesterolemia, diabetes and obesity, among healthy adults; the accuracy of the MedDietScore. *Prev. Med.* **2007**, *44*, 335–340. [CrossRef]
32. Hu, N.; Yu, J.-T.; Tan, L.; Wang, Y.-L.; Sun, L.; Tan, L. Nutrition and the risk of Alzheimer's disease. *Biomed. Res. Int.* **2013**, *2013*, 524820. [CrossRef] [PubMed]
33. Korb, D.R.; Blackie, C.A.; Finnemore, V.M.; Douglass, T. Effect of using a combination of lid wipes, eye drops, and omega-3 supplements on meibomian gland functionality in patients with lipid deficient/evaporative dry eye. *Cornea* **2015**, *34*, 407–412. [CrossRef] [PubMed]
34. Epitropoulos, A.T.; Donnenfeld, E.D.; Shah, Z.A.; Holland, E.J.; Gross, M.; Faulkner, W.J.; Matossian, C.; Lane, S.S.; Toyos, M.; Bucci, F.A.; et al. Effect of oral re-esterified omega-3 nutritional supplementation on dry eyes. *Cornea* **2016**, *35*, 1185–1191. [CrossRef] [PubMed]
35. Asbell, P.A.; Maguire, M.G.; Pistilli, M.; Ying, G.S.; Szczotka-Flynn, L.B.; Hardten, D.R.; Lin, M.C.; Shtein, R.M. n-3 fatty acid supplementation for the treatment of dry eye disease. *N. Engl. J. Med.* **2018**, *378*, 1681–1690. [PubMed]
36. Orsavova, J.; Misurcova, L.; Ambrozova, J.V.; Vicha, R.; Mlcek, J. Fatty acids composition of vegetable oils and its con-tribution to dietary energy intake and dependence of cardiovascular mortality on dietary intake of fatty acids. *Int. J. Mol. Sci.* **2015**, *16*, 12871–12890. [CrossRef]
37. Dougherty, J.M.; McCulley, J.P. Analysis of the free fatty acid component of meibomian secretions in chronic blepharitis. *Investig. Ophthalmol. Vis. Sci.* **1986**, *27*, 52–56.
38. Joffre, C.; Souchier, M.; Gregoire, S.; Viau, S.; Bretillon, L.; Acar, N.; Bron, A.M.; Creuzot-Garcher, C. Differences in meibomian fatty acid composition in patients with meibomian gland dysfunction and aqueous-deficient dry eye. *Br. J. Ophthalmol.* **2008**, *92*, 116–119. [CrossRef]
39. Gillingham, L.G.; Harris-Janz, S.; Jones, P.J. Dietary monounsaturated fatty acids are protective against metabolic syndrome and cardiovascular disease risk factors. *Lipids* **2011**, *46*, 209–228. [CrossRef]
40. Knop, E.; Knop, N.; Millar, T.; Obata, H.; Sullivan, D.A. The International workshop on meibomian gland dysfunction: Report of the subcommittee on anatomy, physiology, and pathophysiology of the meibomian gland. *Investig. Ophthalmol. Vis. Sci.* **2011**, *52*, 1938–1978. [CrossRef] [PubMed]
41. Shine, W.E.; McCulley, J.P. Association of meibum oleic acid with meibomian seborrhea. *Cornea* **2000**, *19*, 72–74. [CrossRef]
42. Bowen, K.J.; Kris-Etherton, P.M.; West, S.G.; Fleming, J.A.; Connelly, P.W.; Lamarche, B.; Couture, P.; Jenkins, D.J.A.; Taylor, C.G.; Zahradka, P.; et al. Diets enriched with conventional or high-oleic acid canola oils lower atherogenic lipids and lipoproteins compared to a diet with a western fatty acid profile in adults with central adiposity. *J. Nutr.* **2019**, *149*, 471–478. [CrossRef] [PubMed]
43. Dao, A.H.; Spindle, J.D.; Harp, B.A.; Jacob, A.; Chuang, A.Z.; Yee, R.W. Association of dyslipidemia in moderate to severe meibomian gland dysfunction. *Am. J. Ophthalmol.* **2010**, *150*, 371–375.e1. [CrossRef]
44. Módulo, C.M.; Machado Filho, E.B.; Malki, L.T.; Dias, A.C.; de Souza, J.C.; Oliveira, H.C.; Jorge, Í.C.; Santos Gomes, I.B.; Meyrelles, S.S.; Rocha, E.M. The role of dyslipidemia on ocular surface, lacrimal and meibomian gland structure and function. *Curr. Eye Res.* **2012**, *37*, 300–308. [CrossRef] [PubMed]

45. Bukhari, A.A. Associations between the grade of meibomian gland dysfunction and dyslipidemia. *Ophthalmic Plast. Reconstr. Surg.* **2013**, *29*, 101–103. [CrossRef] [PubMed]
46. Braich, P.S.; Howard, M.K.; Singh, J.S. Dyslipidemia and its association with meibomian gland dysfunction. *Int. Ophthalmol.* **2016**, *36*, 469–476. [CrossRef] [PubMed]
47. Naik, M.; Guliani, B.P.; Bhalla, A. Association of the severity of meibomian gland dysfunction with dyslipidemia in Indian population. *Indian J. Ophthalmol.* **2018**, *66*, 1411–1416. [CrossRef]
48. Liu, Y.; Kam, W.R.; Sullivan, D.A. Influence of omega 3 and 6 fatty acids on human meibomian gland epithelial cells. *Cornea* **2016**, *35*, 1122–1126. [CrossRef]
49. Sullivan, B.D.; Cermak, J.M.; Sullivan, R.M.; Papas, A.S.; Evans, J.E.; Dana, M.R.; Sullivan, D.A. Correlations between nutrient intake and the polar lipid profiles of meibomian gland secretions in women with Sjogren's syndrome. *Adv. Exp. Med. Biol.* **2002**, *506 Pt A*, 441–447.
50. Lichtenstein, A.H.; Appel, L.J.; Brands, M.; Carnethon, M.; Daniels, S.; Franch, H.A.; Franklin, B.; Kris-Etherton, P.; Harris, W.S.; Howard, B.; et al. Diet and lifestyle recommendations revision 2006: A scientific statement from the American Heart Association Nutrition Committee. *Circulation* **2006**, *114*, 82–96. [CrossRef]
51. McGuire, S.U.S. Department of Agriculture and U.S. Department of Health and Human Services, dietary guidelines for Americans, 2010. 7th Edition, Washington, DC: U.S. Government Printing Office, January 2011. *Adv. Nutr.* **2011**, *2*, 293–294. [CrossRef]
52. De Souza, R.J.; Mente, A.; Maroleanu, A.; Cozma, A.I.; Ha, V.; Kishibe, T.; Uleryk, E.; Budylowski, P.; Schunemann, H.J.; Beyene, J.; et al. Intake of saturated and trans unsaturated fatty acids and risk of all cause mortality, cardiovascular disease, and type 2 diabetes: Systematic review and meta-analysis of observational studies. *BMJ* **2015**, *351*, h3978. [CrossRef] [PubMed]
53. Zhu, Y.; Bo, Y.; Liu, Y. Dietary total fat, fatty acids intake, and risk of cardiovascular disease: A dose-response meta-analysis of cohort studies. *Lipids Health Dis.* **2019**, *18*, 91. [CrossRef] [PubMed]
54. Cao, Y.; Hou, L.; Wang, W. Dietary total fat and fatty acids intake, serum fatty acids and risk of breast cancer: A meta-analysis of prospective cohort studies. *Int. J. Cancer* **2016**, *138*, 1894–1904. [CrossRef] [PubMed]
55. Huang, L.-H.; Lin, J.-S.; Yang, G.; Aris, I.M.; Aris, I.M.; Chen, W.-Q.; Li, L.-J. Circulating saturated fatty acids and incident type 2 diabetes: A systematic review and meta-analysis. *Nutrients* **2019**, *11*, 998. [CrossRef] [PubMed]
56. Yildirim, P.; Garip, Y.; Karci, A.A.; Guler, T. Dry eye in vitamin D deficiency: More than an incidental association. *Int. J. Rheum. Dis.* **2016**, *19*, 49–54. [CrossRef]
57. Yoon, S.Y.; Bae, S.H.; Shin, Y.J.; Park, S.G.; Hwang, S.-H.; Hyon, J.Y.; Wee, W.R. Low Serum 25-Hydroxyvitamin D Levels Are Associated with Dry Eye Syndrome. *PLoS ONE* **2016**, *11*, e0147847. [CrossRef]
58. Shetty, R.; Deshpande, K.; Deshmukh, R.; Jayadev, C.; Shroff, R. Bowman break and subbasal nerve plexus changes in a patient with dry eye presenting with chronic ocular pain and vitamin D deficiency. *Cornea* **2016**, *35*, 688–691. [CrossRef]
59. Christakos, S.; Dhawan, P.; Verstuyf, A.; Verlinden, L.; Carmeliet, G. Vitamin D: Metabolism, molecular mechanism of action, and pleiotropic effects. *Physiol. Rev.* **2016**, *96*, 365–408. [CrossRef]
60. Jester, J.V.; Parfitt, G.J.; Brown, D.J. Meibomian gland dysfunction: Hyperkeratinization or atrophy? *BMC Ophthalmol.* **2015**, *15*, 156. [CrossRef]
61. Morimoto, S.; Kumahara, Y. A patient with psoriasis cured by 1 alpha-hydroxyvitamin D3. *Med. J. Osaka Univ.* **1985**, *35*, 51–54.
62. Kragballe, K.; Beck, H.I.; Søgaard, H. Improvement of psoriasis by a topical vitamin D3 analogue (MC 903) in a double-blind study. *Br. J. Dermatol.* **1988**, *119*, 223–230. [CrossRef] [PubMed]
63. Bikle, D.D. Vitamin D: A calciotropic hormone regulating calcium-induced keratinocyte differentiation. *J. Am. Acad. Dermatol.* **1997**, *37 3 Pt 2*, 42–52.
64. Cianferotti, L.; Cox, M.; Skorija, K.; DeMay, M.B. Vitamin D receptor is essential for normal keratinocyte stem cell function. *Proc. Natl. Acad. Sci. USA* **2007**, *104*, 9428–9433. [CrossRef] [PubMed]
65. Prietl, B.; Treiber, G.; Pieber, T.R.; Amrein, K. Vitamin D and immune function. *Nutrients* **2013**, *5*, 2502–2521. [CrossRef] [PubMed]

66. Savastano, S.B.L.; Barrea, L.; Savanelli, M.C.; Nappi, F.; Di Somma, C.; Orio, F.; Colao, A. Low vitamin D status and obesity: Role of nutritionist. *Rev. Endocr. Metab. Disord.* **2017**, *18*, 215–225. [CrossRef] [PubMed]
67. Zittermann, A.; Gummert, J.F.; Börgermann, J. The role of vitamin D in dyslipidemia and cardiovascular disease. *Curr. Pharm. Des.* **2011**, *17*, 933–942. [CrossRef] [PubMed]
68. Pannu, P.K.; Calton, E.K.; Soares, M.J. Calcium and vitamin D in obesity and related chronic disease. *Adv. Food Nutr. Res.* **2016**, *77*, 57–100. [CrossRef]

Publisher's Note: MDPI stays neutral with regard to jurisdictional claims in published maps and institutional affiliations.

 © 2021 by the authors. Licensee MDPI, Basel, Switzerland. This article is an open access article distributed under the terms and conditions of the Creative Commons Attribution (CC BY) license (http://creativecommons.org/licenses/by/4.0/).

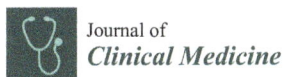

Article

Multicenter Study of Intense Pulsed Light for Patients with Refractory Aqueous-Deficient Dry Eye Accompanied by Mild Meibomian Gland Dysfunction

Reiko Arita [1,2,*], Shima Fukuoka [2,3], Takanori Mizoguchi [2,4] and Naoyuki Morishige [2,5]

1. Department of Ophthalmology, Itoh Clinic, 626-11 Minami-Nakano, Minumaku, Saitama, Saitama 337-0042, Japan
2. Lid and Meibomian Gland Working Group (LIME), Tokyo 112-0006, Japan; fshima3271@gmail.com (S.F.); t-mizo@siren.ocn.ne.jp (T.M.); morishig@corneajp.com (N.M.)
3. Omiya Hamada Eye Clinic, 1-169-1, Sakuragicho, Omiyaku, Saitama 330-0854, Japan
4. Mizoguchi Eye Clinic, 6-13, Tawaramachi, Sasebo, Nagasaki 857-0016, Japan
5. Division of Cornea and Ocular Surface, Ohshima Eye Hospital, 11-8, Kamigofukumachi, Hakataku, Fukuoka 812-0036, Japan
* Correspondence: ritoh@za2.so-net.ne.jp; Tel.: +81-48-686-5588

Received: 20 September 2020; Accepted: 26 October 2020; Published: 28 October 2020

Abstract: Aqueous-deficient dry eye (ADDE) and meibomian gland dysfunction (MGD) can be refractory to therapy. Intense pulsed light (IPL) was recently introduced as an effective treatment for MGD. We here evaluated the efficacy of IPL combined with MG expression (MGX) compared with MGX alone (n = 23 and 20, respectively) for patients with refractory ADDE with mild MGD at three sites. Symptom score, visual acuity (VA), noninvasive breakup time (NIBUT) and lipid layer thickness (LLT) of the tear film, lid margin abnormalities, fluorescein BUT (FBUT), fluorescein staining, tear meniscus height (TMH), meibum grade, meiboscore, and Schirmer's test value were assessed at baseline and 1 and 3 months after treatment. LLT, plugging, vascularity, FBUT and NIBUT were improved only in the IPL-MGX group at three months compared with baseline. All parameters with the exception of VA, meiboscore, TMH, Schirmer's test value were also improved in the IPL-MGX group compared with the control group at three months, as was VA in patients with central corneal epitheliopathy. Although IPL-MGX does not affect aqueous layer, the induced improvement in quality and quantity of the lipid layer may increase tear film stability and ameliorate symptoms not only for evaporative dry eye but for ADDE.

Keywords: aqueous-deficient dry eye; meibomian gland dysfunction; meibomian gland; intense pulsed light

1. Introduction

Dry eye disease is a common condition that causes ocular discomfort [1]. Although it generally does not reduce conventionally tested visual acuity (VA), most individuals with this condition manifest impairment of functional visual acuity, with higher-order aberrations in particular leading to disturbance of quality of vision [2]. Dry eye disease is classified into two major subtypes—aqueous-deficient dry eye (ADDE) and evaporative dry eye (EDE) [3]—both of which can involve pathology of meibomian glands, lacrimal glands, the eyelids, the tear film, and ocular surface cells [4]. ADDE and EDE tend to coexist, in part because the lacrimal gland defects associated with ADDE can lead to meibomian gland dysfunction (MGD) [5], and consequent EDE as a result of friction between the lid margin and the cornea and conjunctiva [6].

Common therapies for patients with ADDE include various topical medications such as cyclosporine, diclofenac sodium, steroids, loteprednol etabonate, resolvin E1, tacrolimus, autologous serum, and vitamin A [7,8]. In addition, punctal plug insertion, oral systemic antibiotics, surgery, dietary modification, local environmental changes, and alternative medicines have been applied [8]. Common therapies for patients with MGD, which is a major cause of EDE, include the application of a warm compress [9], the practice of lid hygiene [9], dietary supplementation with omega-3 fatty acids [9], forced meibum expression [9], intraductal probing [10], automated thermal pulsation [11], and the administration of topical steroids [9], topical and oral antibiotics including topical cyclosporine and azithromycin [9], preservative-free artificial tears [9], lipid-containing eyedrops [9], and topical diquafosol [12,13]. Despite the varied treatment options available, however, some patients with ADDE or MGD are refractory to therapy and therefore do not experience complete or long-term relief of symptoms.

Intense pulsed light (IPL) therapy based on the delivery of intense pulses of noncoherent light with wavelengths of 500 to 1200 nm has been applied in dermatology to treat various conditions, including benign cavernous hemangiomas or venous malformations, telangiectasia, port wine stains, and other pigmented lesions [14,15]. The efficacy of IPL therapy for patients with dry eye due to MGD was discovered during IPL treatment of facial rosacea [16]. Subsequent studies found that IPL, with or without concomitant meibomian gland expression (MGX), is effective for improvement of subjective symptoms and objective findings in patients with mild to moderate MGD or dry eye [17–28]. The combination of IPL and MGX was also shown to be effective in patients with refractory MGD [28,29]. In addition, it ameliorated dry eye symptoms and improved meibomian gland function in patients with refractory dry eye, including not only individuals with MGD but also those with graft-versus-host disease or Sjögren syndrome [20] or those with keratoconjunctivitis sicca [30]. However, as far as we are aware, no previous study has evaluated the effects of IPL on tear fluid–related parameters in addition to meibomian gland–related parameters in patients with refractory ADDE accompanied by mild MGD. We have therefore now performed a multicenter, retrospective, controlled study to evaluate the efficacy of IPL combined with MGX in comparison with MGX alone in patients with refractory ADDE and mild MGD who had been treated with conventional therapies.

2. Experimental Section

2.1. Patients

This retrospective controlled study was approved by the Institutional Review Boards of Itoh Clinic (approval code: IRIN201903-03), Mizoguchi Eye Clinic, and Ohshima Eye Hospital on March 11th, 2019, and it adhered to the tenets of the Declaration of Helsinki. Patients with refractory ADDE associated with mild MGD who were treated with either IPL and MGX or MGX alone between April and December 2017 at three sites in Japan (Itoh Clinic, Mizoguchi Eye Clinic, and Ohshima Eye Hospital) were enrolled in the study. Informed consent to study participation was obtained from each patient.

Inclusion criteria were as follows: (1) an age of at least 20 years; (2) a diagnosis of ADDE based on the diagnostic criteria for ADDE in Japan [31], which encompass ocular symptoms, a fluorescein tear film breakup time (FBUT) of ≤5 s, a Schirmer's test value of ≤5 mm, and the presence of conjunctival or corneal epithelial damage as evidenced by a fluorescein staining (Fluo) score of ≥1 (on a scale of 0 to 9) according to the van Bijsterveld method [32]; (3) a diagnosis of mild MGD based on the diagnostic criteria for MGD in Japan [33], which encompass ocular symptoms, plugged gland orifices (plugging grade [34] of ≥1, which corresponds to plugging of fewer than three gland orifices with a distribution of less than half of the full length of the lid), vascularity and irregularity of lid margins, reduced meibum expression (meibum grade of ≥2, on a scale of 0 to 3, where 0 = clear meibum easily expressed, 1 = cloudy meibum expressed with mild pressure, 2 = cloudy meibum expressed with more than moderate pressure, and 3 = meibum cannot be expressed even with strong pressure) [35], and a meiboscore of ≥3 (on a scale of 0 to 6) [36]; (4) refractoriness of ADDE as defined by the failure to respond over a period of ≥2 years to at least three types of conventional therapy prescribed in Japan, including tear replacement therapy, tear conservation, and anti-inflammatory eyedrops; and (5) a Fitzpatrick skin type of 1 to 4 based on sun sensitivity and appearance [37]. Exclusion criteria included the presence of active skin lesions, skin cancer, or other specific skin pathology or of active ocular infection or ocular inflammatory disease.

2.2. Experimental Design

Each patient underwent a series of four IPL-MGX treatment sessions or four sessions of MGX alone at 3-week intervals and was subjected to clinical assessment as described below both before treatment as well as 4 and 12 weeks after the final treatment session. All patients were asked to continue their current ocular medications as well as not to initiate therapy with a new topical or systemic agent for dry eye or MGD during the treatment course.

2.3. Clinical Assessment

The thickness of the lipid layer of the tear film (LLT), noninvasive breakup time of the tear film (NIBUT), and interferometric fringe pattern of the tear film were determined with a DR-1α tear interferometer (Kowa, Tokyo, Japan) as described previously [38]. Lid margin abnormalities (plugging of meibomian gland orifices and vascularity of lid margins) [34], FBUT, the Fluo score [32], tear meniscus height (TMH) based on fluorescein staining, and meibum grade [35] were evaluated with a slitlamp microscope. For determination of TMH, the center of the lower tear meniscus stained with fluorescein was photographed with a CCD camera attached to the slitlamp microscope, with a magnification of 10 × and under lighting with a blue-free filter. The photographs were examined by an ocular surface expert (R.A.) for semiquantitative grading of TMH as low, normal or high. Morphological changes of meibomian glands were assessed on the basis of the meiboscore [36] as determined by noninvasive meibography. Tear fluid production was measured by Schirmer's test as performed without anesthesia [39]. Symptoms were assessed with the standard patient evaluation of eye dryness (SPEED) validated questionnaire (scale of 0 to 28) [40,41]. VA was also measured with the use of Landolt C charts, and best corrected Landolt VA was converted to logarithm of the minimum angle of resolution (logMAR) VA.

2.4. IPL-MGX Procedure

Before the first treatment, each patient underwent Fitzpatrick skin typing [37] and the IPL machine (M22; Lumenis, Yokneam, Israel) was adjusted to the appropriate setting (Toyos setting: 590-nm cutoff filter, triple pulses of 6.0 ms with an interval of 50 ms, and total fluence range of 13 to 15 J/cm^2). At each treatment session, both eyes of the patient were closed and sealed with IPL-Aid disposable eye shields (Honeywell Safety Products, Smithfield, RI, USA). After generous application of ultrasonic gel to the targeted skin area, each patient received ~13 pulses of light (with slightly overlapping applications) from the right preauricular area, across the cheeks and nose, to the left preauricular area, reaching up to the inferior boundary of the eye shields. This procedure was then repeated in a second pass. Immediately after the IPL treatment, MGX was performed on both upper and lower eyelids of each eye with an Arita Meibomian Gland Compressor (Katena, Denville, NJ, USA). Pain was minimized during MGX by the application of 0.4% oxybuprocaine hydrochloride to each eye. Patients in the control group underwent the MGX procedure alone, without IPL.

2.5. Statistical Analysis

Data were found to be non-normally distributed with the Shapiro–Wilk test ($p < 0.05$), and nonparametric testing was therefore applied. The Mann–Whitney U test was used to compare numerical variables between the control (MGX alone) and the IPL-MGX groups. The Wilcoxon signed-rank test was used to compare numerical variables between baseline and either 1 or 3 months after the final treatment session. Fisher's exact test was used to compare categorical variables between the control and IPL-MGX groups. The chi-square test was used to compare lipid layer grade and TMH between before and either 1 or 3 months after the final treatment session. Adjusted p values were calculated by multiplication of obtained p values by the number of comparisons in Bonferroni's correction. The outcome variables of the study were the SPEED score and NIBUT before and after treatment. We performed a statistical power analysis for both the SPEED score and NIBUT at 3 months after the final treatment session in the control and IPL-MGX groups. The power (1-β) was >0.90 at the level of $\alpha = 0.025$, and the sample size was sufficient. Statistical analysis was performed with JMP Pro version 15 software (SAS, Cary, NC, USA). All statistical tests were two sided, and a p value of <0.05 was considered statistically significant.

3. Results

3.1. Patient Characteristics

The characteristics of the 43 study subjects with refractory ADDE and mild MGD, including 23 individuals in the IPL-MGX group and 20 in the MGX group, are presented in Table 1. Approximately 40% of patients had Sjögren syndrome or rheumatoid arthritis.

Table 1. Characteristics of the study subjects with aqueous-deficient dry eye (ADDE) and mild meibomian gland dysfunction in the intense pulsed light (IPL)-meibomian gland expression (MGX) and MGX (control) groups.

Characteristic	Control (MGX) Group (n = 20 Subjects, 40 Eyes)	IPL-MGX Group (n = 23 Subjects, 46 Eyes)	p
Age (years), mean ± SD (range)	61.4 ± 15.1 (31–78)	59.0 ± 15.0 (43–84)	0.64
Sex (male/female)	7/13	9/14	0.78
Duration of ADDE (years), mean ± SD (range)	8.8 ± 5.1 (2–20)	8.1 ± 6.7 (2–24)	0.60
History of contact lens wear	22 eyes of 11 patients (55.0%)	24 eyes of 12 patients (52.2%)	0.85
Previous ocular surgery	24 eyes of 12 patients (60.0%)	18 eyes of 9 patients (39.1%)	0.17
Sjögren syndrome	6 patients (30.0%)	7 patients (30.4%)	1
Rheumatoid arthritis	2 patients (10.0%)	2 patients (8.7%)	1

p values were determined with Mann–Whitney U test (displayed in gray) or Fisher's exact test. SD, standard deviations.

The frequency of other ADDE therapies previously administered is shown in Table 2, with most patients having been treated with diquafosol eyedrops, topical steroids, hyaluronic acid eyedrops, or punctal plugs.

Table 2. Previous therapies for the study patients in the intense pulsed light (IPL)-meibomian gland expression (MGX) and MGX (control) groups.

Therapy	No. (%) of Patients	
	Control Group (n = 20)	IPL-MGX Group (n = 23)
Diquafosol eyedrops	19 (95.0)	22 (95.7)
Topical steroids	10 (50.0)	21 (91.3)
Rebamipide eyedrops	9 (45.0)	15 (65.2)
Hyaluronic acid eyedrops	8 (40.0)	18 (78.3)
Punctal plugs	8 (40.0)	16 (69.6)
Preservative-free artificial tears	8 (40.0)	10 (43.5)
Omega-3 fatty acid supplementation	3 (15.0)	6 (26.1)

3.2. Efficacy of IPL-MGX

The SPEED score was significantly reduced at 4 weeks after the final treatment session compared with baseline in both IPL-MGX group and MGX groups, and this difference was maintained for up to 3 months (Table 3). LLT was significantly increased at both 1 and 3 months after the final treatment session in the IPL-MGX group but not in the control group (Table 3).

Both NIBUT and FBUT were significantly prolonged at both 1 and 3 months after the final treatment session in the IPL-MGX group, whereas they were significantly improved only at 1 month in the control group (Table 3). Changes in interferometric fringe pattern (lipid layer grade) from one typical of aqueous deficiency (Jupiter like) to the normal condition (pearl like) were apparent in 61% and 35% of eyes in the IPL-MGX group as well as in 30% and 5% of those in the control group at 1 and 3 months, respectively, after the final treatment session compared with baseline (Table 4). Lipid layer grade was thus significantly better in the IPL-MGX group compared to the control group at both 1 and 3 months after the final treatment session. The Fluo score had decreased significantly at both 1 and 3 months after the final treatment session in both groups, with the value being significantly lower in the IPL-MGX group than in the control group at both posttreatment assessment points (Table 3).

The logMAR VA of eyes in the IPL-MGX group was significantly improved at both 1 and 3 months after treatment completion compared with baseline, although the values that did not differ between the two groups either before or 1 or 3 months after treatment (Table 5). Eleven of 40 (27.5%) and 12 of 46 (26.1%) eyes in the control and IPL-MGX groups, respectively, manifested central corneal epitheliopathy central corneal epitheliopathy (CCE) with these frequencies not differing significantly between the two groups ($p = 1$, Fisher's exact test). A significantly improvement in log MAR VA was apparent for the eyes with CCE in the IPL-MGX group compared with those in the control group, both after amerilration of the CCE at 1 month and at 3 months after treatment completion (Table 5, Figure 1).

Meibum grade was significantly decreased in both groups at both 1 and 3 months after treatment completion compared with baseline, whereas vascularity score was significantly decreased at both time points only in the IPL-MGX group (Table 3). Plugging score was significantly decreased in both groups at 1 month after treatment completion compared with baseline, whereas only in the IPL-MGX at 3 months (Table 3). The IPL-MGX group showed a significant difference in meibum grade and lid margin abnormality (plugging and vascularity) scores compared with the control group at both 1 and 3 months after the treatment (Table 3). The meiboscore was not significantly changed at either 1 or 3 months in the IPL-MGX or control group (Table 3). Schirmer's test value also remained unchanged at 1 and 3 months after the final treatment session in both the IPL-MGX and control groups (Table 3). Finally, TMH was low at baseline and remained so after treatment in both groups (Table 4).

Table 3. Characteristics of the study subjects with aqueous-deficient dry eye and mild meibomian gland dysfunction in intense pulsed light (IPL)-meibomian gland expression (MGX) and MGX (control) groups before as well as 1 and 3 months after the final treatment session.

Characteristic	Group	Baseline		1 Month after the Final Treatment Session				3 Months after the Final Treatment Session			
		Mean ± SD	Adjusted p Value for IPL-MGX vs. Control	Mean ± SD	Mean Change ± SE	Adjusted p Value vs. Baseline	Adjusted p Value for IPL-MGX vs. Control	Mean ± SD	Mean Change ± SE	Adjusted p Value vs. Baseline	Adjusted p Value for IPL-MGX vs. Control
SPEED score (0–28)	Control	14.2 ± 4.6	0.53	10.1 ± 3.9	−4.2 ± 0.6	<0.001 **	0.003 *	10.4 ± 4.1	−3.8 ± 0.6	<0.001 **	<0.001 **
	IPL-MGX	15.9 ± 4.2		6.0 ± 4.6	−9.9 ± 0.7	<0.001 **		4.2 ± 3.9	−11.7 ± 0.9	<0.001 **	
LLT (mm)	Control	63.1 ± 16.2	0.72	56.1 ± 11.2	−7.0 ± 2.6	0.055	<0.001 **	57.9 ± 11.8	−5.2 ± 2.7	0.14	<0.001 **
	IPL-MGX	66.6 ± 24.1		78.6 ± 21.5	14.7 ± 3.2	<0.001 **		84.2 ± 20.6	18.3 ± 2.9	<0.001 **	
Plugging (0–3)	Control	1.0 ± 0.2	0.88	0.8 ± 0.4	−0.3 ± 0.1	0.002 *	<0.001 **	1.1 ± 0.3	0.1 ± 0.1	0.37	<0.001 **
	IPL-MGX	1.0 ± 0.0		0.3 ± 0.4	−0.7 ± 0.1	<0.001 **		0.3 ± 0.5	−0.7 ± 0.1	<0.001 **	
Vascularity (0–3)	Control	1.7 ± 0.6	0.85	1.7 ± 0.6	0.0 ± 0.0	1	<0.001 **	1.7 ± 0.6	0.0 ± 0.0	1	<0.001 **
	IPL-MGX	1.9 ± 0.8		0.8 ± 0.7	−1.1 ± 0.1	<0.001 **		0.9 ± 0.7	−1.0 ± 0.1	<0.001 **	
Meiboscore (0–6)	Control	1.7 ± 0.6	0.69	1.7 ± 0.6	0.0 ± 0.0	1	0.32	1.7 ± 0.6	0.0 ± 0.0	1	0.69
	IPL-MGX	1.5 ± 1.0		1.5 ± 1.0	−0.1 ± 0.0	0.088		1.5 ± 1.0	0.0 ± 0.0	1	
Meibum grade (0–3)	Control	2.0 ± 0.0	1	1.6 ± 0.5	−0.4 ± 0.1	<0.001 **	<0.001 **	1.9 ± 0.4	−0.2 ± 0.1	0.025 *	<0.001 **
	IPL-MGX	2.0 ± 0.0		0.5 ± 0.6	−1.5 ± 0.1	<0.001 **		0.4 ± 0.6	−1.6 ± 0.1	<0.001 **	
NIBUT (s)	Control	2.2 ± 1.1	1	3.6 ± 1.6	1.4 ± 0.2	<0.001 **	0.002 *	2.4 ± 1.2	0.2 ± 0.1	0.22	<0.001 **
	IPL-MGX	2.1 ± 1.3		5.3 ± 2.2	3.2 ± 0.3	<0.001 **		5.5 ± 2.0	3.4 ± 0.3	<0.001 **	
FBUT (s)	Control	2.4 ± 1.1	0.84	3.4 ± 1.5	1.1 ± 0.2	<0.001 **	0.001 *	2.5 ± 1.3	0.1 ± 0.1	0.17	<0.001 **
	IPL-MGX	2.2 ± 1.3		5.2 ± 2.0	3.0 ± 0.4	<0.001 **		5.4 ± 2.1	3.2 ± 0.4	<0.001 **	
Fluo score (0–9)	Control	3.2 ± 0.8	0.75	2.7 ± 0.9	−0.5 ± 0.1	<0.001 **	<0.001 **	2.9 ± 0.9	−0.3 ± 0.1	<0.001 **	<0.001 **
	IPL-MGX	3.4 ± 2.2		0.5 ± 0.9	−3.0 ± 0.3	<0.001 **		0.3 ± 0.6	−3.1 ± 0.3	<0.001 **	
Schirmer's test value (mm)	Control	2.4 ± 1.5	1	2.4 ± 1.5	0.0 ± 0.2	1	1	2.5 ± 1.4	0.1 ± 0.1	1	0.89
	IPL-MGX	2.3 ± 1.5		2.2 ± 1.4	−0.1 ± 0.2	1		2.2 ± 1.4	−0.1 ± 0.1	0.84	

SPEED score: control group (n = 20); IPL-MGX group (n = 23). Other characteristics: control group (n = 40 eyes); IPL-MGX group (n = 46 eyes). p values were determined with the Wilcoxon signed-rank test vs. baseline or Mann–Whitney U test vs. control with Bonferroni's correction (* adjusted p < 0.05, ** adjusted p < 0.001). SPEED, standard patient evaluation of eye dryness; LLT, lipid layer thickness; NIBUT, noninvasive breakup time; FUBT, fluorescein breakup time; Fluo, fluorescein staining; SE, standard errors; SD, standard deviations.

Table 4. Lipid layer grade and tear meniscus height (TMH) of the study subjects with aqueous-deficient dry eye and mild meibomian gland dysfunction in the intense pulsed light (IPL)—meibomian gland expression (MGX) group (n = 46 eyes) and MGX (control) group (n = 40 eyes) at baseline as well as 1 and 3 months after the treatment completion.

Characteristic		Group	Baseline		1 Month after the Final Treatment Session			3 Months after the Final Treatment Session		
			No. (%) of Eyes	Adjusted p Value for IPL-MGX vs. Control	No. (%) of Eyes	Adjusted p Value vs. Baseline	Adjusted p Value for IPL-MGX vs. Control	No. (%) of Eyes	Adjusted p Value vs. Baseline	Adjusted p Value for IPL-MGX vs. Control
Interferometric pattern	Jupiter-like	Control	40 (100.0%)		28 (70.0%)			38 (95.0%)		
	Pearl-like		0 (0.0%)		12 (30.0%)	<0.001 **		2 (5.0%)	<0.001 **	
	Crystal-like		0 (0.0%)	1	0 (0.0%)		0.016 *	0 (0.0%)		0.003 *
	Jupiter-like	IPL-MGX	46 (100.0%)		18 (39.1%)			30 (65.2%)		
	Pearl-like		0 (0.0%)		28 (60.9%)	<0.001 **		16 (34.8%)	<0.001 **	
	Crystal-like		0 (0.0%)		0 (0.0%)			0 (0.0%)		
TMH	Low	Control	40 (100.0%)		40 (100.0%)			40 (100.0%)		
	Normal		0 (0.0%)		0 (0.0%)	1		0 (0.0%)	1	
	High		0 (0.0%)	1	0 (0.0%)		1	0 (0.0%)		1
	Low	IPL-MGX	46 (100.0%)		46 (100.0%)			46 (100.0%)		
	Normal		0 (0.0%)		0 (0.0%)	1		0 (0.0%)	1	
	High		0 (0.0%)		0 (0.0%)			0 (0.0%)		

p values were determined with the chi-square test vs. baseline and Fisher's exact test vs. control with Bonferroni's correction (* adjusted p < 0.05, ** adjusted p < 0.001).

Table 5. Logarithm of the minimum angle of resolution (logMAR) visual acuity of the study subjects with or without central corneal epitheliopathy (CCE) in the intense pulsed light (IPL)—meibomian gland expression (MGX) group (n = 12 and 32, respectively) and MGX (control) group (n = 11 and 29, respectively) at baseline as well as 1 and 3 months after the final treatment session.

Group		Baseline		1 Month after the Final Treatment Session				3 Months after the Final Treatment Session			
		Mean ± SD	Adjusted p Value for IPL-MGX vs. Control	Mean ± SD	Mean Change ± SE	Adjusted p Value vs. Baseline	Adjusted p Value for IPL-MGX vs. Control	Mean ± SD	Mean Change ± SE	Adjusted p Value vs. Baseline	Adjusted p Value for IPL-MGX vs. Control
Total	Control	0.23 ± 0.22	1	0.23 ± 0.22	0.00 ± 0.00	1	1	0.23 ± 0.22	0.01 ± 0.01	0.8	1
	IPL-MGX	0.22 ± 0.21		0.20 ± 0.21	−0.02 ± 0.01	<0.001 **		0.20 ± 0.21	−0.02 ± 0.01	0.003 *	
Without CCE	Control	0.20 ± 0.24	1	0.19 ± 0.24	−0.01 ± 0.00	0.62	1	0.20 ± 0.23	0.00 ± 0.01	1	1
	IPL-MGX	0.23 ± 0.22		0.22 ± 0.23	−0.01 ± 0.00	0.089		0.22 ± 0.22	−0.01 ± 0.01	0.34	
With CCE	Control	0.31 ± 0.14	0.26	0.31 ± 0.13	0.01 ± 0.01	1	0.036 *	0.32 ± 0.15	0.01 ± 0.02	1	0.030 *
	IPL-MGX	0.19 ± 0.17		0.14 ± 0.16	−0.05 ± 0.01	0.016 *		0.14 ± 0.14	−0.05 ± 0.01	0.016 *	

p values were determined with the Wilcoxon signed-rank test vs. baseline or Mann–Whitney U test vs. control with Bonferroni's correction (* adjusted p < 0.05, ** adjusted p < 0.001). SE; standard errors, SD; standard deviations.

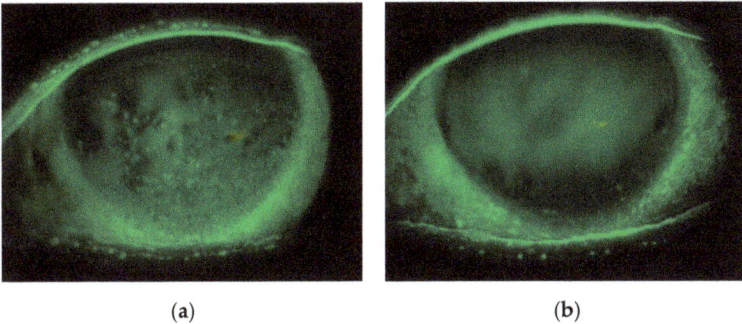

(a) (b)

Figure 1. Representative case of a 72-year-old woman treated with intense pulsed light-meibomian gland expression. Slitlamp images of fluorescein staining of the left eye obtained before (**a**) and 3 months after completion of (**b**) treatment showed amelioration of central corneal epitheliopathy. The logMAR visual acuity also improved from 0.15 to 0.09 in association with improvement in the lipid layer of the tear film, whereas tear meniscus height was unchanged.

4. Discussion

This is the first multicenter study to show an improvement in subjective symptoms and objective signs in patients with refractory ADDE (including those with Sjögren syndrome or rheumatoid arthritis) with mild MGD by treatment with a series of IPL sessions combined with MGX compared to MGX alone. Clinical parameters including ocular symptoms, tear film stability, fluorescein staining, and meibomian gland function were significantly improved by IPL-MGX treatment compared with MGX alone, although tear fluid parameters remained unchanged. Moreover, eyes with CCE showed an improvement in VA associated with IPL-MGX after amelioration of the epitheliopathy. Our results thus suggest that IPL-MGX might be an effective treatment not only for EDE but also for ADDE and mixed EDE-ADDE, although the present study examined only patients with refractory ADDE accompanied by mild MGD. Given that homeostasis of the lipid and tear fluid components of the tear film appears to be important for tear film health, IPL-MGX may have a role as a supportive treatment for ADDE.

We found that IPL-MGX therapy was more effective for the management of refractory ADDE accompanied by mild MGD than was MGX alone, and it was associated with an improvement in meibomian gland-related parameters but not with a change in tear fluid-related parameters. Although >30 studies have indicated that IPL is safe and effective for the treatment of MGD, as far as we are aware only one previous study included patients with Sjögren syndrome [20]. However, this previous study did not evaluate tear fluid-related parameters such as TMH or Schirmer's test value, but instead assessed only ocular symptoms and meibomian gland expressibility [20]. Five previous studies determined the Schirmer's test value [30,42–44], but all of these studies with the exception of one [43] found no significant change in this parameter in response to IPL therapy. The one exception among these five studies showed that the median Schirmer's test value increased from 13 to 15 mm ($p = 0.046$) after IPL therapy [43]. The one previous study that measured TMH found no significant difference in this parameter between before and after IPL treatment [21]. Our present results are thus largely consistent with those of previous studies and suggest that IPL does not affect lacrimal glands, but rather influences meibomian glands alone.

With regard to the mechanism of action of IPL in MGD, the treatment likely warms meibomian glands by increasing the temperature of the thin periocular skin and thereby promotes the melting of meibum [16,23]. In addition, the IPL device emits energy that is absorbed by chromophores in hemoglobin and likely thereby promotes closing of abnormal vessels in the lid margin and adjacent conjunctiva as well as attenuates the local release of inflammatory factors from the abnormal vessels [45,46]. A recent study found that the concentrations of various inflammatory factors—including interleukin-17A, interleukin-6, and prostaglandin E_2—in tear fluid were reduced after IPL therapy [25].

IPL treatment is also likely able to reduce bacterial load of the eyelid margin and the number of *Demodex* mites surrounding adnexa [44] as well as to ameliorate the associated inflammation [47].

Our present results show that MGX alone was also effective for the treatment of refractory ADDE accompanied by mild MGD with regard not only to subjective symptoms but also objective parameters with the exception of LLT, vascularity of lid margins, the meiboscore, TMH and Schirmer value. MGX alone likely does not have anti-inflammatory and meibum-melting effects or improve the condition of the aqueous layer of the tear film. In contrast, IPL-MGX showed significant effects on all of the parameters measured with the exception of the meiboscore, TMH and Schirmer's test value compared with MGX alone. Our findings suggest that IPL alone might be effective for the treatment of refractory ADDE, although the present study did not examine the effects of IPL without MGX.

The improvement of ADDE by IPL-MGX is consistent with the notion that tear film homeostasis is required for maintenance of tear film health. Self-reported ocular symptoms covered by the SPEED questionnaire were significantly ameliorated after IPL-MGX treatment in the present study, similar to the results of previous studies [20,23,25,29,42,48]. Twenty-two of the 23 study patients (96%) thus showed a decrease in the SPEED score of ≥ 8 points at both one and three months after the final IPL-MGX treatment session. The Fluo score was also significantly reduced after IPL-MGX therapy, again consistent with previous data [21,23,28–30,42–44,49]. Of note, eyes with CCE showed a significant improvement in VA after IPL-MGX compared with those receiving MGX alone. The targeting of MGD by IPL-MGX may thus improve the quality and quantity of lipids in the tear film and thereby result in a decline in the concentrations of inflammatory cytokines in tear fluid. Such an action might break the vicious cycle of corneal-conjunctival epitheliopathy and ocular surface inflammation.

The patients treated with IPL-MGX therapy in the present study had experienced ADDE for 8.1 ± 6.7 years (range of 2–24 years), and conventional therapies had proven insufficient of amelioration of ocular symptoms and improvement of tear film–related parameters. A recent study found that most patients with ADDE due to Sjögren syndrome and a disease duration of >3 years also developed MGD, likely because the early destruction of lacrimal glands eventually begins to affect meibomian glands [50]. Indeed, ~40% of patients in the present study also had systemic diseases such as Sjögren syndrome or rheumatoid arthritis. The conditions of such patients may be too severe to manage even with a combination of several conventional therapies. Our study has now demonstrated an improvement in clinical parameters of patients with refractory ADDE and mild MGD by treatment with IPL-MGX or MGX alone, suggesting that therapy targeted to the lipid layer of the tear film may be necessary for such patients who do not respond to conventional therapies. The efficacy of MGX alone in the present study was essentially apparent only one month after treatment completion, whereas that of IPL-MGX remained manifest at three months. The combination of therapies that target both aqueous and lipid layers may thus improve homeostasis of the tear film, resulting in amelioration of corneal-conjunctival epitheliopathy and subjective symptoms as well as an increase in VA.

Previous studies have found that ADDE and EDE occur frequently together, given that not only lacrimal glands but also meibomian glands can be affected in ADDE. A reduced production of tear fluid can increase friction between the eyelid and the ocular surface and thereby promote eyelid inflammation [4,5]. We propose that IPL therapy can increase the quality and quantity of lipid in the tear film, dampen the inflammatory reaction due to abnormal vessels, and thereby block the vicious circle underlying the pathophysiology of dry eye. It ameliorates ocular surface epitheliopathy and increases tear film stability, leading to an improvement in ocular symptoms (Figure 2). Together, our results suggest that it is important to treat not only the aqueous layer but also the lipid layer of the tear film in order to restore ocular surface health in patients with ADDE including those with refractory ADDE associated with mild MGD.

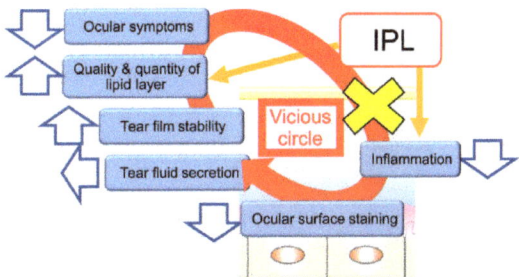

Figure 2. Proposed mechanism of action of IPL therapy on the vicious cycle of dry eye. IPL increases the quality and quantity of the lipid layer of the tear film as well as reduces inflammation of the ocular surface and lid margin. These effects result in amelioration of ocular surface epitheliopathy (ocular surface staining) and an increase in tear film stability, followed by improvement of ocular symptoms without any change in tear fluid secretion. IPL can block the vicious cycle (yellow x) underlying the pathophysiology of dry eye. IPL, Intense pulsed light.

Limitations of the present study include its retrospective nature and the relatively small sample size. In addition, both eyes of the study subjects were included, although the two eyes of each patient are not independent. Moreover, the study was not randomized or performed in a masked manner. Finally, osmolarity of tear fluid was not measured as an indicator of the efficacy of IPL-MGX treatment. Our data nevertheless suggest that prospective case-control studies with long-term follow-up are warranted for IPL-MGX treatment of patients with refractory ADDE associated with mild MGD. Further studies should also investigate the effectiveness of such treatment for patients with ADDE alone. Guidelines for IPL therapy based on disease severity are also needed for dry eye patients.

In conclusion, our results suggest that IPL-MGX therapy is effective for patients with refractory ADDE accompanied by mild MGD, with the severe disease of such patients being difficult to manage with conventional therapies. IPL-MGX thus has the potential to improve the condition of not only patients with MGD but also those with refractory ADDE and mild MGD.

Author Contributions: Conceptualization, R.A. and S.F.; formal analysis, S.F.; investigation, R.A., T.M. and N.M.; writing—original draft preparation, R.A.; writing—review and editing, N.M., S.F. and T.M.; supervision, N.M.; project administration, R.A. All authors have read and agreed to the published version of the manuscript.

Funding: This research received no external funding.

Conflicts of Interest: R.A. has the patent of the non-invasive meibography system (JP Patent Registration No. 5281846, US Patent Publication No.2011-0273550A1, EP Patent Publication No. 2189108A1). R.A. is a consultant for Lumenis Japan, KOWA company and TOPCON Japan. No conflicting relationship exists for the other authors.

References

1. McGinnigle, S.; Naroo, S.A.; Eperjesi, F. Evaluation of dry eye. *Surv. Ophthalmol.* **2012**, *57*, 293–316. [CrossRef] [PubMed]
2. Koh, S. Mechanisms of Visual Disturbance in Dry Eye. *Cornea* **2016**, *35*, S83–S88. [CrossRef] [PubMed]
3. Craig, J.P.; Nichols, K.K.; Akpek, E.K.; Caffery, B.; Dua, H.S.; Joo, C.K.; Liu, Z.; Nelson, J.D.; Nichols, J.J.; Tsubota, K.; et al. TFOS DEWS II Definition and Classification Report. *Ocul. Surf.* **2017**, *15*, 276–283. [CrossRef] [PubMed]
4. Bron, A.J.; de Paiva, C.S.; Chauhan, S.K.; Bonini, S.; Gabison, E.E.; Jain, S.; Knop, E.; Markoulli, M.; Ogawa, Y.; Perez, V.; et al. TFOS DEWS II pathophysiology report. *Ocul. Surf.* **2017**, *15*, 438–510. [CrossRef] [PubMed]
5. Shimazaki, J.; Goto, E.; Ono, M.; Shimmura, S.; Tsubota, K. Meibomian gland dysfunction in patients with Sjogren syndrome. *Ophthalmology* **1998**, *105*, 1485–1488. [CrossRef]

6. Vu, C.H.V.; Kawashima, M.; Yamada, M.; Suwaki, K.; Uchino, M.; Shigeyasu, C.; Hiratsuka, Y.; Yokoi, N.; Tsubota, K.; Dry Eye Cross-Sectional Study in Japan Study Group. Influence of Meibomian Gland Dysfunction and Friction-Related Disease on the Severity of Dry Eye. *Ophthalmology* **2018**, *125*, 1181–1188. [CrossRef] [PubMed]
7. Sy, A.; O'Brien, K.S.; Liu, M.P.; Cuddapah, P.A.; Acharya, N.R.; Lietman, T.M.; Rose-Nussbaumer, J. Expert opinion in the management of aqueous Deficient Dry Eye Disease (DED). *BMC Ophthalmol.* **2015**, *15*, 133. [CrossRef]
8. Jones, L.; Downie, L.E.; Korb, D.; Benitez-Del-Castillo, J.M.; Dana, R.; Deng, S.X.; Dong, P.N.; Geerling, G.; Hida, R.Y.; Liu, Y.; et al. TFOS DEWS II Management and Therapy Report. *Ocul. Surf.* **2017**, *15*, 575–628. [CrossRef]
9. Geerling, G.; Tauber, J.; Baudouin, C.; Goto, E.; Matsumoto, Y.; O'Brien, T.; Rolando, M.; Tsubota, K.; Nichols, K.K. The international workshop on meibomian gland dysfunction: Report of the subcommittee on management and treatment of meibomian gland dysfunction. *Investig. Ophthalmol. Vis. Sci.* **2011**, *52*, 2050–2064. [CrossRef]
10. Maskin, S.L. Intraductal meibomian gland probing relieves symptoms of obstructive meibomian gland dysfunction. *Cornea* **2010**, *29*, 1145–1152. [CrossRef]
11. Greiner, J.V. A single LipiFlow(R) Thermal Pulsation System treatment improves meibomian gland function and reduces dry eye symptoms for 9 months. *Curr. Eye Res.* **2012**, *37*, 272–278. [CrossRef] [PubMed]
12. Arita, R.; Suehiro, J.; Haraguchi, T.; Maeda, S.; Maeda, K.; Tokoro, H.; Amano, S. Topical diquafosol for patients with obstructive meibomian gland dysfunction. *Br. J. Ophthalmol.* **2013**, *97*, 725–729. [CrossRef] [PubMed]
13. Fukuoka, S.; Arita, R. Increase in tear film lipid layer thickness after instillation of 3% diquafosol ophthalmic solution in healthy human eyes. *Ocul. Surf.* **2017**, *15*, 730–735. [CrossRef] [PubMed]
14. Raulin, C.; Greve, B.; Grema, H. IPL technology: A review. *Lasers Surg. Med.* **2003**, *32*, 78–87. [CrossRef] [PubMed]
15. Wat, H.; Wu, D.C.; Rao, J.; Goldman, M.P. Application of intense pulsed light in the treatment of dermatologic disease: A systematic review. *Dermatol. Surg.* **2014**, *40*, 359–377. [CrossRef] [PubMed]
16. Toyos, R.; McGill, W.; Briscoe, D. Intense pulsed light treatment for dry eye disease due to meibomian gland dysfunction; a 3-year retrospective study. *Photomed. Laser Surg.* **2015**, *33*, 41–46. [CrossRef] [PubMed]
17. Craig, J.P.; Chen, Y.H.; Turnbull, P.R. Prospective trial of intense pulsed light for the treatment of meibomian gland dysfunction. *Investig. Ophthalmol. Vis. Sci.* **2015**, *56*, 1965–1970. [CrossRef]
18. Vora, G.K.; Gupta, P.K. Intense pulsed light therapy for the treatment of evaporative dry eye disease. *Curr. Opin. Ophthalmol.* **2015**, *26*, 314–318. [CrossRef]
19. Gupta, P.K.; Vora, G.K.; Matossian, C.; Kim, M.; Stinnett, S. Outcomes of intense pulsed light therapy for treatment of evaporative dry eye disease. *Can. J. Ophthalmol.* **2016**, *51*, 249–253. [CrossRef]
20. Vegunta, S.; Patel, D.; Shen, J.F. Combination Therapy of Intense Pulsed Light Therapy and Meibomian Gland Expression (IPL/MGX) Can Improve Dry Eye Symptoms and Meibomian Gland Function in Patients With Refractory Dry Eye: A Retrospective Analysis. *Cornea* **2016**, *35*, 318–322. [CrossRef]
21. Jiang, X.; Lv, H.; Song, H.; Zhang, M.; Liu, Y.; Hu, X.; Li, X.; Wang, W. Evaluation of the Safety and Effectiveness of Intense Pulsed Light in the Treatment of Meibomian Gland Dysfunction. *J. Ophthalmol.* **2016**, *2016*, 1910694. [CrossRef] [PubMed]
22. Dell, S.J. Intense pulsed light for evaporative dry eye disease. *Clin. Ophthalmol.* **2017**, *11*, 1167–1173. [CrossRef] [PubMed]
23. Dell, S.J.; Gaster, R.N.; Barbarino, S.C.; Cunningham, D.N. Prospective evaluation of intense pulsed light and meibomian gland expression efficacy on relieving signs and symptoms of dry eye disease due to meibomian gland dysfunction. *Clin. Ophthalmol.* **2017**, *11*, 817–827. [CrossRef]
24. Rong, B.; Tu, P.; Tang, Y.; Liu, R.X.; Song, W.J.; Yan, X.M. Evaluation of short-term effect of intense pulsed light combined with meibomian gland expression in the treatment of meibomian gland dysfunction. *Zhonghua Yan Ke Za Zhi* **2017**, *53*, 675–681. [PubMed]
25. Liu, R.; Rong, B.; Tu, P.; Tang, Y.; Song, W.; Toyos, R.; Toyos, M.; Yan, X. Analysis of Cytokine Levels in Tears and Clinical Correlations After Intense Pulsed Light Treating Meibomian Gland Dysfunction. *Am. J. Ophthalmol.* **2017**, *183*, 81–90. [CrossRef] [PubMed]

26. Guilloto Caballero, S.; Garcia Madrona, J.L.; Colmenero Reina, E. Effect of pulsed laser light in patients with dry eye syndrome. *Arch. Soc. Esp. Oftalmol.* **2017**, *92*, 509–515. [CrossRef] [PubMed]
27. Yin, Y.; Liu, N.; Gong, L.; Song, N. Changes in the Meibomian Gland After Exposure to Intense Pulsed Light in Meibomian Gland Dysfunction (MGD) Patients. *Curr. Eye Res.* **2018**, *43*, 308–313. [CrossRef] [PubMed]
28. Albietz, J.M.; Schmid, K.L. Intense pulsed light treatment and meibomian gland expression for moderate to advanced meibomian gland dysfunction. *Clin. Exp. Optom.* **2018**, *101*, 23–33. [CrossRef]
29. Arita, R.; Fukuoka, S.; Morishige, N. Therapeutic efficacy of intense pulsed light in patients with refractory meibomian gland dysfunction. *Ocul. Surf.* **2019**, *17*, 104–110. [CrossRef]
30. Ruan, F.; Zang, Y.; Sella, R.; Lu, H.; Li, S.; Yang, K.; Jin, T.; Afshari, N.A.; Pan, Z.; Jie, Y. Intense Pulsed Light Therapy with Optimal Pulse Technology as an Adjunct Therapy for Moderate to Severe Blepharitis-Associated Keratoconjunctivitis. *J. Ophthalmol.* **2019**, *2019*, 3143469. [CrossRef]
31. Shimazaki, J. Definition and diagnosis of dry eye. *Atarashii Ganka (J. Eye)* **2006**, *24*, 181–184.
32. Van Bijsterveld, O.P. Diagnostic tests in the Sicca syndrome. *Arch. Ophthalmol.* **1969**, *82*, 10–14. [CrossRef] [PubMed]
33. Amano, S.; Arita, R.; Kinoshita, S.; Japanese Dry Eye Society MGD Working Group. Definition and diagnostic criteria for meibomian gland dysfunction. *Atarashii Ganka (J. Eye)* **2010**, *27*, 627–631.
34. Arita, R.; Minoura, I.; Morishige, N.; Shirakawa, R.; Fukuoka, S.; Asai, K.; Goto, T.; Imanaka, T.; Nakamura, M. Development of Definitive and Reliable Grading Scales for Meibomian Gland Dysfunction. *Am. J. Ophthalmol.* **2016**, *169*, 125–137. [CrossRef] [PubMed]
35. Shimazaki, J.; Sakata, M.; Tsubota, K. Ocular surface changes and discomfort in patients with meibomian gland dysfunction. *Arch. Ophthalmol.* **1995**, *113*, 1266–1270. [CrossRef] [PubMed]
36. Arita, R.; Itoh, K.; Inoue, K.; Amano, S. Noncontact infrared meibography to document age-related changes of the meibomian glands in a normal population. *Ophthalmology* **2008**, *115*, 911–915. [CrossRef]
37. Fitzpatrick, T.B. The validity and practicality of sun-reactive skin types I through VI. *Arch. Dermatol.* **1988**, *124*, 869–871. [CrossRef]
38. Arita, R.; Morishige, N.; Fujii, T.; Fukuoka, S.; Chung, J.L.; Seo, K.Y.; Itoh, K. Tear Interferometric Patterns Reflect Clinical Tear Dynamics in Dry Eye Patients. *Investig. Ophthalmol. Vis. Sci.* **2016**, *57*, 3928–3934. [CrossRef] [PubMed]
39. Shirmer, O. Studiun zur Physiologie und Pathologie der Tranenabsonderung und Tranenabfuhr. *Albrecht Graefes Arch. Ophthalmol.* **1903**, *56*, 197–291. [CrossRef]
40. Korb, D.R.; Blackie, C.A.; McNally, E.N. Evidence suggesting that the keratinized portions of the upper and lower lid margins do not make complete contact during deliberate blinking. *Cornea* **2013**, *32*, 491–495. [CrossRef]
41. Ngo, W.; Situ, P.; Keir, N.; Korb, D.; Blackie, C.; Simpson, T. Psychometric properties and validation of the Standard Patient Evaluation of Eye Dryness questionnaire. *Cornea* **2013**, *32*, 1204–1210. [CrossRef] [PubMed]
42. Arita, R.; Mizoguchi, T.; Fukuoka, S.; Morishige, N. Multicenter Study of Intense Pulsed Light Therapy for Patients with Refractory Meibomian Gland Dysfunction. *Cornea* **2018**, *37*, 1566–1571. [CrossRef]
43. Mejia, L.F.; Gil, J.C.; Jaramillo, M. Intense pulsed light therapy: A promising complementary treatment for dry eye disease. *Arch. Soc. Esp. Oftalmol.* **2019**, *94*, 331–336. [CrossRef] [PubMed]
44. Cheng, S.N.; Jiang, F.G.; Chen, H.; Gao, H.; Huang, Y.K. Intense Pulsed Light Therapy for Patients with Meibomian Gland Dysfunction and Ocular Demodex Infestation. *Curr. Med. Sci.* **2019**, *39*, 800–809. [CrossRef] [PubMed]
45. Schroeter, C.A.; Haaf-von Below, S.; Neumann, H.A. Effective treatment of rosacea using intense pulsed light systems. *Dermatol. Surg.* **2005**, *31*, 1285–1289. [CrossRef] [PubMed]
46. De Godoy, C.H.; Silva, P.F.; de Araujo, D.S.; Motta, L.J.; Biasotto-Gonzalez, D.A.; Politti, F.; Mesquita-Ferrari, R.A.; Fernandes, K.P.; Albertini, R.; Bussadori, S.K. Evaluation of effect of low-level laser therapy on adolescents with temporomandibular disorder: Study protocol for a randomized controlled trial. *Trials* **2013**, *14*, 229. [CrossRef]
47. Farrell, H.P.; Garvey, M.; Cormican, M.; Laffey, J.G.; Rowan, N.J. Investigation of critical inter-related factors affecting the efficacy of pulsed light for inactivating clinically relevant bacterial pathogens. *J. Appl. Microbiol.* **2010**, *108*, 1494–1508. [CrossRef] [PubMed]

48. Rong, B.; Tang, Y.; Tu, P.; Liu, R.; Qiao, J.; Song, W.; Toyos, R.; Yan, X. Intense Pulsed Light Applied Directly on Eyelids Combined with Meibomian Gland Expression to Treat Meibomian Gland Dysfunction. *Photomed. Laser Surg.* **2018**, *36*, 326–332. [CrossRef]
49. Choi, M.; Han, S.J.; Ji, Y.W.; Choi, Y.J.; Jun, I.; Alotaibi, M.H.; Ko, B.Y.; Kim, E.K.; Kim, T.I.; Nam, S.M.; et al. Meibum Expressibility Improvement as a Therapeutic Target of Intense Pulsed Light Treatment in Meibomian Gland Dysfunction and Its Association with Tear Inflammatory Cytokines. *Sci. Rep.* **2019**, *9*, 7648. [CrossRef]
50. Wang, Y.; Qin, Q.; Liu, B.; Fu, Y.; Lin, L.; Huang, X.; Jin, X. Clinical Analysis: Aqueous-Deficient and Meibomian Gland Dysfunction in Patients With Primary Sjogren's Syndrome. *Front. Med.* **2019**, *6*, 291. [CrossRef] [PubMed]

Publisher's Note: MDPI stays neutral with regard to jurisdictional claims in published maps and institutional affiliations.

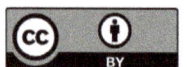

© 2020 by the authors. Licensee MDPI, Basel, Switzerland. This article is an open access article distributed under the terms and conditions of the Creative Commons Attribution (CC BY) license (http://creativecommons.org/licenses/by/4.0/).

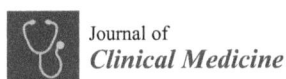

Article

The HYLAN M Study: Efficacy of 0.15% High Molecular Weight Hyaluronan Fluid in the Treatment of Severe Dry Eye Disease in a Multicenter Randomized Trial

Gysbert-Botho van Setten [1], Christophe Baudouin [2], Jutta Horwath-Winter [3], Daniel Böhringer [4], Oliver Stachs [5], Ebru Toker [6], Sultan Al-Zaaidi [7], Jose M. Benitez-del-Castillo [8], Ria Beck [5], Osama Al-Sheikh [9], Berthold Seitz [10], Stefano Barabino [11], Herbert A. Reitsamer [12] and Wolfgang G.K. Müller-Lierheim [13],*

1. Karolinska Institutet, Department of Clinical Neuroscience, St. Eriks Eye Hospital, 11282 Stockholm, Sweden; gysbert.van.setten@ki.se
2. Quinze-Vingts National Eye Hospital & Vision Institute, IHU Foresight, 75571 Paris, France; cbaudouin@15-20.fr
3. Department of Ophthalmology, Medical University Graz, 8036 Graz, Austria; jutta.horwath@medunigraz.at
4. Eye Center, University Eye Hospital Freiburg and Medical Faculty, Albert Ludwigs University, 79106 Freiburg, Germany; daniel.boehringer@uniklinik-freiburg.de
5. Department of Ophthalmology, University Medical Center Rostock, 18057 Rostock, Germany; oliver.stachs@uni-rostock.de (O.S.); ria.beck@gewebenetzwerk.de (R.B.)
6. Department of Ophthalmology, Marmara University School of Medicine, 34899 Istanbul, Turkey; dretoker@gmail.com
7. Department of Ophthalmology, PSMMC Prince Sultan Military Medical City, MSD Medical Services Department, MODA Ministry of Defense and Aviation, Riyadh 12233, Saudi Arabia; alzaaidi_s@yahoo.com
8. Universidad Complutense de Madrid, Hospital Clinico San Carlos, Clinica Rementeria, 28040 Madrid, Spain; jbenitez.hcsc@salud.madrid.org
9. KKESH–King Khaled Eye Specialist Hospital, Riyadh 11462, Saudi Arabia; oshaikh@kkesh.med.sa
10. Department of Ophthalmology, Saarland University Medical Center, 66421 Homburg/Saar, Germany; berthold.seitz@uks.eu
11. Ocular Surface & Dry Eye Center, Ospedale L. Sacco, University of Milan, 20157 Milan, Italy; stebarabi@gmail.com
12. Department of Ophthalmology & Department of Experimental Ophthalmology and Glaucoma Research, University Clinic Salzburg, Paracelsus Medical University, 5020 Salzburg, Austria; h.reitsamer@salk.at
13. CORONIS GmbH, 81241 Munich, Germany
* Correspondence: ml@coronis.net

Received: 3 October 2020; Accepted: 31 October 2020; Published: 2 November 2020

Abstract: The aim of the HYLAN M study was to investigate if symptoms and/or signs of patients suffering from severe dry eye disease (DED) can be improved by substituting individually optimized artificial tear therapy by high molecular weight hyaluronan (HMWHA) eye drops. In this international, multicenter study, patients with symptoms of at least ocular surface disease index (OSDI) 33 and corneal fluorescein staining (CFS) of at least Oxford grade 3 were included. A total of 84 per-protocol patients were randomized in two study arms. The control group continued to use their individual optimum artificial tears over the study period of eight weeks; in the verum group, the artificial tears were substituted by eye drops containing 0.15% HMWHA. At the week 8 visit, the average OSDI of the verum group had improved by 13.5 as compared to the control group ($p = 0.001$). The best corrected visual acuity (BCVA) had improved by 0.04 logMAR ($p = 0.033$). CFS, tear film break-up time (TBUT), Schirmer I, lid wiper epitheliopathy (LWE), mucocutaneous junction (Yamaguchi score), and tear osmolarity were not significantly different between the verum and control groups ($p > 0.050$). We conclude that for most patients with severe DED, 0.15% HMWHA eye drops provide excellent improvement of symptoms without impairment of dry eye signs.

Keywords: dry eye disease; severe keratitis; hyaluronan; hylan A; multicenter; randomized trial

1. Introduction

Dry eye disease (DED) is a multifactorial disorder affecting 5% to 35% of the world population [1]. In cases of severe DED, patients experience symptoms of ocular discomfort and visual instability, resulting in a considerable loss of quality of life. Ocular burning or stinging, ocular discomfort, and ocular pain are rated as the most important symptoms by patients [2]. The loss of visual stability additionally causes a negative impact on quality of life and is attributed to an instable tear film [3]. DED has a significant socio-economic effect due to considerable direct treatment costs as well as indirect costs due to a loss of work productivity [4–6].

The Tear Film and Ocular Surface Society (TFOS) summarizes the current concepts as a staged management and treatment for DED. Lubricating, hydrating eye drops not targeting the underlying pathophysiology of DED are the standard long-term treatment for DED [7]. Secretagogues may have an initial effect, but this may fade over time. If ocular lubricants and secretagogues are not providing acceptable relief from symptoms, immunomodulatory eye drops such as cyclosporine may be tried [7]. This treatment approach reflects the current model of pathophysiology of DED. Other models can either reflect a different understanding or the existence of regional differences. The Asia Dry Eye Society, e.g., proposes a tear film-oriented therapy distinguishing between lipid layer, aqueous/secretory mucin deficiency, and corneal epithelial surface/membrane bound mucin deficiency [8,9]. It is assumed that the instability of the tear film increases the friction between the eyelids and the eye, which will result in ocular inflammation and epithelial damage [9–11]. Persistent systemic conditions of the patient or environmental adverse conditions may lead to a self-maintaining vicious circle of inflammation, which may result in chronic, eventually irreversible forms of severe dry eye [12]. Hence, a prerequisite for successful therapy is personalized clinical assessment and treatment [13]. Inflammation caused by autoimmune diseases or elevated osmolarity of the tear film due to excess evaporation have been pointed out as driving forces of the vicious circle of inflammation. Here, the treatment of inflammation as a driving force within the vicious circle plays a key role [14–16]. Although hyperosmolarity measured in the tear meniscus has been proposed for diagnosing DED, the level of osmolarity and its absolute value apparently plays a minor role as a local stress factor compared to the extent of diurnal variation [17–19]. Severe discomfort as a symptom of DED may transit to changes in neuroception, reflecting nerve damage. Nerve damage itself may be another underlying pathophysiological mechanism in severe chronic DED [20]. Not only does nerve damage result in a reduction of trophic support for the corneal epithelium, it could also initiate and maintain inflammation, and thus the interplay between nerve damage and inflammation needs to be taken into consideration [21,22]. This might contribute to the well-known discordance between dry eye signs and symptoms [23–26]. Although some substances have recently demonstrated certain potential in the treatment of neuropathic keratopathy, there is currently no therapy that directly addresses the underlying nerve damage [27,28]. Additionally, patients suffering from neuropathic ocular pain frequently respond poorly to treatment with lubricant eye drops [29,30].

High molecular weight hyaluronan (HMWHA) has in contrast to the majority of lubricating eye drops anti-inflammatory activity and the capability to reduce the activity of the pain transducing channel TRPV1 in nociceptive nerves, thus reducing neuropathic pain [31–35]. HMWHA in eye drops provides excellent lubrication due to shear-thinning properties such as the natural tear film, good hydrating and water-binding properties resulting in reduced evaporation, and stabilization of the ocular surface barrier function to recover the protection against infection [36]. A recent study demonstrated in an environmental dry eye stress model in mice that HMWHA eye drops protect the ocular surface from mechanical damage and inflammation better than low molecular weight hyaluronan (LMWHA) [37].

The aim of the presented study (HYLAN M study) was to investigate the effect of HMWHA eye drops in comparison with other tear substitutes in an international multicenter prospective open label clinical investigation.

2. Experimental Section

2.1. Study Design

The HYLAN M study, a multicenter prospective randomized open label study, was performed in 11 centers in eight countries. Details of the study centers, administrative structure, planning, and conduct are provided in Appendix A. The study adhered to the Declaration of Helsinki, was approved by ethics committees of all eight countries involved, and registered as outlined in Appendix B.

Patients identified as having severe DED were randomized in two parallel arms. The control group continued with the currently used therapy as by the time of inclusion. In the verum group, the individual lubricant eye drops used by each patient by the time of inclusion were replaced by preservative-free eye drops containing 0.15% HMWHA dissolved in isotonic saline solution buffered with 120 mmol/L phosphate (Comfort Shield® eye drops; i.com medical GmbH, Munich, Germany; see Appendix C). Concomitant treatment for dry eye such as cyclosporine eye drops remained unchanged in both arms.

Demographic data and medical history were recorded during the baseline visits. Symptoms and signs associated with DED were assessed at the baseline visit and at the week 4 and week 8 follow-up visits, respectively (see Table 1).

Table 1. Diagnostic testing schedule with optional tests in round brackets.

Test	Baseline	Week 4	Week 8
OSDI	X	X	X
dropping frequency	X	X	X
BCVA	X	X	X
CFS	X	X	X
TBUT	X	X	X
Schirmer 1	X		X
Tear osmolarity	X		X
IOP	X		X
LWE Korb score	(X)		(X)
Yamaguchi score	(X)		(X)
Confocal microscopy	(X)		(X)

2.2. Participants

Patients over 18 years suffering from DED of any underlying etiology were eligible for inclusion. The patients had to be under stable, unchanged dry eye therapy for at least two months (in case of concomitant cyclosporine therapy three month) by the time of inclusion. Patients were excluded if they participated in any other clinical trial, suffered from eye diseases other than dry eyes, had ocular surgery less than three months prior to study inclusion, were using punctual plugs, or had masquerading conditions as identified by Karpecki [38]. Masquerading conditions are conjunctivochalasis, recurrent corneal erosions, epithelial basement membrane dystrophy, mucin fishing syndrome, floppy eyelid syndrome, giant papillary conjunctivitis, Salzmann's nodular degeneration, and ocular rosacea.

As inclusion criteria for severe dry eye, the primary criteria according to Baudouin et al. were chosen [39]. The dry eye symptoms were assessed using the ocular surface disease index (OSDI) questionnaire [40]. For inclusion, patients had to have an OSDI score of 33 or more [39]. As dry eye sign, corneal fluorescein staining (CFS) was chosen [41]. For inclusion, patients had to have at least one eye with CFS Oxford grade 3 or more, but no confluent CFS.

Based on the OSDI score and visually assessed CFS grade, the study centers decided on preliminary enrollment. CFS images were transferred to the reading center for quantitative electronic evaluation of corneal fluorescein staining (RC1), as described in Appendix D. The reading center was masked for the assigned treatment to minimize bias. If the submitted images met the criteria for automated assessment, the staining was not confluent, and at least one eye of the patient met the CFS inclusion criteria, the reading center confirmed the definite enrollment of the patient. Otherwise the patient was excluded as "screen fail".

The eyes with the higher staining score were defined as study eyes. However, the fellow eye was retrospectively redefined as a study eye if the masked reading center determined that the images from the fellow eye had significantly better contrast than those of the designated eye, given that the follow eye fulfilled all inclusion criteria at the baseline visit.

2.3. Efficacy Assessment

TFOS recommends to formally assess dry eye disease by symptoms using a questionnaire such as the OSDI in combination with at least one test for homeostasis markers (signs) such as tear break-up time (TBUT), tear osmolarity, or ocular surface staining [42]. Accordingly, the OSDI questionnaire was used to assess dry eye symptoms throughout the HYLAN M Study. Due to the variable and controversial association between dry eye signs and symptoms, the following standardized battery of tests for dry eye signs was applied in the HYLAN M study. Best corrected visual acuity (BCVA) was used as an indicator of visual stability. CFS, TBUT, and the Schirmer test without topical anesthesia (Schirmer I) were used to assess the lubricating properties, stability, and quantity of the tear film [43–47]. Tear film osmolarity in the lower tear meniscus was additionally measured using the TearLab osmolarity system (TearLab Corporation, San Diego, CA, USA). Specific training of the correct test performance and daily calibration of the test instrument was performed at every study center. Intraocular pressure (IOP) was determined by Goldman applanation tonometry or Icare® tonometry at the baseline and week 8 visits as a safety parameter to rule out uncontrolled glaucoma or ocular hypertension.

Additionally, most but not all study centers additionally performed lissamine green staining of the lid rim to assess lid wiper epitheliopathy (LWE) as the Korb score and the mucocutaneous junction (Marx line) as the Yamaguchi score [48–50]. Moreover, four out of 11 study centers assessed the subbasal nerve plexus by confocal laser scanning microscopy and provided images to a second masked reading center (RC2) for evaluation [51].

Table 1 provides the testing schedule of the HYLAN M study. For more details on diagnostic test methods and assessment of results by reading centers, see Appendices A and D.

2.4. Statistical Analysis

The primary endpoint for the demonstration of superiority of Comfort Shield eye drops (verum group) over other ocular lubricants currently used by the patients (control group) was the difference between CFS at week 8 and at baseline visits as quantitatively determined by RC1 (see Appendix D).

The key secondary endpoint was the difference between OSDI scores at week 8 and baseline [40]. To further analyze the improvement of symptoms, OSDI subscores for the questions related to pain $OSDI_{pain}$ (OSDI questions 1–3) and OSDI subscore for questions related to visual stability $OSDI_{vision}$ (OSDI questions 4–9) were analyzed according to the following formulas:

$$OSDI_{pain} = \frac{\text{sensitive to light} + \text{feeling gritty} + \text{pain score eye}}{n} \times 25 \qquad (1)$$

$$OSDI_{vision} = \frac{\text{blurred vision} + \text{poor vision} + \text{reading} + \text{driving at night} + \text{computer ATM} + \text{watch TV}}{n} \times 25 \qquad (2)$$

n = number of questions answered (at most, 3 for the pain, and 6 for vision subscores, respectively)

Additional secondary endpoints were the differences between BCVA, TBUT, Schirmer I value, tear osmolarity, Korb score, and Yamaguchi score at week 8 and baseline, respectively.

The full analysis set (FAS) was defined as all patients who were not in "screen fail" status, have at least once used their eye drops, have data for the primary endpoint (CFS from reading center RC1) or the key secondary endpoint OSDI, and have had at least one follow-up visit. The per-protocol set (PPS) comprised all patients of the FAS without any major protocol deviation that could substantially affect the evaluation of the randomized treatment. One patient who had not taken lubricant eye drops before the time of inclusion and patients who did not show up for the week 8 follow-up visit were excluded from the PPS.

Considering the potential influence of climatic differences, two subgroups of the verum and control groups were defined: Desert = all patients from the two study centers in Riyadh, Saudi Arabia, and Europe = all other patients. For these subgroups, the results of CFS and OSDI were separately analyzed [52].

3. Results

3.1. Participant Flow

Figure 1 summarizes the participant flow. In total, 148 patients were pre-screened for severe dry eye disease. Out of these, eight patients were excluded at the initial interview and not randomized, and 121 patients have at least once taken their eye drops (= safety set SS). In total, 140 patients were preliminarily included by the study centers and randomized (= randomized set RS), out of these 75 in the Comfort Shield group and 65 in the control group. Out of the 140 randomized patients, 47 were classified as "screen fails" by the reading center or did not use their eye drops. Of the remaining 93 patients, 49 had been randomized to the Comfort Shield group and 44 had been randomized to the control group (=full analysis set FAS). Out of these, five patients of the Comfort Shield group and four patients of the control group did not show up for the week 8 visit. Therefore, the per-protocol set (PPS) comprises 44 patients in the Comfort Shield group and 40 patients in the control group (see Figure 1).

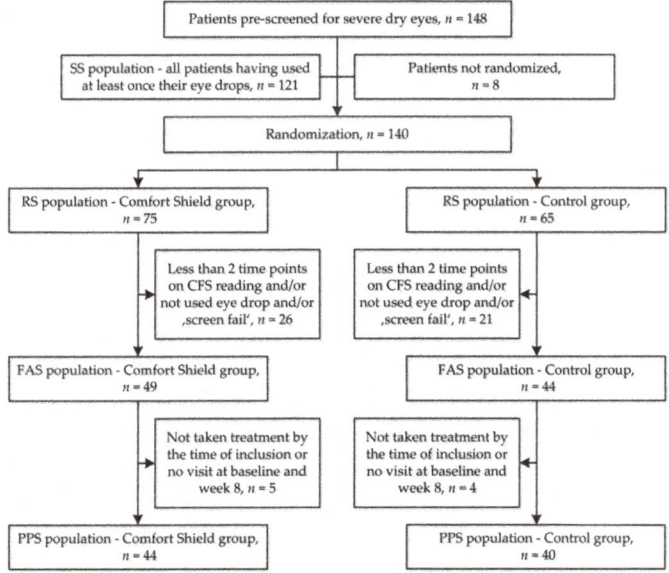

Figure 1. Participant flowchart.

3.2. Demographic Data

The full analysis set (FAS) of the HYLAN M study comprises 93 patients. Out of these, 84 belonged to the per-protocol set (PPS), 44 belonged to the Comfort Shield group, and 40 were in the control group. The study was performed in different climate zones, and patients from different ethnicities were enrolled. Table 2 provides an overview of the socio-demographic data of the study.

Table 2. Climate zone and socio-demographic characteristics according to the treatment arm–per-protocol set (PPS) population ($n = 84$).

		Comfort Shield ($n = 44$)	Control ($n = 40$)	Total ($n = 84$)
climate zone	n	44	40	84
	Desert	6 (13.6)	7 (17.5)	13 (15.5)
	Europe	38 (86.4)	33 (82.5)	71 (84.5)
	missing	0	0	0
age (years)	n	44	40	84
	mean (sd)	57.66 (14.39)	59.45 (12.48)	58.51 (13.46)
	median (iqr)	61.5 (50.75, 65.25)	60 (51.5, 69.0)	61 (50.75, 67.00)
	min, max	26, 81	27, 84	26, 84
	missing	0	0	0
age (years)	n	44	40	84
	<40	6 (13.6)	2 (5.0)	8 (9.5)
	[40–65[	25 (56.8)	23 (57.5)	48 (57.1)
	≥65	13 (29.5)	15 (37.5)	28 (33.3)
	missing	0	0	0
sex n (%)	n	44	40	84
	female	35 (79.5)	34 (85.0)	69 (82.1)
	male	9 (20.5)	6 (15.0)	15 (17.9)
	missing	0	0	0
ethnicity n (%)	n	44	40	84
	Arabian	7 (15.9)	8 (20.0)	15 (17.9)
	Caucasian	36 (81.8)	31 (77.5)	67 (79.8)
	other	1 (2.3)	1 (2.5)	2 (2.4)
	missing	0	0	0

Abbreviations: sd = standard deviation; iqr = interquartile range; min = minimum; max = maximum [53].

An overview of the medical history for the PPS set is provided in Appendix E, Table A1.

3.3. Efficacy Results

The results presented below refer to the 84 per-protocol patients in the study (PPS population in Figure 1).

3.3.1. Corneal Fluorescein Staining

The difference in corneal fluorescein staining (CFS) between baseline and week 8 determined by the masked reading center RC1 was the primary endpoint of the HYLAN M Study. The test method, electronic assessment, and calculation are described in Appendix D. Figure 2 and Table 3 describe the test results for the Comfort Shield group and the control group.

The changes from baseline to week 4 and to week 8 are documented in Table 4.

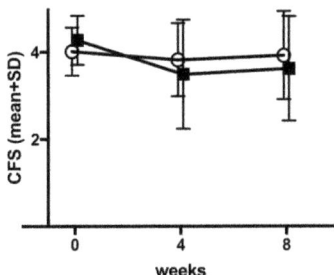

Figure 2. Mean (±SD) of corneal fluorescein staining (CFS) (central reading value, transformed into grade exact value) by group according time—PPS (*n* = 84). Open circles = Comfort Shield group, filled squares = control group.

Table 3. CFS: Value at baseline and at each post-baseline visit—PPS (*n* = 84)—Descriptive analysis, by group.

		Comfort Shield (*n* = 44)	Control (*n* = 40)	Total (*n* = 84)
value at baseline	n	44	40	84
	mean (sd)	4.01 (0.55)	4.27 (0.56)	4.13 (0.57)
	median (iqr)	3.92 (3.55, 4.37)	4.39 (3.72, 4.67)	4.18 (3.6, 4.6)
	min, max	3.0, 5.0	3.12, 5.00	3.0, 5.0
	missing	0	0	0
value at week 4	n	41	38	
	mean (sd)	3.82 (0.84)	3.49 (1.25)	
	median (iqr)	4 (3.26, 4.46)	3.8 (2.82, 4.36)	
	min, max	1.35, 5.0	0.0, 5.0	
	missing	3	2	
value at week 8	n	41	38	
	mean (sd)	3.91 (1.04)	3.62 (1.2)	
	median (iqr)	4.31 (3.38, 4.68)	3.82 (3.27, 4.43)	
	min, max	0.0, 5.0	0.0, 5.0	
	missing	3	2	

Table 4. CFS: Value at baseline and change from baseline to each post-baseline visit—PPS (*n* = 84)—Descriptive analysis, by group.

		Comfort Shield (*n* = 44)	Control (*n* = 40)	Total (*n* = 84)
baseline	n	44	40	84
	mean (sd)	4.01 (0.55)	4.27 (0.56)	4.13 (0.57)
	median (iqr)	3.92 (3.55, 4.37)	4.39 (3.72, 4.67)	4.18 (3.6, 4.6)
	min,max	3.0, 5.0	3.12, 5.00	3.0, 5.0
	missing	0	0	0
change from baseline to week 4	n	41	38	
	mean (sd)	−0.22 (0.76)	−0.76 (1.02)	
	median (iqr)	−0.06 (−0.70, 0.28)	−0.68 (−1.02, −0.20)	
	min,max	−2.54, 1.13	−4.41, 0.90	
	missing	3	2	
change from baseline to week 8	n	41	38	
	mean (sd)	−0.13 (1.08)	−0.63 (1.05)	
	median (iqr)	−0.07 (−0.57, 0.58)	−0.33 (−0.99, 0.10)	
	min,max	−4.73, 1.45	−3.60, 0.84	
	missing	3	2	

There was no significant (*p*-value < 0.05) difference between the two groups for the primary endpoint CFS, as documented in Table 5.

Table 5. CFS: multivariate analysis on change from baseline to week 8—mixed-effects model for repeated measures—PPS population (n = 84). n used = 79.

Parameter	Comparison	E[1]	CI 95% Low	CI 95% High	*p*-Value [2]
Change from baseline to week 8	Control vs. Comfort Shield	−0.411	−0.865	0.043	0.075

[1] Estimate (E) and associated 95% two-sided confidence interval (CI) of the difference between treatment group adjusted means: mixed-effects model for repeated measures (MMRM) with the fixed, categorical effects of treatment, visit, and treatment-by-visit interaction, the random categorical effect of center, as well as the continuous, fixed covariates of baseline and baseline-by-visit interaction. A positive estimate of the difference between treatment group adjusted means is in favour of the Comfort Shield, a negative ones in disfavor of the Comfort Shield. [2] two-sided *p*-value associated with the test of treatment effect.

3.3.2. Ocular Surface Disease Index

The key secondary endpoint of the HYLAN M study was the difference in ocular surface disease index (OSDI) between baseline and week 8 assessed by a questionnaire to be filled by the patients at the beginning of each visit. The Comfort Shield group had experienced at the end of the study (week 8 visit) significantly more relief from dry eye symptoms than the control group as documented in Figure 3a and Tables 6–8 (*p*-value 0.001).

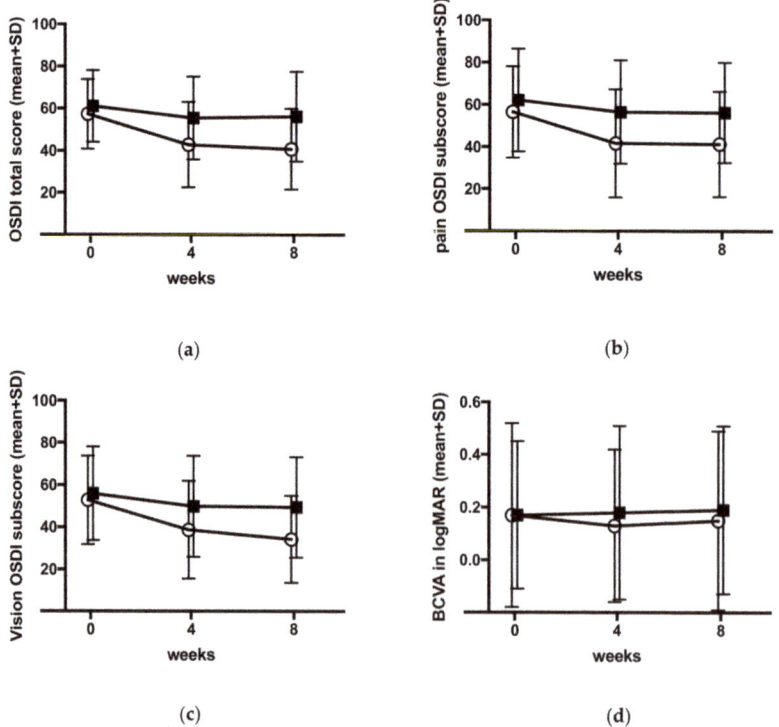

Figure 3. (a) Mean (±SD) OSDI total score; (b) mean (±SD) OSDI pain subscore; (c) mean (±SD) OSDI vision subscore; (d) mean (±SD) best corrected visual acuity (BCVA). Open circles = Comfort Shield group, filled squares = control group.

Table 6. Ocular surface disease index (OSDI): value at baseline and at each post-baseline visit—PPS (n = 84)—descriptive analysis, by group.

		Comfort Shield (n = 44)	Control (n = 40)	Total (n = 84)
value at baseline	n	44	40	84
	mean (sd)	57.41 (16.5)	61.13 (16.99)	59.18 (16.74)
	median (iqr)	54.55 (43.61, 68.75)	61.8 (51.56, 75.00)	57.91 (43.75, 70.45)
	min, max	34.09, 91.67	34.09, 95.45	34.09, 95.45
	missing	0	0	0
value at week 4	n	44	40	
	mean (sd)	42.82 (20.34)	55.49 (19.64)	
	median (iqr)	39.2 (29.79, 56.96)	54.03 (38.07, 68.50)	
	min, max	7.14, 85.42	22.22, 95.45	
	missing	0	0	
value at week 8	n	44	40	
	mean (sd)	40.7 (19.18)	56.16 (21.39)	
	median (iqr)	40.91 (28.13, 52.81)	57.91 (36.11, 75.00)	
	min, max	0.0, 87.5	9.09, 93.18	
	missing	0	0	

Table 7. OSDI: value at baseline and change from baseline to each post-baseline visit—PPS (n = 84)—Descriptive analysis, by group.

		Comfort Shield (n = 44)	Control (n = 40)	Total (n = 84)
value at baseline	n	44	40	84
	mean (sd)	57.41 (16.5)	61.13 (16.99)	59.18 (16.74)
	median (iqr)	54.55 (43.61, 68.75)	61.8 (51.56, 75.00)	57.91 (43.75, 70.45)
	min, max	34.09, 91.67	34.09, 95.45	34.09, 95.45
	missing	0	0	0
change from baseline to week 4	n	44	40	
	mean (sd)	−14.6 (20.71)	−5.63 (12.66)	
	median (iqr)	−10.21 (−25.80, −2.09)	−3.98 (−12.5, 0.0)	
	min, max	−70.83, 27.27	−37.92, 25.76	
	missing	0	0	
change from baseline to week 8	n	44	40	
	mean (sd)	−16.71 (22.25)	−4.96 (16.95)	
	median (iqr)	−13.41 (−29.66, −0.68)	−3.82 (−13.02, 6.99)	
	min, max	−84.09, 27.08	−43.06, 40.91	
	missing	0	0	

Table 8. OSDI: Multivariate analysis on change from baseline to week 8—mixed-effects model for repeated measures—PPS population (n = 84)—n used = 84.

Parameter	Comparison	E [1]	CI 95% Low	CI 95% High	p-Value [2]
Change from baseline to week 8	Control vs. Comfort Shield	13.511	5.586	21.437	0.001

[1] Estimate (E) and associated 95% two-sided confidence interval (CI) of the difference between treatment group adjusted means: MMRM with the fixed, categorical effects of treatment, visit, and treatment-by-visit interaction, the random categorical effect of center, as well as the continuous, fixed covariates of baseline and baseline-by-visit interaction. A positive estimate of the difference between treatment group adjusted means is in favor of the Comfort Shield, a negative one in disfavor of the Comfort Shield. [2] two-sided p-value associated with the test of treatment effect.

The subscores for pain and visual stability-related symptoms were calculated and analyzed as described in the section on statistical analysis. The results are provided in Figure 3b,c and in Tables 9 and 10. Both subscores OSDI$_{pain}$ and OSDI$_{vision}$ improved significantly in the Comfort Shield group as compared to the control group (p-values 0.002 and 0.003, respectively).

Table 9. Pain OSDI subscore: multivariate analysis on change from baseline to week 8—mixed-effects model for repeated measures—PPS population (n = 84)—n used = 84.

Parameter	Comparison	E [1]	95% CI Low [1]	95% CI High [1]	p-Value [2]
Change from baseline to week 8	Comfort Shield vs. Control	14.503	5.517	23.49	0.002

[1] Estimate (E) and associated 95% two-sided confidence interval (CI) of the difference between treatment group adjusted means: MMRM with the fixed, categorical effects of treatment, visit, and treatment-by-visit interaction, the random categorical effect of center, as well as the continuous, fixed covariates of baseline and baseline-by-visit interaction. A positive estimate of the difference between treatment group adjusted means is in favour of the Comfort Shield, a negative one in disfavour of the Comfort Shield. [2] two-sided p-value associated with the test of treatment effect.

Table 10. Vision OSDI subscore: Multivariate analysis on change from baseline to week 8—mixed-effects model for repeated measures—PPS population (n = 84)–n used = 84.

Parameter	Comparison	E [1]	95% CI Low [1]	95% CI High [1]	p-Value [2]
Change from baseline to week 8	Comfort Shield vs. Control	13.999	5.011	22.986	0.003

[1] Estimate (E) and associated 95% two-sided confidence interval (CI) of the difference between treatment group adjusted means: MMRM with the fixed, categorical effects of treatment, visit, and treatment-by-visit interaction, the random categorical effect of center, as well as the continuous, fixed covariates of baseline and baseline-by-visit interaction. A positive estimate of the difference between treatment group adjusted means is in favour of the Comfort Shield, a negative one in disfavor of the Comfort Shield. [2] two-sided p-value associated with the test of treatment effect.

3.3.3. Best Corrected Visual Acuity

The BCVA slightly improved after eight weeks of Comfort Shield treatment as compared to the control group (p-value 0.033). Details are provided in Figure 3d and Table 11.

Table 11. BCVA: value at baseline and change from baseline to each post-baseline visit—PPS (n = 84)—descriptive analysis, by treatment arm.

		Comfort Shield (n = 44)	Control (n = 40)	Total (n = 84)	p-Value
baseline	n	44	40	84	
	mean (sd)	0.17 (0.35)	0.17 (0.28)	0.17 (0.31)	
	median (iqr)	0 (0.0, 0.2)	0.1 (0.00, 0.22)	0 (0.0, 0.2)	
	min, max	−0.1, 1.5	−0.2, 1.3	−0.2, 1.5	
	missing	0	0	0	
change from baseline to week 4	n	41	39		
	mean (sd)	0 (0.11)	0.02 (0.11)		
	median (iqr)	0 (0, 0)	0 (0.00, 0.05)		
	min, max	−0.4, 0.3	−0.2, 0.5		
	missing	3	1		
change from baseline to week 8	n	44	40		0.033
	mean (sd)	−0.02 (0.14)	0.02 (0.1)		
	median (iqr)	0 (−0.1, 0.0)	0 (0.0, 0.1)		
	min, max	−0.4, 0.6	−0.2, 0.3		
	missing	0	0		

3.3.4. Other Secondary Endpoints

The secondary endpoints TBUT, Schirmer I, lid wiper epitheliopathy Korb score, Yamaguchi score, and tear film osmolarity are summarized in Table 12. No significant differences between the Comfort Shield group and control group were observed (all p-values > 0.05).

Table 12. Values at baseline and change from baseline to week 8 for tear film break-up time (TBUT), Schirmer I, lid wiper epitheliopathy (LWE) Korb score, Yamaguchi score, and tear osmolarity—PPS ($n = 84$).

	Comfort Shield Group $n = 44$		Control Group $n = 40$		p-Value Change from Baseline to Week 8
	Baseline Mean (SD)	Change at Week 8 Mean (SD)	Baseline Mean (SD)	Change at Week 8 Mean (SD)	
TBUT (s)	$n = 44$ 2.90 (1.87)	$n = 42$ 0.66 (2.32)	$n = 40$ 2.76 (1.44)	$n = 40$ 0.24 (1.47)	0.468
Schirmer I (mm/5 min)	$n = 44$ 5.19 (5.99)	$n = 43$ −0.43 (4.72)	$n = 40$ 6.50 (7.52)	$n = 40$ 0.55 (4.61)	0.343
LWE Korb score	$n = 37$ 1.22 (1.00)	$n = 37$ −0.19 (0.92)	$n = 37$ 0.91 (0.96)	$n = 37$ 0.12 (0.71)	0.153
Yamaguchi score	$n = 37$ 5.05 (2.33)	$n = 37$ −0.14 (2.42)	$n = 37$ 4.14 (2.41)	$n = 37$ 0.19 (1.97)	0.498
tear osmolarity * (mOsm/L)	$n = 40$ 297.12 (14.47)	$n = 37$ 2.11 (14.54)	$n = 37$ 299.16 (12.11)	$n = 35$ 0.94 (17.59)	0.294

* See Appendix F for details of statistical handling of measurement values below the detection limit of the TearLab test instrument.

3.3.5. Observation of the Subbasal Nerve Plexus by Confocal Microscopy

Confocal laser scanning microscopy was performed on 16 patients (eight patients each in the Comfort Shield group and in the control group) at four out of 11 study centers. Images of the subbasal nerve plexus were taken at baseline and week 8 and assessed at RC2. There was a significant increase of total nerve fiber length in the Comfort Shield group (51% growth; p-value 0.030), whereas in the control group, the total subbasal corneal nerve fiber length did not significantly change from baseline to week 8. Detailed results will be subject to a separate publication.

3.3.6. Dropping Frequency

The patients were instructed to use their lubricant eye drops whenever ocular discomfort occured. They recorded the dropping daily. The average dropping frequency was not significantly different in the two treatment arms. By the time of inclusion into the study, the patients reported using 7.6 (minimum: 2; maximum: 36) artificial tear drops or autologous serum eye drops per day in the control group, and 8.2 (minimum: 3; maximum: 20) in the Comfort Shield Group. During week 8 of the study, the average dropping frequency was 6.5 (minimum: 1; maximum: 24.6) per day in the control group and 7.1 (minimum: 2; maximum: 23.8) in the Comfort Shield group.

3.3.7. Influence of Climate on CFS and OSDI

In order to investigate whether or not climate has a significant impact on the study results, the primary endpoint CFS and the key secondary endpoint OSDI were analyzed separately for the nine study centers located in Europe and the two study centers in Riyadh in the desert region of Saudi Arabia. There were no significant differences between these two subgroups. The complete results are presented in Appendix G, Tables 6–8 and A5.

3.4. Safety Results

The assessment of safety results refers to the safety set (SS), i.e., all patient that had at least once received eye drops ($n = 121$).

The average intraocular pressure in both study arms at baseline and week 8 was 14 mmHg. All values were between 8 and 23 mmHg. There were no patients suspect of uncontrolled glaucoma or ocular hypertension.

Of the Comfort Shield group, one patient discontinued the participation in the study after one week because the dry eye symptoms had worsened. Two patients reported during the week 4 visit about blurred vision for 10 min after the instillation of Comfort Shield eye drops, but they wanted to continue to participate in the study. One patient reported during the week 4 visit about persistent redness but wanted to continue to participate in the study. One patient reported during the week 4 visit about burning sensation, but they wanted to continue to participate in the study. One patient reported during the week 4 visit an episode of three days of red, painful, itching left eye, but they wanted to continue to participate in the study.

Of the control group, three patients had experienced not device-related adverse events between the week 4 and week 8 visits. One patient had nausea for two days, one patient had a mild viral conjunctivitis, and one patient had to be admitted to the hospital with cervical pain and was treated for six days with analgesics.

4. Discussion

The population of this study shows the typical predominance of age and female gender in dry eye disease, as the majority of patients was older than 45 years (90.4%, respectively, 65 years (33.3%) and most patients were female (82.1%) [54]. There was no significant difference between the verum and the control group.

The design of clinical trials on dry eye disease needs to consider symptoms, namely ocular discomfort and visual disturbance, as well as signs, such as tear film instability, damage of the ocular surface, increased tear osmolarity, and inflammation of the ocular surface [55]. International regulatory agencies rely on ocular surface staining as a primary endpoint for new drug approvals [56]. The ODISSEY European Consensus Group recommended CFS as the primary sign for severity of DED [39]. For this reason, the HYLAN M study used CFS as the primary endpoint of the study and standardized the test method as well as the objective assessment of staining as far as reasonably possible. Other dry eye signs, such as tear osmolarity, TBUT, Schirmer I, lid wiper epitheliopathy, and position of the mucocutaneous junction at the lid rim were chosen as secondary endpoints, having in mind the well-known poor correlation between symptoms and signs in DED. As corneal nerve damage has in recent years been recognized as an important pathomechanism in severe ocular surface disease, the assessment of the subbasal nerve plexus using confocal laser scanning microscopy had been included as an additional optional test in the study design. OSDI was chosen as the key secondary endpoint for the assessment of dry eye symptoms as it is widely used and easy to interpret.

The HYLAN M study did not find a statistically significant difference between the Comfort Shield group and the control group at the week 8 visit for the primary endpoint CFS or any of the following secondary endpoints: TBUT, Schirmer I, lid wiper epitheliopathy, and tear osmolarity. This emphasizes that in patients with severe dry eyes, a change from the therapy with individualized lubricant eye drops to HMWHA eye drops does not result in a worsening of dry eye signs.

The primary endpoint of the HYLAM M study, CFS, did not show any significant difference between the two study arms. The value of CFS as an absolute number to judge the improvement or deterioration of the corneal surface condition has been questioned. As it is known that the difference in grading between different investigators may limit the sensitivity of detectable changes in CFS over time, the CFS test method within the HYLAN M study had been highly standardized, and a reading center performing electronic assessment of CFS images has been involved (see Appendix D). The well-known, possibly even physiological variation of CFS between measurements has been supported by the present study. Moreover, it is known that CFS is sensitive to effects of quenching and pooling, which may affect the repeatability and accuracy of measurement. A post hoc analysis of the control group demonstrated that there is a significant fluctuation in CFS over time even in the best treated patients under stable optimum treatment (see Appendix H). This variation emphasizes the difficulty of judging the ocular surface condition from surface staining intensity. Similar fluctuations such as the one experienced for CFS are known for other dry eye signs [17,52,57–63]. Originally enthusiastically welcomed as a highly reliable parameter for DED and used as a major decision maker with respect to the severity of DED, the diagnostic significance of tear osmolarity determined in the lower tear meniscus has recently been questioned [64]. The average osmolarity of 298 mOsm/L found in the HYLAN M study for patients suffering from severe DED is not hyperosmotic, as expected for severe DED.

OSDI was the key secondary endpoint of the HYLAN M study. The OSDI questionnaire is one of the most commonly used tests to assess dry eye symptoms [42]. The OSDI score was assessed at the baseline visit, after four weeks, and after eight weeks. Whereas, in the control group, the OSDI score slightly improved in the first four weeks, which was presumably due to better compliance of the patients with their treatment regimen, but it did not further improve beyond the four-week study participation. Contrarily, the OSDI score significantly improved under Comfort Shield treatment in the first four weeks and continued to improve in the second four-week period (see Figure 3a). Such improvement applies also to the subscore for discomfort and pain, as well as for the subscore for visual instability (see Figure 3b,c). After eight weeks treatment, the difference between the Comfort Shield group and the control group were for the total OSDI score 13.5 (p-value 0.001), for the pain subscore 14.5 (p-value 0.002), and for the vision subscore 14.0 (p-value 0.003). This unexpectedly great improvement in dry eye symptoms under the treatment with HMWHA eye drops deserves further investigation. The Asia Dry Eye Society recently concluded that subjective severity (symptoms) could be used as a marker for therapeutic efficacy in dry eye treatment [9].

The improvement of the symptoms of visual stability in the HYLAN M study was reflected by a minor but significant improvement of BCVA. Whereas, BCVA determines the best visual acuity within a certain period of time, functional visual acuity continuously determines visual acuity and, therefore, better reflects the subjective stability of vision [65–67]. Therefore, in future clinical studies on dry eye disease, functional visual acuity rather than BCVA might be used as an endpoint.

As an optional test within the HYLAN M study, the subbasal nerve plexus was analyzed in a subgroup of 16 patients. There was a significant increase of total nerve fiber length in the Comfort Shield group as compared to the control group after eight weeks of treatment. This observation correlates well with the significant improvement of pain symptoms. The fact that at the same time there was no significant change of other dry eye signs suggests that the observed therapeutic effect cannot be attributed to a physical effect of the eye drops such as hydration or lubrication, but it is likely to result from a pharmacological effect downregulating ocular inflammation and supporting corneal nerve recovery.

5. Conclusions

In an international multicenter randomized clinical study on patients suffering from severe dry eye disease, 0.15% high molecular weight hyaluronan (HMWHA) eye drops have been compared with lubricant eye drops individually selected as optimum therapy. HMWHA eye drops have shown superior potential to significantly ameliorate symptoms including discomfort and pain, as well as visual instability without affecting dry eye signs.

Author Contributions: See Appendix A. Authors have confirmed that format for that Section.

Funding: The HYLAN M study received unrestricted funding from i.com medical GmbH, Munich, Germany.

Acknowledgments: The principle investigators wish to acknowledge the great support by their study teams, in particular Bernadette Matijak-Kronschachner and Andrea Heidinger in Graz, Semra Akkaya Turhan in Istanbul, Anoud Saati and Nouf Aljwaiser at PSMMC, Jose Vargas, Gharam Al Zahrani and Sarah Al Harbi at KKESH, Anita Koschmieder in Rostock, and Laurence Quérat and Christine Åkerstedt in Stockholm.

Conflicts of Interest: The study director Wolfgang G.K. Müller-Lierheim is also CEO of the company i.com medical GmbH, Munich, Germany. The remaining authors declare no conflict of interest.

Appendix A. Study Centers, Administrative Structure of the Study, and Author Contributions

Eleven study centers in eight countries with different climate zones and different ethnicities participated in the HYLAN M Study:

(1) Centre Hospitalier National d'Ophtalmologie—Quinze-Vingts, Paris, France, principle investigator (PI) Christophe Baudouin
(2) St. Erik Eye Hospital, Stockholm, Sweden, PI Gysbert-Botho van Setten
(3) Department of Ophthalmology, University Medical Center Rostock, Rostock, Germany, PI Ria Beck
(4) Department of Ophthalmology, Medical University Graz, Graz, Austria, PI Jutta Horwath-Winter
(5) Department of Ophthalmology, University Clinic Salzburg, Paracelsus Medical University, Salzburg, Austria, PI Herbert A. Reitsamer
(6) Department of Ophthalmology, Saarland University Medical Center, Homburg/Saar, Germany, PI Berthold Seitz
(7) KKESH—King Khaled Eye Specialist Hospital, Riyadh, Saudi Arabia, PI Osama Al-Sheikh
(8) Marmara University Pendik Training and Research Hospital, Marmara University Medical School, Department of Ophthalmology, Istanbul, Turkey, PI Ebru Toker
(9) Department of Ophthalmology, PSMMC Prince Sultan Military Medical City, MSD Medical Services Department, MODA Ministry of Defense and Aviation, Riyadh, Saudi Arabia, PI Sultan Al-Zaaidi
(10) Universidad Complutense de Madrid, Hospital Clinico San Carlos, Departamentos de Oftalmologia, Madrid, Spain, PI Jose M. Benitez-del-Castillo
(11) Ocular Surface & Dry Eye Center, Ospedale L. Sacco, University of Milan, Milan, Italy, PI Stefano Barabino

The HYLAN M Study was designed in accordance with the international standard ISO 14155:2012 by the sponsor CORONIS GmbH (Munich, Germany) in close cooperation with the PIs Christophe Baudouin, Gysbert van Setten, and Jutta Horwath-Winter, the representatives of the reading centers, Daniel Böhringer for RC1 and Oliver Stachs for RC2, the biostatistician Sébastien Marque (IQVIA, France), and the randomization center (C2R, Paris, France). CORONIS is operating under a quality management system including clinical research, which was certified according to the international standard 13485:2016 and annually supervised by the European notified body mdc medical device certification GmbH (Stuttgart, Germany).

The representative of the sponsor, Wolfgang G.K. Müller-Lierheim, had overall responsibility as study director (SD). In obtaining local ethics committee approval, registering the study with national authorities, and monitoring the study, he was supported by

- IPR—International Pharmaceutical Consultancy, Paris, France
- OPIS, Desio, Italy
- Monitor Medikal Araştırma ve Danışmanlık Tic. Ltd. Şti., Istanbul, Turkey
- KKESH Research Department, Riyadh, Kingdom of Saudi Arabia.

The medical scientific management of the HYLAN M Study was under the overall responsibility of the coordinating investigator (CI) Gysbert-Botho van Setten, who was supported by Jutta Horwath-Winter with respect to the lissamine green staining procedure and diagnostic judgement, and Oliver Stachs regarding confocal microscopy.

The HYLAN M Study used detailed work instructions including the diagnostic procedures corneal fluorescein staining (see Appendix D), tear film break-up time, lissamine green staining (including assessment of lid wiper epitheliopathy and mucocutaneous junction), tear film osmolarity using the TearLab osmolarity system (TearLab Corporation, San Diego, CA, USA), and taking and evaluating confocal microscopy images of the subbasal nerve plexus using the Heidelberg Retina Tomograph HRT in combination with the Rostock Cornea Module RCM (Heidelberg Engineering GmbH, Heidelberg, Germany).

Paper case report forms (CRF) were used by the study centers throughout the study and were archived by each study center for a minimum of 10 years beyond the completion of the HYLAN M study. The contents of the case report forms were anonymously transferred to electronic case report forms (eCRF) using a web-based system allowing electronic transfer to the HYLAN M study database hosted at the University Eye Hospital in Freiburg, Germany. For monitoring purposes, the SD had online access to the HYLAN M database. Printouts of the eCRFs were used to assure the correct and complete data transfer from the paper CRFs to the eCRFs during regular monitoring visits of the study centers. At the closure visits of each study center, printouts of all eCRFs were signed by the responsible PI and provided to the sponsor who scanned and electronically archived the signed eCRFs. After the closing the last study center and monitoring the reading centers and the host of the study database, the database was locked on 26 March 2020, and exported for statistical analysis.

The company C2R (Paris, France) under the responsibility of the data managers Pascale Croix and Mélinda Ezzedine provided the electronic block randomization of patients of the HYLAN M study in two equally sized study arms A (control group) and B (Comfort Shield group = verum group). The investigators were kept unaware of block randomization and the block size of four. For the randomization, the module CSRandomization of the ENNOV CLINICAL® software (version 7.5) was used. The clinical data management system had been developed and validated to meet all regulatory requirements of data management and create a non-modifiable audit trail. The study centers had password-protected secure CS Online internet interface access to the randomization tool. After entering the patient number, the system automatically created the result of randomization. Then, the study centers printed the patient number and result of randomization and filed this together with their CRFs to be controlled during monitoring visits.

The HYLAN M Study used two masked reading centers for the analysis of digital images provided by the study centers. The cornea reading center located at the Eye Center, University Hospital Freiburg, Germany, in the text referred to as RC1, analyzed the corneal fluorescein staining (see Appendix D). Oliver Stachs (Department of Ophthalmology, University Medical Center, Rostock, Germany), in the text referred to as RC2, analyzed the subbasal nerve fibers in confocal microscopy images, which were taken as an additional optional diagnostic test at the baseline and week 8 visits of the HYLAN M study (the results of this subgroup analysis will be published separately).

The statistical analysis plan (SAP) for the HYLAN M Study was developed by IQVIA, Bordeaux, France in cooperation with the SD. IQVIA performed the statistical analysis by using the software R version 3.5.3 (The R Foundation for Statistical Computing, Vienna, Austria) after database lock and provided the statistical analysis report (SAR) of the HYLAN M study. Upon request, the sponsor of the HYLAN M study will provide a copy of the SAR.

The statistical analysis of the results from the optional assessment of the subbasal nerve plexus by confocal laser scanning microscopy was performed by RC2.

The manuscript of this report was prepared by Gysbert-Botho van Setten, Jutta Horwath-Winter, Daniel Böhringer, Oliver Stachs, and Wolfgang G.K. Müller-Lierheim.

Appendix B. Ethics Committee Approval, Compliance with the Declaration of Helsinki, and Registration of the Study

The HYLAN M study was approved by ethics committees in all eight countries where study centers were located:

- Austria: Medical University Graz, Ethic Committee, reg. no. 28-458 ex 15/16
- France: Comite de protection des Persones Ile de France V, reg. no. 16138
- Germany: Ärztekammer des Saarlandes, Ethik-Kommission, reg. no. 176/16

- Italy: Comitato Etico Milano Area 1, protocol no. 47068/2018
- Kingdom of Saudi Arabia: King Khaled Eye Specialist Hospital, Research Department, reference RSCH/665/5957-16 and Prince Sultan Military Medical City, Research Ethics Committee, reg. no. HAP-01-R-015
- Spain: CEIC Hospital Clinico San Carlos, reg. no. 18/016-R_P
- Sweden: EPN Regionala etikprövningsnämnden I Stockholm protocol 19 October 2016
- Turkey: Marmara University Hospital, Klinik Arastirmalar Etik Kurulu, form 2013-KAEK-60

All subjects gave their informed consent for inclusion before they participated in the HYLAN M Study. The study was conducted in accordance with the Declaration of Helsinki.

The HYLAN M study was registered on the database of the European Commission for medical devices EUDAMED under the registration number CIV-16-06-015964. Moreover, the study was registered with national competent authorities in Austria, France, Germany, Italy, Sweden, and Turkey.

Appendix C. Investigational Device

The control group of the HYLAN M study continued to use the lubricant eye drops which the individual participant had been using by the time of inclusion. In the verum group (Comfort Shield group), the lubricant eye drops which the individual participant had been using by the time of inclusion were replaced by Comfort Shield® eye drops (i.com medical GmbH, Munich, Germany). Comfort Shield® eye drops were available to the participants in two dosage forms with identical preservative-free composition, as Comfort Shield® SD in boxes containing 15 monodoses each, and as Comfort Shield® MDS in 10 mL bottles. Comfort Shield® contains 0.15% high molecular weight hyaluronan (Hylan A; intrinsic viscosity 2.9 m^3/kg) dissolved in isotonic saline solution with 1.20 mmol/L phosphate buffer.

Comfort Shield® eye drops are approved in Europe as Class IIb medical device and were used within the HYLAN M study in accordance with the labeling.

Appendix D. Corneal Fluorescein Staining and Electronic Analysis Method

Sterile, preservative-free 0.5% sodium fluorescein solution in 0.4 mL monodose containers (FLUORESCEINE FAURE 0.5 PER CENT ophthalmic solution in unit dose, SERB SAS, Paris, France) and Eppendorf Reference 2 pipettes with 10 µL fixed volume (Eppendorf AG, Hamburg, Germany) were provided by the sponsor to each study center.

Then, 10 µL fluorescein solution was released in the cul-de-sac of the patient's eye without touching the ocular surface. The patient blinked five times to evenly distribute the fluorescein on the ocular surface. After 20 to 120 s, the corneal and conjunctival fluorescein staining was judged visually at 16× magnification using the slitlamp with "cobalt" blue light illumination and a yellow barrier filter in the observation beam and graded using the Oxford score [41]. Digital images are taken. The images are electronically transferred to the reading center RC1 with the file names containing the patient number, visit, and eye (OD = right eye or OS = left eye).

During the qualification of the study centers, each study center submitted images of corneas with fluorescein staining together with their visual Oxford grading of staining to ensure and verify that RC1 will correctly assess the staining grade. Then, the settings of slitlamp, illumination, filters, and camera were fixed and kept constant throughout the HYLAN M study.

RC1 analyzed the staining in two steps. Figure A1a shows a typical image that is uploaded to the reading center. First, the region of interest comprising the cornea to be analyzed is segmented manually. In the second step, the CSF-positive lesions are electronically segmented using a threshold-based image processing algorithm. Figure A1b shows the image after electronic processing. The final readout is the percentage of total green pixels divided by the total pixels of the cornea area. The parameters for the automated segmentation were carefully set up for each study center individually as part of the center certification procedure.

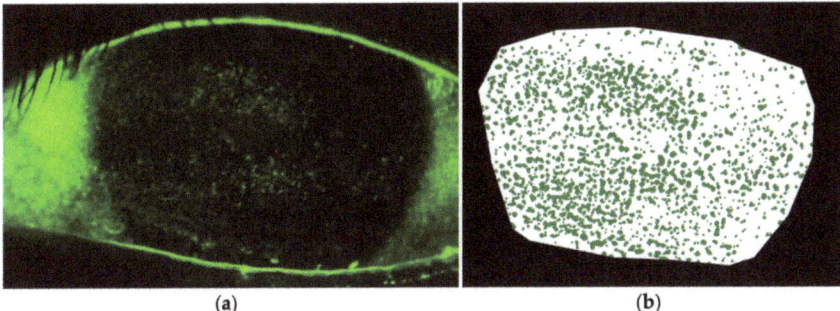

Figure A1. (**a**) CFS image as uploaded by the trial sites to the reading center; (**b**) CFS image after manually segmenting the cornea and application of a threshold-based segmentation of the CFS-positive lesions. The final readout is the percentage of total green pixels divided by the total pixels of the cornea area.

RC1 had empirically found that 2.00% staining correlates well with Oxford grade 3, and therefore, this was used as the inclusion criteria to be met at least by one eye of the patient. Patients with confluent staining were excluded because the staining cannot be electronically quantified.

The Oxford grading is based on 0.5 log units difference between grade 1 and grade 5 [41]. Therefore, for the transformation percentage of fluorescein staining into "continuous Oxford grades", the following formula was used:

If staining $< 0.2\% \rightarrow$ Grade $= 0$
If staining $[0.2\text{–}20\%] \rightarrow$ Grade $= 2.398 + 2 \times \log_{10}(\%\ \text{staining})$
If staining $> 20\% \rightarrow$ Grade $= 5$.

Appendix E. Medical History

Table A1. Tabular overview of the medical history according to the treatment arm—PPS population ($n = 84$).

		Comfort Shield ($n = 44$)	Control ($n = 40$)	Total ($n = 84$)
Rheumatoid disease n (%)	n	43	40	83
	no	21 (48.8)	20 (50.0)	41 (49.4)
	yes	22 (51.2)	20 (50.0)	42 (50.6)
	missing	1	0	1
Thyroid disease n (%)	n	43	40	83
	no	27 (62.8)	33 (82.5)	60 (72.3)
	yes	16 (37.2)	7 (17.5)	23 (27.7)
	missing	1	0	1
Trachoma n (%)	n	43	40	83
	no	43 (100.0)	40 (100.0)	83 (100.0)
	missing	1	0	1
Other disease n (%)	n	43	39	82
	no	23 (53.5)	17 (43.6)	40 (48.8)
	yes	20 (46.5)	22 (56.4)	42 (51.2)
	missing	1	1	2
History betablocker n (%)	n	43	40	83
	no	33 (76.7)	33 (82.5)	66 (79.5)
	yes	10 (23.3)	7 (17.5)	17 (20.5)
	missing	1	0	1

Table A1. Tabular overview of the medical history according to the treatment arm—PPS population ($n = 84$).

		Comfort Shield ($n = 44$)	Control ($n = 40$)	Total ($n = 84$)
Antidepressants n (%)	n	43	40	83
	no	36 (83.7)	34 (85.0)	70 (84.3)
	yes	7 (16.3)	6 (15.0)	13 (15.7)
	missing	1	0	1
Other drugs n (%)	n	42	38	80
	no	20 (47.6)	11 (28.9)	31 (38.8)
	yes	22 (52.4)	27 (71.1)	49 (61.2)
	missing	2	2	4
History contact lenses n (%)	n	43	40	83
	no	42 (97.7)	40 (100.0)	82 (98.8)
	yes	1 (2.3)	0 (0.0)	1 (1.2)
	missing	1	0	1
Conjunctival injection n (%)	n	43	39	82
	no	25 (58.1)	20 (51.3)	45 (54.9)
	yes	18 (41.9)	19 (48.7)	37 (45.1)
	missing	1	1	2
Inflammation of lid rim n (%)	n	43	39	82
	no	30 (69.8)	28 (71.8)	58 (70.7)
	yes	13 (30.2)	11 (28.2)	24 (29.3)
	missing	1	1	2

Six patients of the Comfort Shield group and two patients of the control group had received autologous serum eye drops by the time of inclusion into the study. In the Comfort Shield group, the autologous serum therapy was substituted by Comfort Shield eye drops.

Fifteen (34.1%) of 44 patients in the Comfort Shield group and 15 (37.5%) of 40 patients in the control group received cyclosporine eye drops and continued their application throughout the study.

Twenty-five (56.8%) of 44 patients in the Comfort Shield group and 23 (57.5%) of 40 patients in the control group were using hyaluronan containing artificial tears by the time of inclusion into the HYLAN M study.

Appendix F. Tear Osmolarity Test Results

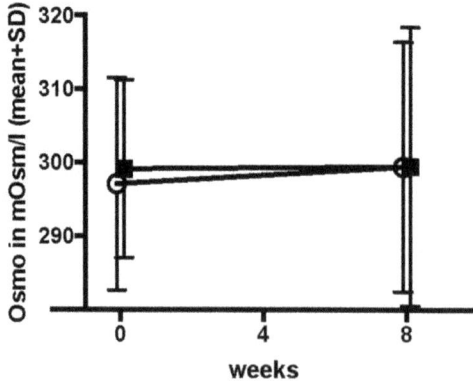

Figure A2. Mean (±SD) of osmolarity by treatment arm according time—PPS ($n = 84$). Open circles = Comfort Shield group, filled squares = control group.

Table A2. Osmolarity: value in mOsm/L at baseline and at week 8—PPS (n = 84)—Descriptive analysis, by treatment arm.

		Comfort Shield (n = 44)	Control (n = 40)	Total (n = 84)
value at baseline	n	40	37	77
	mean (sd)	297.12 (14.47)	299.16 (12.11)	298.1 (13.34)
	median (iqr)	295.5 (287.75, 304.25)	299 (292, 307)	298 (289, 306)
	min, max	277, 337	275, 336	275, 337
	* <275 mOsm/L	2	2	4
	missing	2	1	3
value at week 8	n	40	37	
	mean (sd)	299.43 (16.99)	299.49 (18.94)	
	median (iqr)	300 (286, 308)	299 (291, 304)	
	min, max	275, 353	276, 395	
	* <275 mOsm/L	1	3	
	missing	3	0	

* values below detection limit (<275 mOsm/L) were not included in the statistical analysis.

Table A3. Osmolarity: Value in mOsm/L at baseline and at week 8—PPS (n = 84)–Descriptive analysis, by treatment arm.

		Comfort Shield (n = 44)	Control (n = 40)	Total (n = 84)
value at baseline	n	42	39	81
	<275 mOsm/L	2 (4.8)	2 (5.1)	4 (4.9)
	≥275 mOsm/L	40 (95.2)	37 (94.9)	77 (95.1)
	missing	2	1	3
value at week 8	n	41	40	
	<275 mOsm/L	1 (2.4)	3 (7.5)	
	* ≥275 mOsm/L	40 (97.6)	37 (92.5)	
	missing	3	0	

* values below detection limit (<275 mOsm/L) were not included in the statistical analysis.

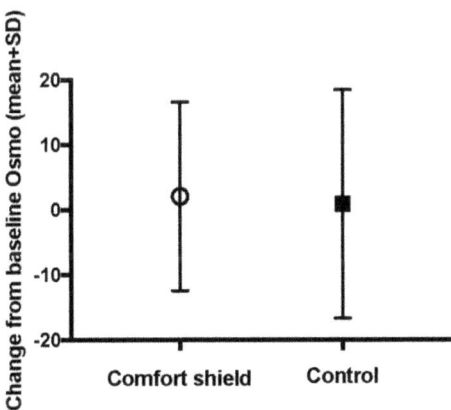

Figure A3. Mean (±SD) change from baseline to week 8 (week 8–baseline) of osmolarity by group—PPS (n = 84). Open circle = Comfort Shield group, filled square = control group.

Table A4. Osmolarity: value in mOsm/L at baseline and change from baseline to week 8–PPS ($n = 84$)–Descriptive analysis, by treatment arm.

		Comfort Shield ($n = 44$)	Control ($n = 40$)	Total ($n = 84$)	p-Value
value at baseline	n	40	37	77	
	mean (sd)	297.12 (14.47)	299.16 (12.11)	298.1 (13.34)	
	median (iqr)	295.5 (287.75, 304.25)	299 (292, 307)	298 (289, 306)	
	min, max	277, 337	275, 336	275, 337	
	* <275 mOsm/L	2	2	4	
	missing	2	1	3	
change from baseline to week 8	n	37	35		0.294
	mean (sd)	2.11 (14.54)	0.94 (17.59)		
	median (iqr)	2 (−6, 12)	−1 (−7.0, 7.5)		
	min, max	−29, 27	−30, 80		
	* <275 mOsm/L	1	3		
	** missing	6	2		

* No missing value but at least one value below detection limit (<275 mOsm/L). ** At least one missing value at baseline or Week 8.

Appendix G. Influence of Climate on CFS and OSDI

The primary endpoint CFS and the key secondary endpoint were separately assessed for two subgroups: "Europe" (patients from all European study centers, including Istanbul) and "Desert" (patients from the two study centers in Riyadh, Saudi Arabia). The results are summarized in the following tables.

Table A5. CFS: value at baseline and at each post-baseline visit—PPS ($n = 84$)—descriptive analysis by subgroup.

		Comfort Shield		Control	
		Desert ($n = 6$)	Europe ($n = 38$)	Desert ($n = 7$)	Europe ($n = 33$)
value at baseline	n	6	38	7	33
	mean (sd)	3.79 (0.71)	4.04 (0.52)	4.11 (0.61)	4.30 (0.55)
	median (iqr)	3.62 (3.37, 4.05)	3.94 (3.59, 4.39)	3.95 (3.60, 4.56)	4.41 (3.80, 4.65)
	min, max	3, 5	3, 5	3, 5	3, 5
	missing	0	0	0	0
value at week 4	n	5	36	6	32
	mean (sd)	3.37 (0.89)	3.89 (0.82)	2.22 (1.53)	3.72 (1.05)
	median (iqr)	3.74 (2.81, 4.09)	4.00 (3.43, 4.54)	2.15 (1.41, 3.36)	3.93 (3.25, 4.48)
	min, max	2, 4	1, 5	0, 4	0, 5
	missing	1	2	1	1
value at week 8	n	6	35	6	32
	mean (sd)	3.79 (1.30)	3.94 (0.97)	2.21 (1.91)	3.88 (0.83)
	median (iqr)	4.20 (2.60, 4.84)	4.31 (3.38, 4.68)	2.56 (0.58, 3.22)	3.99 (3.37, 4.45)
	min, max	2, 5	0, 5	0, 5	2, 5
	missing	0	3	1	1

Table A6. CFS: value at baseline and change from baseline to each post-baseline visit—PPS (n = 84)—descriptive analysis by subgroup.

		Comfort Shield		Control	
		Desert (n = 6)	Europe (n = 38)	Desert (n = 7)	Europe (n = 33)
baseline	n	6	38	7	33
	mean (sd)	3.79 (0.71)	4.04 (0.52)	4.11 (0.61)	4.30 (0.55)
	median (iqr)	3.62 (3.37, 4.05)	3.94 (3.59, 4.39)	3.95 (3.60, 4.56)	4.41 (3.80, 4.65)
	min, max	3, 5	3, 5	3, 5	3, 5
	missing	0	0	0	0
change from baseline to week 4	n	5	36	6	32
	mean (sd)	−0.43 (0.59)	−0.18 (0.78)	−1.74 (1.16)	−0.57 (0.90)
	median (iqr)	−0.70 (−0.91, −0.06)	−0.03 (−0.52, 0.31)	−1.51 (−2.29, −0.82)	−0.35 (−0.92, −0.14)
	min, max	−1, 0	−3, 1	−4, −1	−4, 1
	missing	1	2	1	1
change from baseline to week 8	n	6	35	6	32
	mean (sd)	0.00 (0.98)	−0.14 (1.06)	−1.79 (1.48)	−0.42 (0.82)
	median (iqr)	−0.02 (−0.62, 0.64)	−0.07 (−0.56, 0.56)	−1.33 (−3.11, −0.75)	−0.23 (−0.64, 0.12)
	min, max	−1, 1	−4, 1	−4, 0	−3, 1
	missing	0	3	1	1

Table A7. OSDI: value at baseline and at each post-baseline visit—PPS (n = 84)—descriptive analysis by subgroup.

		Comfort Shield		Control	
		Desert (n = 6)	Europe (n = 38)	Desert (n = 7)	Europe (n = 33)
baseline	n	6	38	7	33
	mean (sd)	62.34 (18.55)	56.63 (16.29)	62.98 (20.34)	60.73 (16.53)
	median (iqr)	63.63 (51.14, 76.14)	54.36 (43.32, 68.44)	70.45 (46.93, 77.71)	61.11 (52.08, 75.00)
	min, max	35, 84	34, 92	36, 85	34, 95
	missing	0	0	0	0
value at week 4	n	6	38	7	33
	mean (sd)	36.89 (31.71)	43.75 (18.39)	49.74 (15.73)	56.71 (20.37)
	median (iqr)	20.45 (19.18, 61.36)	40.91 (32.71, 55.31)	43.18 (36.82, 64.02)	55.56 (41.67, 69.44)
	min, max	7, 80	9, 85	33, 70	22, 95
	missing	0	0	0	0
value at week 8	n	6	38	7	33
	mean (sd)	26.45 (20.34)	42.95 (18.26)	65.85 (12.65)	54.11 (22.42)
	median (iqr)	32.95 (9.38, 40.91)	41.67 (29.27, 55.94)	65.91 (58.62, 74.75)	52.08 (35.42, 75.00)
	min, max	0, 48	15, 88	46, 82	9, 93
	missing	0	0	0	0

Table A8. OSDI: Value at baseline and change from baseline to each post-baseline visit—PPS ($n = 84$)—descriptive analysis by subgroup.

		Comfort Shield		Control	
		Desert ($n = 6$)	Europe ($n = 38$)	Desert ($n = 7$)	Europe ($n = 33$)
baseline	n	6	38	7	33
	mean (sd)	62.34 (18.55)	56.63 (16.29)	62.98 (20.34)	60.73 (16.53)
	median (iqr)	63.63 (51.14, 76.14)	54.36 (43.32, 68.44)	70.45 (46.93, 77.71)	61.11 (52.08, 75.00)
	min, max	35, 84	34, 92	36, 85	34, 95
	missing	0	0	0	0
change from baseline to week 4	n	6	38	7	33
	mean (sd)	−25.45 (33.48)	−12.88 (18.03)	−13.24 (12.94)	−4.02 (12.19)
	median (iqr)	−34.59 (−45.60, −7.07)	−9.66 (−19.69, −2.61)	−12.50 (−16.32, −5.93)	−2.50 (−8.61, 0.00)
	min, max	−64, 27	−71, 17	−38, 2	−31, 26
	missing	0	0	0	0
change from baseline to week 8	n	6	38	7	33
	mean (sd)	−35.89 (27.94)	−13.68 (20.02)	2.88 (18.26)	−6.63 (16.47)
	median (iqr)	−34.95 (−40.34, −23.15)	−12.50 (−20.98, −0.23)	−2.50 (−7.41, 4.52)	−3.86 (−18.75, 6.82)
	min, max	−84, 0	−69, 27	−12, 41	−43, 15
	missing	0	0	0	0

Appendix H. Fluctuation of Corneal Fluorescein Staining in the Control Group

The HYLAN M study included patients with severe dry eye, whose optimum therapy had not changed within the two months (in the case of concomitant cyclosporine therapy, three months) prior to inclusion. Therefore, it was assumed that the corneal fluorescein staining in the control group, where the therapy remained unchanged, will remain fairly constant over the eight-week study period. To prove this assumption, we post hoc analyzed the changes in corneal fluorescein staining of the study eyes of the control group from the baseline to the week 4 visit and from the week 4 to the week 8 visit. We found that from the baseline visit to the week 4 visit, the CFS Oxford grade improved on average by 0.69 with a standard deviation of 1.05, and from the week 4 visit to the week 8 visit, it worsened on the average by 0.23 with a standard deviation of 1.12. An improvement from the baseline to the week 4 visit might be attributable to the fact that the patients participated in a study with controlled dropping frequency and, therefore, adhered more strictly to the prescribed therapy. However, this argument should not apply to the differences observed between the week 8 visit and the week 4 visit.

We interpret our findings in the sense that CFS as an endpoint is subject to significant fluctuation in patients suffering from severe dry eye disease.

References

1. Stapleton, F.; Alves, M.; Bunya, V.Y.; Jalbert, I.; Lekhanont, K.; Malet, F.; Na, K.S.; Schaumberg, D.; Uchino, M.; Vehof, J.; et al. TFOS DEWS II Epidemiology Report. *Ocul. Surf.* **2017**, *15*, 334–365. [CrossRef] [PubMed]
2. Saldanha, I.J.; Petris, R.; Han, G.; Dickersin, K.; Akpek, E.K. Research Questions and Outcomes Prioritized by Patients With Dry Eye. *JAMA Ophthalmol.* **2018**, *136*, 1170–1179. [CrossRef] [PubMed]
3. Benítez-del-Castillo, J.; Labetoulle, M.; Baudouin, C.; Rolando, M.; Akova, Y.A.; Aragona, P.; Geerling, G.; Merayo-Lloves, J.; Messmer, E.M.; Boboridis, K. Visual acuity and quality of life in dry eye disease: Proceedings of the OCEAN group meeting. *Ocul. Surf.* **2017**, *15*, 169–178. [CrossRef] [PubMed]
4. Patel, V.; Watanabe, J.; Strauss, J.; Dubey, A. Work productivity loss in patients with dry eye disease: An online survey. *Curr. Med Res. Opin.* **2011**, *27*, 1041–1048. [CrossRef] [PubMed]

5. Yu, J.; Asche, C.V.; Fairchild, C.J. The economic burden of dry eye disease in the United States: A decision tree analysis. *Cornea* **2011**, *30*, 379–387. [CrossRef]
6. Uchino, M. What We Know About the Epidemiology of Dry Eye Disease in Japan. *Investig. Ophthalmol. Vis. Sci.* **2018**, *59*, DES1–DES6. [CrossRef]
7. Jones, L.; Downie, L.E.; Korb, D.; Benitez-Del-Castillo, J.M.; Dana, R.; Deng, S.X.; Dong, P.N.; Geerling, G.; Hida, R.Y.; Liu, Y.; et al. TFOS DEWS II Management and Therapy Report. *Ocul. Surf.* **2017**, *15*, 575–628. [CrossRef]
8. Tsubota, K.; Yokoi, N.; Shimazaki, J.; Watanabe, H.; Dogru, M.; Yamada, M.; Kinoshita, S.; Kim, H.M.; Tchah, H.W.; Hyon, J.Y.; et al. New Perspectives on Dry Eye Definition and Diagnosis: A Consensus Report by the Asia Dry Eye Society. *Ocul. Surf.* **2017**, *15*, 65–76. [CrossRef]
9. Tsubota, K.; Yokoi, N.; Watanabe, H.; Dogru, M.; Kojima, T.; Yamada, M.; Kinoshita, S.; Kim, H.M.; Tchah, H.W.; Hyon, J.Y.; et al. A New Perspective on Dry Eye Classification: Proposal by the Asia Dry Eye Society. *Eye Contact Lens* **2020**, *46* (Suppl. 1), S2–S13. [CrossRef]
10. van Setten, G.B.; Mueller-Lierheim, W.; Baudouin, C. Dry Eye Etiology: Focus on Friction. *Klin. Mon. Augenheilkd.* **2019**, *237*, 1235–1236. [CrossRef]
11. van Setten, G.-B. Impact of Attrition, Intercellular Shear in Dry Eye Disease: When Cells are Challenged and Neurons are Triggered. *Int. J. Mol. Sci.* **2020**, *21*, 4333. [CrossRef] [PubMed]
12. Stern, M.E.; Pflugfelder, S.C. Inflammation in dry eye. *Ocul. Surf.* **2004**, *2*, 124–130. [CrossRef]
13. Aragona, P.; Giannaccare, G.; Mencucci, R.; Rubino, P.; Cantera, E.; Rolando, M. Modern approach to the treatment of dry eye, a complex multifactorial disease: A P.I.C.A.S.S.O. board review. *Br. J. Ophthalmol.* **2020**, 32703782. [CrossRef] [PubMed]
14. Baudouin, C. A new approach for better comprehension of diseases of the ocular surface. *J. Fr. Ophtalmol.* **2007**, *30*, 239–246. [CrossRef]
15. Baudouin, C.; Irkec, M.; Messmer, E.M.; Benitez-Del-Castillo, J.M.; Bonini, S.; Figueiredo, F.C.; Geerling, G.; Labetoulle, M.; Lemp, M.; Rolando, M.; et al. Clinical impact of inflammation in dry eye disease: Proceedings of the ODISSEY group meeting. *Acta Ophthalmol.* **2018**, *96*, 111–119. [CrossRef]
16. Bron, A.J.; de Paiva, C.S.; Chauhan, S.K.; Bonini, S.; Gabison, E.E.; Jain, S.; Knop, E.; Markoulli, M.; Ogawa, Y.; Perez, V.; et al. TFOS DEWS II pathophysiology report. *Ocul. Surf.* **2017**, *15*, 438–510. [CrossRef]
17. van Setten, G.B. Osmokinetics: A new dynamic concept in dry eye disease. *J. Fr. Ophtalmol.* **2019**, *42*, 221–225. [CrossRef]
18. Craig, J.P.; Nelson, J.D.; Azar, D.T.; Belmonte, C.; Bron, A.J.; Chauhan, S.K.; de Paiva, C.S.; Gomes, J.A.P.; Hammitt, K.M.; Jones, L.; et al. TFOS DEWS II Report Executive Summary. *Ocul. Surf.* **2017**, *15*, 802–812. [CrossRef]
19. van Setten, G.B. Osmokinetics: Defining the Characteristics of Osmotic Challenge to the Ocular Surface. *Klin. Mon. Augenheilkd.* **2020**, *237*, 644–648. [CrossRef]
20. Belmonte, C. Pain, Dryness, and Itch Sensations in Eye Surface Disorders Are Defined By a Balance Between Inflammation and Sensory Nerve Injury. *Cornea* **2019**, *38* (Suppl. 1), S11–S24. [CrossRef]
21. Shaheen, B.S.; Bakir, M.; Jain, S. Corneal nerves in health and disease. *Surv. Ophthalmol.* **2014**, *59*, 263–285. [CrossRef] [PubMed]
22. Al-Aqaba, M.A.; Dhillon, V.K.; Mohammed, I.; Said, D.G.; Dua, H.S. Corneal nerves in health and disease. *Prog. Retin. Eye Res.* **2019**, *73*, 100762. [CrossRef] [PubMed]
23. Schein, O.D.; Tielsch, J.M.; Munoz, B.; Bandeen-Roche, K.; West, S. Relation between signs and symptoms of dry eye in the elderly. A population-based perspective. *Ophthalmology* **1997**, *104*, 1395–1401. [CrossRef]
24. Nichols, K.K.; Nichols, J.J.; Mitchell, G.L. The lack of association between signs and symptoms in patients with dry eye disease. *Cornea* **2004**, *23*, 762–770. [CrossRef] [PubMed]
25. Ong, E.S.; Felix, E.R.; Levitt, R.C.; Feuer, W.J.; Sarantopoulos, C.D.; Galor, A. Epidemiology of discordance between symptoms and signs of dry eye. *Br. J. Ophthalmol.* **2018**, *102*, 674–679. [CrossRef] [PubMed]
26. Bartlett, J.D.; Keith, M.S.; Sudharshan, L.; Snedecor, S.J. Associations between signs and symptoms of dry eye disease: A systematic review. *Clin. Ophthalmol.* **2015**, *9*, 1719–1730. [CrossRef]
27. Galor, A.; Moein, H.R.; Lee, C.; Rodriguez, A.; Felix, E.R.; Sarantopoulos, K.D.; Levitt, R.C. Neuropathic pain and dry eye. *Ocul. Surf.* **2018**, *16*, 31–44. [CrossRef]

28. Dua, H.S.; Said, D.G.; Messmer, E.M.; Rolando, M.; Benitez-Del-Castillo, J.M.; Hossain, P.N.; Shortt, A.J.; Geerling, G.; Nubile, M.; Figueiredo, F.C.; et al. Neurotrophic keratopathy. *Prog. Retin. Eye Res.* **2018**, *66*, 107–131. [CrossRef]
29. Galor, A.; Batawi, H.; Felix, E.R.; Margolis, T.P.; Sarantopoulos, K.D.; Martin, E.R.; Levitt, R.C. Incomplete response to artificial tears is associated with features of neuropathic ocular pain. *Br. J. Ophthalmol.* **2016**, *100*, 745–749. [CrossRef]
30. Galor, A. Painful Dry Eye Symptoms: A Nerve Problem or a Tear Problem? *Ophthalmology* **2019**, *126*, 648–651. [CrossRef]
31. Jiang, D.; Liang, J.; Noble, P.W. Hyaluronan as an immune regulator in human diseases. *Physiol. Rev.* **2011**, *91*, 221–264. [CrossRef]
32. Tavianatou, A.G.; Caon, I.; Franchi, M.; Piperigkou, Z.; Galesso, D.; Karamanos, N.K. Hyaluronan: Molecular size-dependent signaling and biological functions in inflammation and cancer. *FEBS J.* **2019**, *286*, 2883–2908. [CrossRef]
33. Gomis, A.; Pawlak, M.; Balazs, E.A.; Schmidt, R.F.; Belmonte, C. Effects of different molecular weight elastoviscous hyaluronan solutions on articular nociceptive afferents. *Arthritis Rheum.* **2004**, *50*, 314–326. [CrossRef] [PubMed]
34. Caires, R.; Luis, E.; Taberner, F.J.; Fernandez-Ballester, G.; Ferrer-Montiel, A.; Balazs, E.A.; Gomis, A.; Belmonte, C.; de la Pena, E. Hyaluronan modulates TRPV1 channel opening, reducing peripheral nociceptor activity and pain. *Nat. Commun.* **2015**, *6*, 8095. [CrossRef] [PubMed]
35. Ferrari, L.F.; Khomula, E.V.; Araldi, D.; Levine, J.D. CD44 Signaling Mediates High Molecular Weight Hyaluronan-Induced Antihyperalgesia. *J. Neurosci.* **2018**, *38*, 308–321. [CrossRef]
36. Müller-Lierheim, W.G.K. Why Chain Length of Hyaluronan in Eye Drops Matters. *Diagnostics* **2020**, *10*, 511. [CrossRef]
37. Kojima, T.; Nagata, T.; Kudo, H.; Müller-Lierheim, W.G.K.; van Setten, G.-B.; Dogru, M.; Tsubota, K. The Effects of High Molecular Weight Hyaluronic Acid Eye Drop Application in Environmental Dry Eye Stress Mice. *Int. J. Mol. Sci.* **2020**, *21*, 3516. [CrossRef] [PubMed]
38. Karpecki, P.M. Why dry eye trials often fail: From disease variability to confounding underlying conditions, there are countless reasons why new dry eye drugs have come up short in FDA testing. *Rev. Optom.* **2013**, *2013*, 50.
39. Baudouin, C.; Aragona, P.; Van Setten, G.; Rolando, M.; Irkec, M.; Benitez del Castillo, J.; Geerling, G.; Labetoulle, M.; Bonini, S.; Members, O.E.C.G. Diagnosing the severity of dry eye: A clear and practical algorithm. *Br. J. Ophthalmol.* **2014**, *98*, 1168–1176. [CrossRef]
40. Schiffman, R.M.; Christianson, M.D.; Jacobsen, G.; Hirsch, J.D.; Reis, B.L. Reliability and validity of the Ocular Surface Disease Index. *Arch. Ophthalmol.* **2000**, *118*, 615–621. [CrossRef]
41. Bron, A.J.; Evans, V.E.; Smith, J.A. Grading of corneal and conjunctival staining in the context of other dry eye tests. *Cornea* **2003**, *22*, 640–650. [CrossRef]
42. Wolffsohn, J.S.; Arita, R.; Chalmers, R.; Djalilian, A.; Dogru, M.; Dumbleton, K.; Gupta, P.K.; Karpecki, P.; Lazreg, S.; Pult, H.; et al. TFOS DEWS II Diagnostic Methodology report. *Ocul. Surf.* **2017**, *15*, 539–574. [CrossRef]
43. Fuller, D.G.; Potts, K.; Kim, J. Noninvasive tear breakup times and ocular surface disease. *Optom. Vis. Sci. Off. Publ. Am. Acad. Optom.* **2013**, *90*, 1086–1091. [CrossRef]
44. Johnson, M.E.; Murphy, P.J. The Effect of instilled fluorescein solution volume on the values and repeatability of TBUT measurements. *Cornea* **2005**, *24*, 811–817. [CrossRef]
45. Murube, J. The Schirmer test: Celebration of its first centenary. *Ocul. Surf.* **2003**, *1*, 157–159. [CrossRef]
46. Han, S.B.; Liu, Y.C.; Mohamed-Noriega, K.; Tong, L.; Mehta, J.S. Objective Imaging Diagnostics for Dry Eye Disease. *J. Ophthalmol.* **2020**, *2020*, 3509064. [CrossRef]
47. Methodologies to diagnose and monitor dry eye disease: Report of the Diagnostic Methodology Subcommittee of the International Dry Eye WorkShop (2007). *Ocul. Surf.* **2007**, *5*, 108–152. [CrossRef]
48. Hamrah, P.; Alipour, F.; Jiang, S.; Sohn, J.H.; Foulks, G.N. Optimizing evaluation of Lissamine Green parameters for ocular surface staining. *Eye* **2011**, *25*, 1429–1434. [CrossRef]
49. Korb, D.R.; Herman, J.P.; Blackie, C.A.; Scaffidi, R.C.; Greiner, J.V.; Exford, J.M.; Finnemore, V.M. Prevalence of lid wiper epitheliopathy in subjects with dry eye signs and symptoms. *Cornea* **2010**, *29*, 377–383. [CrossRef]

50. Yamaguchi, M.; Kutsuna, M.; Uno, T.; Zheng, X.; Kodama, T.; Ohashi, Y. Marx line: Fluorescein staining line on the inner lid as indicator of meibomian gland function. *Am. J. Ophthalmol.* **2006**, *141*, 669–675. [CrossRef] [PubMed]
51. Kowtharapu, B.S.; Winter, K.; Marfurt, C.; Allgeier, S.; Kohler, B.; Hovakimyan, M.; Stahnke, T.; Wree, A.; Stachs, O.; Guthoff, R.F. Comparative quantitative assessment of the human corneal sub-basal nerve plexus by in vivo confocal microscopy and histological staining. *Eye* **2017**, *31*, 481–490. [CrossRef] [PubMed]
52. van Setten, G.; Labetoulle, M.; Baudouin, C.; Rolando, M. Evidence of seasonality and effects of psychrometry in dry eye disease. *Acta Ophthalmol.* **2016**, *94*, 499–506. [CrossRef] [PubMed]
53. Armitage, P.; Berry, G.; Matthews, J.N.S. *Statistical Methods in Medical Research*, 4th ed.; Wiley-Blackwell: Hoboken, NJ, USA, 2001.
54. Farrand, K.F.; Fridman, M.; Stillman, I.O.; Schaumberg, D.A. Prevalence of Diagnosed Dry Eye Disease in the United States Among Adults Aged 18 Years and Older. *Am. J. Ophthalmol.* **2017**, *182*, 90–98. [CrossRef]
55. Novack, G.D.; Asbell, P.; Barabino, S.; Bergamini, M.V.W.; Ciolino, J.B.; Foulks, G.N.; Goldstein, M.; Lemp, M.A.; Schrader, S.; Woods, C.; et al. TFOS DEWS II Clinical Trial Design Report. *Ocul. Surf.* **2017**, *15*, 629–649. [CrossRef] [PubMed]
56. Begley, C.; Caffery, B.; Chalmers, R.; Situ, P.; Simpson, T.; Nelson, J.D. Review and analysis of grading scales for ocular surface staining. *Ocul. Surf.* **2019**, *17*, 208–220. [CrossRef]
57. Kim, Y.H.; Graham, A.D.; Li, W.; Radke, C.J.; Lin, M.C. Human Lacrimal Production Rate and Wetted Length of Modified Schirmer's Tear Test Strips. *Transl. Vis. Sci. Technol.* **2019**, *8*, 40. [CrossRef]
58. Harper, C.L.; Boulton, M.E.; Bennett, D.; Marcyniuk, B.; Jarvis-Evans, J.H.; Tullo, A.B.; Ridgway, A.E. Diurnal variations in human corneal thickness. *Br. J. Ophthalmol.* **1996**, *80*, 1068–1072. [CrossRef]
59. Niimi, J.; Tan, B.; Chang, J.; Zhou, Y.; Ghanekar, A.; Wong, M.; Lee, A.; Lin, M.C. Diurnal Pattern of Tear Osmolarity and Its Relationship to Corneal Thickness and Deswelling. *Cornea* **2013**, *32*, 1305–1310. [CrossRef]
60. Ayaki, M.; Tachi, N.; Hashimoto, Y.; Kawashima, M.; Tsubota, K.; Negishi, K. Diurnal variation of human tear meniscus volume measured with tear strip meniscometry self-examination. *PLoS ONE* **2019**, *14*, e0215922. [CrossRef]
61. Shen, M.; Wang, J.; Tao, A.; Chen, Q.; Lin, S.; Qu, J.; Lu, F. Diurnal variation of upper and lower tear menisci. *Am. J. Ophthalmol.* **2008**, *145*, 801–806. [CrossRef]
62. Nichols, K.K.; Mitchell, G.L.; Zadnik, K. The repeatability of clinical measurements of dry eye. *Cornea* **2004**, *23*, 272–285. [CrossRef] [PubMed]
63. Holland, E.J.; Darvish, M.; Nichols, K.K.; Jones, L.; Karpecki, P.M. Efficacy of topical ophthalmic drugs in the treatment of dry eye disease: A systematic literature review. *Ocul. Surf.* **2019**, *17*, 412–423. [CrossRef] [PubMed]
64. Tashbayev, B.; Utheim, T.P.; Utheim, O.A.; Raeder, S.; Jensen, J.L.; Yazdani, M.; Lagali, N.; Vitelli, V.; Dartt, D.A.; Chen, X. Utility of Tear Osmolarity Measurement in Diagnosis of Dry Eye Disease. *Sci. Rep.* **2020**, *10*, 5542. [CrossRef] [PubMed]
65. Goto, E.; Yagi, Y.; Matsumoto, Y.; Tsubota, K. Impaired functional visual acuity of dry eye patients. *Am. J. Ophthalmol.* **2002**, *133*, 181–186. [CrossRef]
66. Kaido, M.; Dogru, M.; Ishida, R.; Tsubota, K. Concept of functional visual acuity and its applications. *Cornea* **2007**, *26* (Suppl. 1), S29–S35. [CrossRef] [PubMed]
67. Kaido, M. Functional Visual Acuity. *Investig. Ophthalmol. Vis. Sci.* **2018**, *59*, DES29–DES35. [CrossRef] [PubMed]

Publisher's Note: MDPI stays neutral with regard to jurisdictional claims in published maps and institutional affiliations.

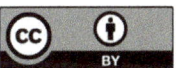 © 2020 by the authors. Licensee MDPI, Basel, Switzerland. This article is an open access article distributed under the terms and conditions of the Creative Commons Attribution (CC BY) license (http://creativecommons.org/licenses/by/4.0/).

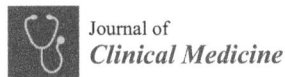

Article

High Molecular Weight Hyaluronan Promotes Corneal Nerve Growth in Severe Dry Eyes

Gysbert-Botho van Setten [1,†], Oliver Stachs [2,†], Bénédicte Dupas [3], Semra Akkaya Turhan [4], Berthold Seitz [5], Herbert Reitsamer [6], Karsten Winter [7], Jutta Horwath-Winter [8], Rudolf F. Guthoff [2] and Wolfgang G. K. Müller-Lierheim [9,*]

1. Department of Clininical Neuroscience, St. Eriks Eye Hospital, Karolinska Institutet, 11282 Stockholm, Sweden; gysbert.van.setten@ki.se
2. Department of Ophthalmology, University Medical Center Rostock, 18057 Rostock, Germany; oliver.stachs@uni-rostock.de (O.S.); rudolf.guthoff@med.uni-rostock.de (R.F.G.)
3. Quinze-Vingts National Eye Hospital & Vision Institute, 75571 Paris, France; bdupas@15-20.fr
4. Department of Ophthalmology, Marmara University School of Medicine, 34899 Istanbul, Turkey; semraakkaya85@hotmail.com
5. Department of Ophthalmology, Saarland University Medical Center, 66421 Homburg/Saar, Germany; berthold.seitz@uks.eu
6. Department of Ophthalmology & Department of Experimental Ophthalmology and Glaucoma Research, University Clinic Salzburg, Paracelsus Medical University, 5020 Salzburg, Austria; h.reitsamer@salk.at
7. Institute of Anatomy, Medical Faculty, University of Leipzig, 04103 Leipzig, Germany; kwinter@rz.uni-leipzig.de
8. Department of Ophthalmology, Medical University Graz, 8036 Graz, Austria; jutta.horwath@medunigraz.at
9. CORONIS GmbH, 81241 Munich, Germany
* Correspondence: ml@coronis.net
† Contributed equally.

Received: 5 October 2020; Accepted: 22 November 2020; Published: 24 November 2020

Abstract: The purpose of this study was to investigate the effect of high molecular weight hyaluronan (HMWHA) eye drops on subbasal corneal nerves in patients suffering from severe dry eye disease (DED) and to evaluate the damage of subbasal corneal nerves associated with severe DED. Designed as an international, multicenter study, 16 patients with symptoms of at least an Ocular Surface Disease Index (OSDI) score of 33, and corneal fluorescein staining (CFS) of at least Oxford grade 3, were included and randomized into two study arms. The control group continued to use their individual optimum artificial tears over the study period of eight weeks; in the verum group, the artificial tears were substituted by eye drops containing 0.15% HMWHA. At the baseline visit, and after eight weeks, the subbasal nerve plexus of 16 patients were assessed by confocal laser scanning microscopy (CSLM). The images were submitted to a masked reading center for evaluation. Results showed a significant increase of total nerve fiber lengths (CNFL) in the HMWHA group ($p = 0.030$) when compared to the control group, where the total subbasal CNFL did not significantly change from baseline to week 8. We concluded that in severe DED patients, HMWHA from topically applied eye drops could cross the epithelial barrier and reach the subbasal nerve plexus, where it exercised a trophic effect.

Keywords: dry eye disease; severe keratitis; diabetes; neuropathic keratopathy; neuropathy; nerve growth; neurotrophic

1. Introduction

Millions of people worldwide are affected by dry eye disease (DED), a heterogeneous, complex disorder of the ocular surface [1]. Within the current concept of a staged treatment, lubricating, hydrating teardrops are the standard long-term therapy for DED [2]. Hyaluronan (HA) eye drops, aiming to increase tear viscosity and enhancing lubrication, are one of the options favored, particularly in Europe and Asia [2]. The combination of concentration and chain length of the HA molecules contained in these eye drops determines their viscoelastic and mucoadhesive properties, resulting in more or less entanglement and rheological synergism with the mucins dissolved in the muco-aqueous layer of the tear film. These physical properties of HA eye drops contribute to minimizing the friction between the moving eyelid and the surface of the eyeball during blinking, thus reducing known stimuli of ocular surface inflammation [3]. High molecular weight hyaluronan (HMWHA) has an anti-inflammatory effect, whereas low molecular weight hyaluronan (LMWHA) promotes inflammation [4,5]. A recent study confirmed in an environmental dry eye stress model in mice that HMWHA eye drops protect the ocular surface from mechanical damage and inflammation better than LMWHA [6]. Future clinical investigations of HMWHA eye drops in humans suffering from chronic ocular surface inflammation should, therefore, include inflammation markers.

The current treatment for severe DED is mainly based on the model of the self-maintaining circle of chronic inflammation [7–10]. The underlying pathomechanism of severe dry eye disease focuses on inflammation in various situations such as in autoimmune diseases, as well as damage of corneal nerves, for example, in diabetes mellitus or aging [11]. The cornea is by far the most densely innervated tissue of the human body [12]. Nerves provide important trophic support to the corneal epithelium and contribute to ocular surface homeostasis [12–16]. Activated corneal nerves release neuropeptides that contribute to neurogenic inflammation [17–19]. Denervation eliminates the neurotrophic support causing neuroparalytic keratitis and breakdown of the corneal epithelium [17,20]. On the other hand, trophic interactions are essential for neuronal survival [21–23]. Moreover, there is cross-talk between glia, the extracellular matrix, and neurons [24]. Attrition within the ocular epithelia has been recognized as a lubrication deficit induced factor, enhancing inflammation [25]. Due to these complex interactions, severe DED is regularly associated with compromised corneal nerves [26–30]. This, in turn, results in dysregulation of tear production and blink reflex [31]. Corneal innervation disorders as a primary pathogenic mechanism are due to the absence of ocular pain only diagnosed in a late-stage, although they are often accompanied by keratopathy and delayed epithelial wound healing, sometimes leading to corneal ulcerations and vision loss [32–34]. There is a lack of treatments targeting nerve regeneration [34,35].

Patients suffering from neuropathic ocular pain tend to respond poorly to the treatment with lubricant eye drops [36,37]. Experimental evidence suggests that HMWHA, but not LMWHA, can suppress pain in nociceptive afferent nerves [38–40], but it is not yet proven whether or not topically applied HMWHA can reduce ocular pain. Moreover, the possible role of hyaluronan in the proliferation of nerve cells has raised attention [24,41,42]. Therefore, we decided to study the potential influence of HMWHA on the corneal nerves within the HYLAN M study. The main intention of the HYLAN M study was to investigate if symptoms and/or signs of patients suffering from severe DED could be improved by substituting the best treatment lubricant eye drops with HMWHA eye drops. In vivo confocal microscopy (IVCM), in particular, when performed as confocal laser scanning microscopy (CSLM), is the gold standard in assessing the subbasal corneal nerve plexus [43–46]. Within the HYLAN M study, CSLM images were taken at baseline and after eight weeks of treatment and were sent to a masked reading center for evaluation.

2. Experimental Section

2.1. Study Design

The HYLAN M study, a multicenter prospective randomized, open-label study, was performed in 11 centers in eight countries. Details have been published elsewhere [47]. The study adhered to the Declaration of Helsinki, was approved by ethics committees of all countries involved, and registered on the database of the European Database for Medical Devices (EUDAMED) under the registration number CIV-16-06-015964.

Patients suffering from severe DED were randomized into two parallel arms. The control group continued with their currently-used therapy by the time of inclusion. In the verum group (Comfort Shield group), the individual lubricant eye drops used by each patient by the time of inclusion were replaced by eye drops containing 0.15% HMWHA (Comfort Shield® eye drops, i.com medical GmbH, Munich, Germany). Concomitant treatment for dry eye, like cyclosporine eye drops, remained unchanged in both arms.

Demographic data and medical history were recorded during the baseline visits. Symptoms and signs associated with DED were assessed at the baseline visit, at week 4, and week 8 follow-up visits, respectively (see Table 1).

Table 1. Diagnostic testing schedule with optional tests in round brackets.

Test	Baseline	Week 4	Week 8
OSDI	X	X	X
Dropping frequency	X	X	X
BCVA	X	X	X
CFS	X	X	X
TBUT	X	X	X
Schirmer 1	X		X
Tear osmolarity	X		X
IOP	X		X
LWE, Korb score [48]	(X)		(X)
Yamaguchi score [49]	(X)		(X)
Confocal microscopy	(X)		(X)

Abbreviations: Ocular Surface Disease Index (OSDI), best corrected visual acuity (BCVA), corneal fluorescein staining (CFS), tear film break-up time (TBUT), intraocular pressure (IOP), and lid wiper epitheliopathy (LWE).

The study centers were suggested to optionally take CSLM images at the baseline and week eight visits and provide them to a masked reading center for assessment. Four out of 11 study centers participated in this optional test. These four study centers provided CSLM images of all their per-protocol patients; thus, the electronic randomization used throughout the HYLAN M study also applied to the optional confocal microscopy study. The results of the assessment of the CSLM images of these four study centers are the subject of this report. The results of the other diagnostic tests performed, such as the Ocular Surface Disease Index (OSDI), dropping frequency, best corrected visual acuity (BCVA), corneal fluorescein staining (CFS), tear film break-up time (TBUT), Schirmer 1, tear osmolarity, intraocular pressure (IOP), lid wiper epitheliopathy (LWE), and Yamaguchi score of all 84 per-protocol patients included in the HYLAN M study have been previously reported [47].

2.2. Participants

Patients over 18 years suffering from DED of any underlying etiology were eligible for inclusion. The patients had to be under stable, unchanged, dry eye therapy for at least two months (in case of concomitant cyclosporine therapy, three months) by the time of inclusion. Patients were excluded if they participated in any other clinical trial, suffered from eye diseases other than dry eyes, had ocular surgery less than three months prior to study inclusion, were using punctual plugs, or had masquerading conditions as identified by Karpecki [50]. Masquerading conditions are conjunctivochalasis, recurrent corneal erosions, epithelial basement membrane dystrophy, mucus fishing syndrome, floppy eyelid syndrome, giant papillary conjunctivitis, Salzmann's nodular degeneration, and ocular rosacea.

As inclusion criteria for severe dry eye, the primary criteria, according to Baudouin et al., were chosen [51]. The dry eye symptoms were assessed using the Ocular Surface Disease Index (OSDI) questionnaire, with an OSDI score of 33 or more being required for inclusion [52]. Corneal fluorescein staining (CFS) was selected as a dry eye sign [53]. For inclusion, patients had to have at least one eye with CFS Oxford grade 3 or more, but no confluent CFS. The eyes with the higher staining score were defined as study eyes.

2.3. Confocal Scanning Laser Microscopy

The Heidelberg Retina Tomograph (HRT 3), in combination with the Rostock Cornea Module (Heidelberg Engineering GmbH, Heidelberg, Germany), was used for the in vivo assessment of the corneal subbasal nerve plexus (SNP), as described previously [54,55]. Both eyes were anesthetized with topical anesthetic and covered with artificial tears. To prevent eye movements, the patients were asked to fixate on a spotlight with the unexamined eye.

Five non-overlapping images were taken in the central region of the cornea, close to the apex and more than 0.5 mm apart from the inferior whorl (see Figure 1A for an example of an image and Figure 1B after image processing by the reading center).

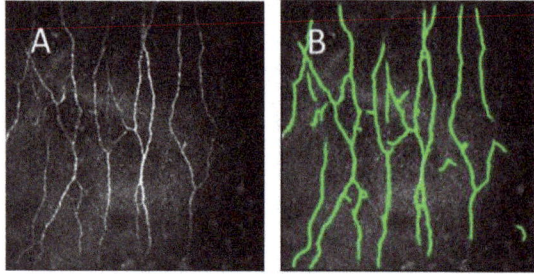

Figure 1. Single image from the subbasal nerve plexus (SNP) in an individual (**A**) and automatically detected nerve fibers used for quantification (**B**).

Image processing and quantitative image analysis were performed by the reading center using Mathematica (Version 11.3, Wolfram Research Inc., Champaign, IL, USA), as previously described [56]. The following SNP parameters were calculated: corneal nerve fiber length (CNFL), defined as the total length of all nerve fibers per unit area (mm/mm^2); corneal nerve fiber density (CNFD), defined as the number of nerve fibers per unit area (n/mm^2); corneal nerve branch density (CNBD), defined as the number of branching points per unit area (n/mm^2); average weighted corneal nerve fiber tortuosity (CNFTo), reflected variability of nerve fiber directions and defined as absolute nerve fiber curvature/nerve fiber length (μm^{-1}); corneal nerve connection points (CNCP), defined as the number of nerve fibers crossing the area boundary (connections/mm^2); average corneal nerve single-fiber length (CNSFL), defined as the average length of nerve fibers (μm); and average weighted corneal nerve fiber thickness (CNFTh), measured as mean thickness perpendicular to the nerve fiber course (μm).

2.4. Statistical Analysis

Statistical analysis was performed using IBM SPSS Statistics (Version 22, IBM Corp., Armonk, NY, USA). Descriptive statistics were calculated, and box plots were generated. Data were examined for normal distribution using the Shapiro–Wilk test. Group comparisons were performed using the Wilcoxon Signed Rank Test and the Mann–Whitney U test, respectively. The significance level was determined to be $p < 0.05$.

3. Results

3.1. Participant Demography

Table 2 contains the socio-demographic characteristics of the patients with the CSLM assessment of the SNP.

Table 2. Socio-demographic characteristics according to the treatment arm ($n = 16$).

		Comfort Shield $n = 8$	Control $n = 8$
Age (years)	n	8	8
	mean (SD)	59.5 (9.2)	61.6 (18.4)
	min, max	36, 77	47, 73
Sex n (%)	n	8	8
	female	6 (75)	6 (75)
	male	2 (25)	2 (25)
Medical History	n	8	8
	Sjögren syndrome	2	3
	rheumatoid disease	3	2
	rheumatoid + thyroid disease	1	
	thyroid disease		1
	Graves disease + betablocker	1	
	diabetes mellitus + betablocker		1
	no dry eye related disease	1	1

3.2. Confocal Microscopy Results

Five CSLM images of eight patients of the control group and eight patients of the Comfort Shield group taken at the end of the baseline visit and at the end of the week 8 visit were analyzed (see examples in Figure 2).

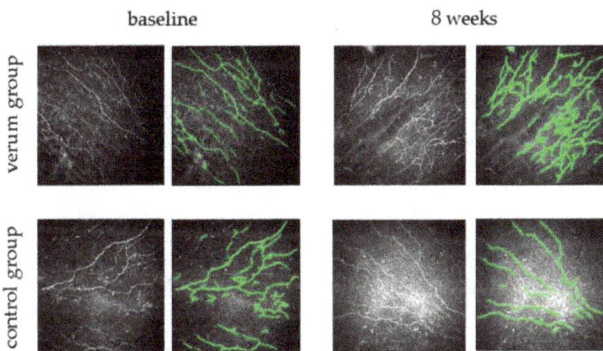

Figure 2. Typical SNP images of subjects from the control and study group, as well as a schematic representation of detected nerve fibers used for characterization of the SNP at baseline and after 8 weeks of treatment.

We found a statistically significant difference in CNFL between baseline and the eight weeks follow-up visit; the Comfort Shield group showed a significant difference in CNFL ($p = 0.030$) contrary to the control group ($p = 0.294$). CNFL was comparable for Comfort Shield and control at baseline ($p = 0.793$) and showed a significant difference after eight weeks ($p = 0.031$). Possibly due to the small number of patients, we did not find significant differences for the other SNP parameters (CNFD, CNBD, CNFTo, CNCP, CNSFL, CNFTh). Moreover, patients suffering from severe dry eye generally do not have a well-developed SNP, and there was a lot of foreign tissue in the vicinity of the SNP that complicated the image analysis. Figure 3 summarized the CNFL findings of the Comfort Shield group and the control group at baseline and eight weeks visit.

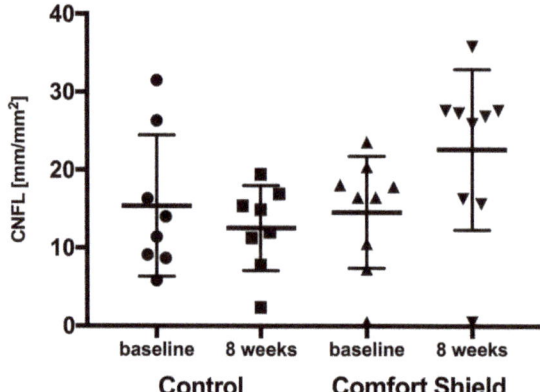

Figure 3. CNFL of the Comfort Shield group and the control group at baseline and eight weeks.

4. Discussion

Due to the heterogeneous, multicausal nature of DED, particularly in patients suffering from severe, chronic DED, a personalized clinical management resulting in an individualized optimum therapy is required [57]. Only patients under stable therapy had been included in the HYLAN M study, and their optimum individual therapy served as a control in comparison to patients in which 0.15% HMWHA eye drops were tested. The assessment of the subbasal corneal nerve plexus was an optional test in addition to the standard diagnostic test battery of the study. Four out of 11 study centers provided CSLM images from 16 per-protocol patients, eight each in the Comfort Shield group and in the control group. The SNP is usually not well structured in severe dry eye disease [58]. Due to the small number of patients, only the results of CNFL showed a significant difference between the two study arms. This is in accordance with other studies reporting that CNFL is the most reproducible parameter in the evaluation of IVCM images of the subbasal nerve plexus [28,59–65].

Until recently, HA eye drops had been applied as a lubricating, hydrating, and mechanically buffering tear substitute [66]. It was known that the apical surface of the superficial epithelial cells of the cornea and conjunctiva have HA receptors (CD44 and HARE), which can bind HA and thus support the antiadhesive properties of the glycocalyx [67–71]. HMWHA, but not LMWHA, can also adhere to the membrane-bound mucins of the glycocalyx, thus strengthening the cellular barrier of the ocular surface [72]. HA is an essential part of the extracellular matrix (ECM) and plays an important molecular weight dependent role in wound healing and immunoregulation [4,73–78]. Disturbed immunoregulation involving chronic inflammation, which triggers a vicious circle, is currently considered the characteristics of severe DED [10]. HMWHA enables cross-bridging between the HA receptors of adjacent cells and can thus contribute to the mechanical stabilization of the wing cell layers of the corneal epithelium [79–81]. Reactive oxygen species (ROS) formed during inflammatory processes effectively cleave HMWHA, which in turn enhances the inflammatory process and weakens the cross-bridging function of HA between epithelial cells [82]. So far, it had been unknown whether HMWHA from topically applied eye drops can, in a situation of chronic ocular inflammation, pass the ocular surface barrier to recover the homeostatic HA weight distribution in the extracellular matrix. The first evidence came from an animal experiment where 0.15% HMWHA eye drops were compared with 0.1% and 0.3% LMWHA eye drops with respect to their ability to prevent and treat DED caused by environmental stress [6]. The 0.15% HMWHA eye drops proved superiority with respect to the prevention and treatment of inflammation and stabilization of aqueous tear secretion and mucin production [6].

The HYLAN M study indicated that topically applied HMWHA could pass the intercellular barrier of the corneal epithelium. By changing the extracellular matrix in the proximity of the subbasal nerve plexus, this could result in trophic effects reflected in the significant regeneration of compromised nerves. This also provided evidence that HMWHA becomes available in the ECM in all cell layers of the corneal epithelium and thus can contribute to regaining ocular surface homeostasis in eyes with chronic inflammation. Further methods detecting specific anti-inflammatory and neurotrophic factors such as nerve growth factor (NGF) in the tear film or in the ocular surface will provide valuable additional information in future clinical studies. On the other hand, the study showed that within eight weeks of treatment, simultaneously with nerve growth, the symptoms of patients with severe DED improved significantly. According to the results of the HYLAN M study, in combination with the animal study [6], we may conclude that 0.15% HMWHA eye drops grant a holistic approach in the treatment of DED, simultaneously addressing the various and complex interacting pathomechanisms of the disease: lubrication, hydration, stabilization of glycocalyx and barrier function, downregulation of inflammation, trophic support to corneal nerves, increasing goblet cell counts and expression of MUC5AC [83], support of aqueous tear production, and reduction of pain.

It needs to be emphasized that the effect of HMWHA on nerve regeneration has only been investigated in a very small number of eyes. Hence, conclusions on significance in numbers cannot be given. Nevertheless, the high incidence of nerve regeneration during treatment with HMWHA was clearly different from the unchanged situation in the control group. Future studies with a higher number of eyes and a primary focus on nerve regeneration will provide further details.

As the HYLAN M study included dry eye patients with any disease etiology, it seems likely that patients with corneal nerve injury or degeneration as an underlying cause for ocular surface disease or neurotrophic keratopathy would benefit from treatment with HMWHA eye drops [11,84]. The causes may include acute nerve injury like in ocular surgery, refractive surgery, corneal cross-linking, chemical burns, or ocular trauma [85,86]. Similarly, HMWHA eye drops may also be effective in promoting neuroregeneration in progressing peripheral neuropathies associated with ocular infections, keratoconus, small-fiber neuropathy, diabetes mellitus, or simply aging [87–90].

The progressive loss of corneal sensory innervation of any etiology may result in neurotrophic keratopathy (NK) [15,16,35,91–94]. NK is characterized by corneal anesthesia and is a condition that is very difficult to treat, especially as for the required regeneration of trigeminal terminal nerve fibers, no such treatment is currently available [35,93,95]. Medical management with lubricating eye drops, anti-inflammatory agents, and anti-proteases provide unspecific temporary relief in NK but do not prevent disease progression [93,96]. Whereas some degree of inflammation promotes nerve regeneration, excessive inflammation may lead to a loss of corneal innervation and subsequent development of NK [15]. As corneal nerve regeneration and inflammation are intertwined, the therapeutic strategy must consider the interaction of both pathways [15]. HMWHA eye drops seem to offer a promising treatment option in this situation.

According to the International Diabetes Federation (IDF), more than 400 million people worldwide suffer from diabetes mellitus (DM). DM is associated with a progressive loss of peripheral nerves. Corneal nerve damage may serve as an early indicator in DM [63,97–99]. The prevalence of corneal neuropathy in diabetic patients is approximately 50% [32,100–103]. However, corneal neuropathy, as a manifestation of DM, is underrated due to the absence of ocular discomfort and pain [33,98,103,104]. Persistent corneal epithelial erosions, superficial punctate keratopathy, delayed epithelial regeneration, and decreased sensitivity are associated with diabetic keratopathy [32,34,105,106]. Diabetic keratopathy is a significant clinical problem and a progressing disease, and currently, no effective treatment is available [34]. IVCM has proven to be a valuable and reliable diagnostic tool to assess nerve fiber damage and assess improvement of risk factors for diabetic neuropathy, thus allowing visualizing treatment success [59,107,108]. Having shown that 0.15% HMWHA eye drops support corneal nerve regeneration allows the assumption that these eye drops will also prove as an effective preventive therapy against the progression of diabetic keratopathy. This may contribute to lower the enormous global economic burden of DM [109]. The results reported here were obtained from a small number of patients. This report is, therefore, intended to encourage further clinical research rather than to provide comprehensive answers or interpretation.

5. Conclusions

This is the first evidence that topically applied HMWHA eye drops induced a significant neurotrophic effect on the subbasal nerve plexus in humans. When applied after any kind of ocular surgery, HMWHA eye drops may serve to support the recovery of damaged nerves. Moreover, HMWHA eye drops offered a new therapeutic option in preventing and treating ocular surface disease, in particular diseases associated with nerve damage like diabetic keratopathy and all forms of neuropathic keratopathy. Future research will focus on the question if patients with diabetic keratopathy and other forms of neuropathic keratopathy could benefit from HMWHA eye drops. HMWHA eye drops provide a holistic approach while simultaneously addressing different interacting pathomechanisms of DED.

Author Contributions: B.D., S.A.T., B.S., and H.R. were the investigators taking IVCM images of their patients within the HYLAN M study; R.F.G. provided advice during the design of the HYLAN M study investigation plan and in the interpretation of the results of IVCM; O.S. provided the precise work instruction for IVCM and served as masked reading center for the IVCM images; K.W. performed the digital assessment of the images; G.-B.v.S. served as the coordinating investigator of the HYLAN M study; W.G.K.M.-L. had an overall responsibility for the HYLAN M study design, organization, regulatory compliance, monitoring, and study report; O.S., K.W., G.-B.v.S., J.H.-W., and W.G.K.M.-L. prepared the manuscript of this publication. All authors have read and agreed to the published version of the manuscript.

Funding: The HYLAN M study received unrestricted funding from i.com medical GmbH, Munich, Germany.

Conflicts of Interest: The study director Wolfgang G.K. Müller-Lierheim is also the CEO of the company i.com medical GmbH, Munich, Germany. The remaining authors declare no conflict of interest.

References

1. Stapleton, F.; Alves, M.; Bunya, V.Y.; Jalbert, I.; Lekhanont, K.; Malet, F.; Na, K.S.; Schaumberg, D.; Uchino, M.; Vehof, J.; et al. TFOS DEWS II Epidemiology Report. *Ocul. Surf.* **2017**, *15*, 334–365. [CrossRef]
2. Jones, L.; Downie, L.E.; Korb, D.; Benitez-Del-Castillo, J.M.; Dana, R.; Deng, S.X.; Dong, P.N.; Geerling, G.; Hida, R.Y.; Liu, Y.; et al. TFOS DEWS II Management and Therapy Report. *Ocul. Surf.* **2017**, *15*, 575–628. [CrossRef] [PubMed]
3. Müller-Lierheim, W.G.K. Why Chain Length of Hyaluronan in Eye Drops Matters. *Diagnostics* **2020**, *10*, 511. [CrossRef] [PubMed]
4. Jiang, D.; Liang, J.; Noble, P.W. Hyaluronan as an immune regulator in human diseases. *Physiol. Rev.* **2011**, *91*, 221–264. [CrossRef] [PubMed]
5. Tavianatou, A.G.; Caon, I.; Franchi, M.; Piperigkou, Z.; Galesso, D.; Karamanos, N.K. Hyaluronan: Molecular size-dependent signaling and biological functions in inflammation and cancer. *FEBS J.* **2019**, *286*, 2883–2908. [CrossRef] [PubMed]
6. Kojima, T.; Nagata, T.; Kudo, H.; Müller-Lierheim, W.G.K.; van Setten, G.-B.; Dogru, M.; Tsubota, K. The Effects of High Molecular Weight Hyaluronic Acid Eye Drop Application in Environmental Dry Eye Stress Mice. *Int. J. Mol. Sci.* **2020**, *21*, 3516. [CrossRef] [PubMed]
7. Stern, M.E.; Pflugfelder, S.C. Inflammation in dry eye. *Ocul. Surf.* **2004**, *2*, 124–130. [CrossRef]
8. Baudouin, C. A new approach for better comprehension of diseases of the ocular surface. *J. Fr. Ophtalmol.* **2007**, *30*, 239–246. [CrossRef]
9. Bron, A.J.; de Paiva, C.S.; Chauhan, S.K.; Bonini, S.; Gabison, E.E.; Jain, S.; Knop, E.; Markoulli, M.; Ogawa, Y.; Perez, V.; et al. TFOS DEWS II pathophysiology report. *Ocul. Surf.* **2017**, *15*, 438–510. [CrossRef]
10. Baudouin, C.; Irkec, M.; Messmer, E.M.; Benitez-Del-Castillo, J.M.; Bonini, S.; Figueiredo, F.C.; Geerling, G.; Labetoulle, M.; Lemp, M.; Rolando, M.; et al. Clinical impact of inflammation in dry eye disease: Proceedings of the ODISSEY group meeting. *Acta Ophthalmol.* **2018**, *96*, 111–119. [CrossRef]
11. Belmonte, C. Pain, Dryness, and Itch Sensations in Eye Surface Disorders Are Defined By a Balance Between Inflammation and Sensory Nerve Injury. *Cornea* **2019**, *38* (Suppl. 1), S11–S24. [CrossRef] [PubMed]

12. Muller, L.J.; Marfurt, C.F.; Kruse, F.; Tervo, T.M. Corneal nerves: Structure, contents and function. *Exp. Eye Res.* **2003**, *76*, 521–542. [CrossRef]
13. Garcia-Hirschfeld, J.; Lopez-Briones, L.G.; Belmonte, C. Neurotrophic influences on corneal epithelial cells. *Exp. Eye Res.* **1994**, *59*, 597–605. [CrossRef] [PubMed]
14. Korsching, S. The neurotrophic factor concept: A reexamination. *J. Neurosci.* **1993**, *13*, 2739–2748. [CrossRef]
15. Shaheen, B.S.; Bakir, M.; Jain, S. Corneal nerves in health and disease. *Surv. Ophthalmol.* **2014**, *59*, 263–285. [CrossRef]
16. Al-Aqaba, M.A.; Dhillon, V.K.; Mohammed, I.; Said, D.G.; Dua, H.S. Corneal nerves in health and disease. *Prog. Retin. Eye Res.* **2019**, *73*, 100762. [CrossRef]
17. Belmonte, C.; Acosta, M.C.; Gallar, J. Neural basis of sensation in intact and injured corneas. *Exp. Eye Res.* **2004**, *78*, 513–525. [CrossRef]
18. Ordovas-Montanes, J.; Rakoff-Nahoum, S.; Huang, S.; Riol-Blanco, L.; Barreiro, O.; von Andrian, U.H. The Regulation of Immunological Processes by Peripheral Neurons in Homeostasis and Disease. *Trends Immunol.* **2015**, *36*, 578–604. [CrossRef]
19. Dastjerdi, M.H.; Dana, R. Corneal nerve alterations in dry eye-associated ocular surface disease. *Int. Ophthalmol. Clin.* **2009**, *49*, 11–20. [CrossRef]
20. Ueno, H.; Ferrari, G.; Hattori, T.; Saban, D.R.; Katikireddy, K.R.; Chauhan, S.K.; Dana, R. Dependence of corneal stem/progenitor cells on ocular surface innervation. *Investig. Ophthalmol. Vis. Sci.* **2012**, *53*, 867–872. [CrossRef]
21. Purves, D. The trophic theory of neural concentrations. *Trends Neurosci.* **1986**, *9*, 486–489. [CrossRef]
22. Di, G.; Qi, X.; Zhao, X.; Zhang, S.; Danielson, P.; Zhou, Q. Corneal Epithelium-Derived Neurotrophic Factors Promote Nerve Regeneration. *Investig. Ophthalmol. Vis. Sci.* **2017**, *58*, 4695–4702. [CrossRef] [PubMed]
23. Sacchetti, M.; Lambiase, A. Neurotrophic factors and corneal nerve regeneration. *Neural Regen Res.* **2017**, *12*, 1220–1224. [PubMed]
24. Song, I.; Dityatev, A. Crosstalk between glia, extracellular matrix and neurons. *Brain Res. Bull.* **2018**, *136*, 101–108. [CrossRef] [PubMed]
25. van Setten, G.-B. Impact of Attrition, Intercellular Shear in Dry Eye Disease: When Cells are Challenged and Neurons are Triggered. *Int. J. Mol. Sci.* **2020**, *21*, 4333. [CrossRef]
26. del Castillo, J.M.B.; Wasfy, M.A.S.; Fernandez, C.; Garcia-Sanchez, J. An In Vivo Confocal Masked Study on Corneal Epithelium and Subbasal Nerves in Patients with Dry Eye. *Investig. Ophthalmol. Vis. Sci.* **2004**, *45*, 3030–3035. [CrossRef]
27. Villani, E.; Galimberti, D.; Viola, F.; Mapelli, C.; Ratiglia, R. The cornea in Sjogren's syndrome: An in vivo confocal study. *Investig. Ophthalmol. Vis. Sci.* **2007**, *48*, 2017–2022. [CrossRef]
28. Labbe, A.; Alalwani, H.; Van Went, C.; Brasnu, E.; Georgescu, D.; Baudouin, C. The relationship between subbasal nerve morphology and corneal sensation in ocular surface disease. *Investig. Ophthalmol. Vis. Sci.* **2012**, *53*, 4926–4931. [CrossRef]
29. Tepelus, T.C.; Chiu, G.B.; Huang, J.; Huang, P.; Sadda, S.R.; Irvine, J.; Lee, O.L. Correlation between corneal innervation and inflammation evaluated with confocal microscopy and symptomatology in patients with dry eye syndromes: A preliminary study. *Graefe's Arch. Clin. Exp. Ophthalmol. Albrecht Von Graefes Arch. Fur Klin. Und Exp. Ophthalmol.* **2017**, *255*, 1771–1778. [CrossRef]
30. Matsumoto, Y.; Ibrahim, O.M.A.; Kojima, T.; Dogru, M.; Shimazaki, J.; Tsubota, K. Corneal In Vivo Laser-Scanning Confocal Microscopy Findings in Dry Eye Patients with Sjogren's Syndrome. *Diagnostics (Basel)* **2020**, *10*, 497. [CrossRef]
31. Belmonte, C.; Nichols, J.J.; Cox, S.M.; Brock, J.A.; Begley, C.G.; Bereiter, D.A.; Dartt, D.A.; Galor, A.; Hamrah, P.; Ivanusic, J.J.; et al. TFOS DEWS II pain and sensation report. *Ocul. Surf.* **2017**, *15*, 404–437. [CrossRef] [PubMed]
32. Ljubimov, A.V. Diabetic complications in the cornea. *Vis. Res.* **2017**, *139*, 138–152. [CrossRef] [PubMed]
33. Kopf, S.; Groener, J.B.; Kender, Z.; Fleming, T.; Bischoff, S.; Jende, J.; Schumann, C.; Ries, S.; Bendszus, M.; Schuh-Hofer, S.; et al. Deep phenotyping neuropathy: An underestimated complication in patients with pre-diabetes and type 2 diabetes associated with albuminuria. *Diabetes Res. Clin. Pract.* **2018**, *146*, 191–201. [CrossRef] [PubMed]
34. Priyadarsini, S.; Whelchel, A.; Nicholas, S.; Sharif, R.; Riaz, K.; Karamichos, D. Diabetic keratopathy: Insights and challenges. *Surv. Ophthalmol.* **2020**, *65*, 513–529. [CrossRef] [PubMed]

35. Mastropasqua, L.; Massaro-Giordano, G.; Nubile, M.; Sacchetti, M. Understanding the Pathogenesis of Neurotrophic Keratitis: The Role of Corneal Nerves. *J. Cell. Physiol.* **2017**, *232*, 717–724. [CrossRef]
36. Galor, A.; Batawi, H.; Felix, E.R.; Margolis, T.P.; Sarantopoulos, K.D.; Martin, E.R.; Levitt, R.C. Incomplete response to artificial tears is associated with features of neuropathic ocular pain. *Br. J. Ophthalmol.* **2016**, *100*, 745–749. [CrossRef]
37. Galor, A.; Moein, H.R.; Lee, C.; Rodriguez, A.; Felix, E.R.; Sarantopoulos, K.D.; Levitt, R.C. Neuropathic pain and dry eye. *Ocul. Surf.* **2018**, *16*, 31–44. [CrossRef]
38. Gomis, A.; Pawlak, M.; Balazs, E.A.; Schmidt, R.F.; Belmonte, C. Effects of different molecular weight elastoviscous hyaluronan solutions on articular nociceptive afferents. *Arthritis Rheum.* **2004**, *50*, 314–326. [CrossRef]
39. Caires, R.; Luis, E.; Taberner, F.J.; Fernandez-Ballester, G.; Ferrer-Montiel, A.; Balazs, E.A.; Gomis, A.; Belmonte, C.; de la Pena, E. Hyaluronan modulates TRPV1 channel opening, reducing peripheral nociceptor activity and pain. *Nat. Commun.* **2015**, *6*, 8095. [CrossRef]
40. Ferrari, L.F.; Khomula, E.V.; Araldi, D.; Levine, J.D. CD44 Signaling Mediates High Molecular Weight Hyaluronan-Induced Antihyperalgesia. *J. Neurosci.* **2018**, *38*, 308–321. [CrossRef]
41. Casini, P.; Nardi, I.; Ori, M. RHAMM mRNA expression in proliferating and migrating cells of the developing central nervous system. *Gene Expr. Patterns* **2010**, *10*, 93–97. [CrossRef] [PubMed]
42. Preston, M.; Sherman, L.S. Neural stem cell niches: Roles for the hyaluronan-based extracellular matrix. *Front. Biosci.* **2011**, *3*, 1165–1179. [CrossRef] [PubMed]
43. Guthoff, R.F.; Zhivov, A.; Stachs, O. In vivo confocal microscopy, an inner vision of the cornea—A major review. *Clin. Exp. Ophthalmol.* **2009**, *37*, 100–117. [CrossRef] [PubMed]
44. Kheirkhah, A.; Dohlman, T.H.; Amparo, F.; Arnoldner, M.A.; Jamali, A.; Hamrah, P.; Dana, R. Effects of corneal nerve density on the response to treatment in dry eye disease. *Ophthalmology* **2015**, *122*, 662–668. [CrossRef]
45. Cruzat, A.; Qazi, Y.; Hamrah, P. In Vivo Confocal Microscopy of Corneal Nerves in Health and Disease. *Ocul. Surf.* **2017**, *15*, 15–47. [CrossRef]
46. Kowtharapu, B.S.; Stachs, O. Corneal Cells: Fine-tuning Nerve Regeneration. *Curr. Eye Res.* **2020**, *45*, 291–302. [CrossRef]
47. van Setten, G.B.; Baudouin, C.; Horwath-Winter, J.; Bohringer, D.; Stachs, O.; Toker, E.; Al-Zaaidi, S.; Benitez-Del-Castillo, J.M.; Beck, R.; Al-Sheikh, O.; et al. The HYLAN M Study: Efficacy of 0.15% High Molecular Weight Hyaluronan Fluid in the Treatment of Severe Dry Eye Disease in a Multicenter Randomized Trial. *J. Clin. Med.* **2020**, *9*, 3536. [CrossRef]
48. Korb, D.R.; Herman, J.P.; Blackie, C.A.; Scaffidi, R.C.; Greiner, J.V.; Exford, J.M.; Finnemore, V.M. Prevalence of lid wiper epitheliopathy in subjects with dry eye signs and symptoms. *Cornea* **2010**, *29*, 377–383. [CrossRef]
49. Yamaguchi, M.; Kutsuna, M.; Uno, T.; Zheng, X.; Kodama, T.; Ohashi, Y. Marx line: Fluorescein staining line on the inner lid as indicator of meibomian gland function. *Am. J. Ophthalmol.* **2006**, *141*, 669–675. [CrossRef]
50. Karpecki, P.M. Why dry eye trials often fail: From disease variability to confounding underlying conditions, there are countless reasons why new dry eye drugs have come up short in FDA testing. *Rev. Optom.* **2013**, *150*, 50–56.
51. Baudouin, C.; Aragona, P.; Van Setten, G.; Rolando, M.; Irkec, M.; Benitez del Castillo, J.; Geerling, G.; Labetoulle, M.; Bonini, S.; ODISSEY European Consensus Group Members. Diagnosing the severity of dry eye: A clear and practical algorithm. *Br. J. Ophthalmol.* **2014**, *98*, 1168–1176. [CrossRef] [PubMed]
52. Schiffman, R.M.; Christianson, M.D.; Jacobsen, G.; Hirsch, J.D.; Reis, B.L. Reliability and validity of the Ocular Surface Disease Index. *Arch. Ophthalmol.* **2000**, *118*, 615–621. [CrossRef] [PubMed]
53. Bron, A.J.; Evans, V.E.; Smith, J.A. Grading of corneal and conjunctival staining in the context of other dry eye tests. *Cornea* **2003**, *22*, 640–650. [CrossRef] [PubMed]
54. Ziegler, D.; Papanas, N.; Zhivov, A.; Allgeier, S.; Winter, K.; Ziegler, I.; Bruggemann, J.; Strom, A.; Peschel, S.; Kohler, B.; et al. Early detection of nerve fiber loss by corneal confocal microscopy and skin biopsy in recently diagnosed type 2 diabetes. *Diabetes* **2014**, *63*, 2454–2463. [CrossRef]
55. Stachs, O.; Guthoff, R.F.; Aumann, S. In Vivo Confocal Scanning Laser Microscopy. In *High Resolution Imaging in Microscopy and Ophthalmology: New Frontiers in Biomedical Optics*; Bille, J.F., Ed.; Springer: Cham, Switzerland, 2019; pp. 263–284.

56. Winter, K.; Scheibe, P.; Kohler, B.; Allgeier, S.; Guthoff, R.F.; Stachs, O. Local Variability of Parameters for Characterization of the Corneal Subbasal Nerve Plexus. *Curr. Eye Res.* **2016**, *41*, 186–198. [CrossRef]
57. Aragona, P.; Giannaccare, G.; Mencucci, R.; Rubino, P.; Cantera, E.; Rolando, M. Modern approach to the treatment of dry eye, a complex multifactorial disease: A P.I.C.A.S.S.O. board review. *Br. J. Ophthalmol.* **2020**. [CrossRef]
58. Giannaccare, G.; Pellegrini, M.; Bernabei, F.; Moscardelli, F.; Buzzi, M.; Versura, P.; Campos, E.C. In Vivo Confocal Microscopy Automated Morphometric Analysis of Corneal Subbasal Nerve Plexus in Patients With Dry Eye Treated With Different Sources of Homologous Serum Eye Drops. *Cornea* **2019**, *38*, 1412–1417. [CrossRef]
59. Malik, R.A.; Kallinikos, P.; Abbott, C.A.; van Schie, C.H.; Morgan, P.; Efron, N.; Boulton, A.J. Corneal confocal microscopy: A non-invasive surrogate of nerve fibre damage and repair in diabetic patients. *Diabetologia* **2003**, *46*, 683–688. [CrossRef]
60. Mocan, M.C.; Durukan, I.; Irkec, M.; Orhan, M. Morphologic alterations of both the stromal and subbasal nerves in the corneas of patients with diabetes. *Cornea* **2006**, *25*, 769–773. [CrossRef]
61. Hertz, P.; Bril, V.; Orszag, A.; Ahmed, A.; Ng, E.; Nwe, P.; Ngo, M.; Perkins, B.A. Reproducibility of in vivo corneal confocal microscopy as a novel screening test for early diabetic sensorimotor polyneuropathy. *Diabet Med.* **2011**, *28*, 1253–1260. [CrossRef]
62. Stem, M.S.; Hussain, M.; Lentz, S.I.; Raval, N.; Gardner, T.W.; Pop-Busui, R.; Shtein, R.M. Differential reduction in corneal nerve fiber length in patients with type 1 or type 2 diabetes mellitus. *J. Diabetes Complicat.* **2014**, *28*, 658–661. [CrossRef] [PubMed]
63. Srinivasan, S.; Dehghani, C.; Pritchard, N.; Edwards, K.; Russell, A.W.; Malik, R.A.; Efron, N. Corneal and Retinal Neuronal Degeneration in Early Stages of Diabetic Retinopathy. *Investig. Ophthalmol. Vis. Sci.* **2017**, *58*, 6365–6373. [CrossRef] [PubMed]
64. Lagali, N.S.; Allgeier, S.; Guimaraes, P.; Badian, R.A.; Ruggeri, A.; Kohler, B.; Utheim, T.P.; Peebo, B.; Peterson, M.; Dahlin, L.B.; et al. Reduced Corneal Nerve Fiber Density in Type 2 Diabetes by Wide-Area Mosaic Analysis. *Investig. Ophthalmol. Vis. Sci.* **2017**, *58*, 6318–6327. [CrossRef]
65. Kalteniece, A.; Ferdousi, M.; Petropoulos, I.; Azmi, S.; Adam, S.; Fadavi, H.; Marshall, A.; Boulton, A.J.M.; Efron, N.; Faber, C.G.; et al. Greater corneal nerve loss at the inferior whorl is related to the presence of diabetic neuropathy and painful diabetic neuropathy. *Sci. Rep.* **2018**, *8*, 3283. [CrossRef] [PubMed]
66. Laurent, T.C.; Laurent, U.B.; Fraser, J.R. The structure and function of hyaluronan: An overview. *Immunol. Cell Biol.* **1996**, *74*, A1–A7. [CrossRef] [PubMed]
67. Asari, A.; Miyauchi, S.; Takahashi, T.; Kohno, K.; Uchiyama, Y. Localization of hyaluronic acid, chondroitin sulfate, and CD44 in rabbit cornea. *Arch. Histol. Cytol.* **1992**, *55*, 503–511. [CrossRef] [PubMed]
68. Lerner, L.E.; Schwartz, D.M.; Hwang, D.G.; Howes, E.L.; Stern, R. Hyaluronan and CD44 in the human cornea and limbal conjunctiva. *Exp. Eye Res.* **1998**, *67*, 481–484. [CrossRef]
69. Zhu, S.N.; Nolle, B.; Duncker, G. Expression of adhesion molecule CD44 on human corneas. *Br. J. Ophthalmol.* **1997**, *81*, 80–84. [CrossRef]
70. Falkowski, M.; Schledzewski, K.; Hansen, B.; Goerdt, S. Expression of stabilin-2, a novel fasciclin-like hyaluronan receptor protein, in murine sinusoidal endothelia, avascular tissues, and at solid/liquid interfaces. *Histochem. Cell Biol.* **2003**, *120*, 361–369. [CrossRef]
71. Harris, E.N.; Baker, E. Role of the Hyaluronan Receptor, Stabilin-2/HARE, in Health and Disease. *Int. J. Mol. Sci.* **2020**, *21*, 3504. [CrossRef]
72. Hansen, I.M.; Ebbesen, M.F.; Kaspersen, L.; Thomsen, T.; Bienk, K.; Cai, Y.; Malle, B.M.; Howard, K.A. Hyaluronic Acid Molecular Weight-Dependent Modulation of Mucin Nanostructure for Potential Mucosal Therapeutic Applications. *Mol. Pharm.* **2017**, *14*, 2359–2367. [CrossRef] [PubMed]
73. Delmage, J.M.; Powars, D.R.; Jaynes, P.K.; Allerton, S.E. The selective suppression of immunogenicity by hyaluronic acid. *Ann. Clin. Lab. Sci.* **1986**, *16*, 303–310. [PubMed]
74. Jiang, D.; Liang, J.; Noble, P.W. Hyaluronan in tissue injury and repair. *Annu. Rev. Cell Dev. Biol.* **2007**, *23*, 435–461. [CrossRef] [PubMed]
75. Petrey, A.C.; de la Motte, C.A. Hyaluronan, a crucial regulator of inflammation. *Front. Immunol.* **2014**, *5*, 101. [CrossRef]
76. Aya, K.L.; Stern, R. Hyaluronan in wound healing: Rediscovering a major player. *Wound Repair Regen. Off. Publ. Wound Health Soc. Eur. Tissue Repair Soc.* **2014**, *22*, 579–593. [CrossRef]

77. Litwiniuk, M.; Krejner, A.; Speyrer, M.S.; Gauto, A.R.; Grzela, T. Hyaluronic Acid in Inflammation and Tissue Regeneration. *Wounds A Compend. Clin. Res. Pract.* **2016**, *28*, 78–88.
78. Ruppert, S.M.; Hawn, T.R.; Arrigoni, A.; Wight, T.N.; Bollyky, P.L. Tissue integrity signals communicated by high-molecular weight hyaluronan and the resolution of inflammation. *Immunol Res.* **2014**, *58*, 186–192. [CrossRef]
79. Toole, B.P. Hyaluronan and its binding proteins, the hyaladherins. *Curr. Opin. Cell Biol.* **1990**, *2*, 839–844. [CrossRef]
80. Knudson, C.B.; Knudson, W. Hyaluronan-binding proteins in development, tissue homeostasis, and disease. *FASEB J.* **1993**, *7*, 1233–1241. [CrossRef]
81. Evanko, S.P.; Tammi, M.I.; Tammi, R.H.; Wight, T.N. Hyaluronan-Dependent Pericellular Matrix. *Adv. Drug Deliv. Rev.* **2007**, *59*, 1351–1365. [CrossRef]
82. Agren, U.M.; Tammi, R.H.; Tammi, M.I. Reactive oxygen species contribute to epidermal hyaluronan catabolism in human skin organ culture. *Free Radic. Biol. Med.* **1997**, *23*, 996–1001. [CrossRef]
83. Di, G.; Qi, X.; Zhao, X.; Zhang, S.; Zhou, Q. Efficacy of Sodium Hyaluronate in Murine Diabetic Ocular Surface Diseases. *Cornea* **2017**, *36*, 1133–1138. [CrossRef]
84. Semeraro, F.; Forbice, E.; Romano, V.; Angi, M.; Romano, M.R.; Filippelli, M.E.; Di Iorio, R.; Costagliola, C. Neurotrophic keratitis. *Ophthalmologica* **2014**, *231*, 191–197. [CrossRef]
85. Ambrósio, R., Jr.; Tervo, T.; Wilson, S.E. LASIK-associated dry eye and neurotrophic epitheliopathy: Pathophysiology and strategies for prevention and treatment. *J. Refract. Surg.* **2008**, *24*, 396–407. [CrossRef]
86. Sarkar, J.; Milani, B.; Kim, E.; An, S.; Kwon, J.; Jain, S. Corneal nerve healing after in situ laser nerve transection. *PLoS ONE* **2019**, *14*, e0218879. [CrossRef] [PubMed]
87. Karacorlu, M.A.; Cakiner, T.; Saylan, T. Corneal sensitivity and correlations between decreased sensitivity and anterior segment pathology in ocular leprosy. *Br. J. Ophthalmol.* **1991**, *75*, 117–119. [CrossRef] [PubMed]
88. Niederer, R.L.; Perumal, D.; Sherwin, T.; McGhee, C.N. Laser scanning in vivo confocal microscopy reveals reduced innervation and reduction in cell density in all layers of the keratoconic cornea. *Investig. Ophthalmol. Vis. Sci.* **2008**, *49*, 2964–2970. [CrossRef]
89. Peters, M.J.; Bakkers, M.; Merkies, I.S.; Hoeijmakers, J.G.; van Raak, E.P.; Faber, C.G. Incidence and prevalence of small-fiber neuropathy: A survey in the Netherlands. *Neurology* **2013**, *81*, 1356–1360. [CrossRef] [PubMed]
90. Erie, J.C.; McLaren, J.W.; Hodge, D.O.; Bourne, W.M. The effect of age on the corneal subbasal nerve plexus. *Cornea* **2005**, *24*, 705–709. [CrossRef] [PubMed]
91. Bonini, S.; Rama, P.; Olzi, D.; Lambiase, A. Neurotrophic keratitis. *Eye* **2003**, *17*, 989–995. [CrossRef] [PubMed]
92. Sacchetti, M.; Lambiase, A. Diagnosis and management of neurotrophic keratitis. *Clin. Ophthalmol.* **2014**, *8*, 571–579. [PubMed]
93. Dua, H.S.; Said, D.G.; Messmer, E.M.; Rolando, M.; Benitez-Del-Castillo, J.M.; Hossain, P.N.; Shortt, A.J.; Geerling, G.; Nubile, M.; Figueiredo, F.C.; et al. Neurotrophic keratopathy. *Prog. Retin. Eye Res.* **2018**, *66*, 107–131. [CrossRef] [PubMed]
94. Soifer, M.; Starr, C.E.; Mousa, H.M.; Savarain, C.; Perez, V.L. Neurotrophic Keratopathy: Current Perspectives. *Curr. Ophthalmol. Rep.* **2020**, *8*, 29–35. [CrossRef]
95. Nishida, T.; Yanai, R. Advances in treatment for neurotrophic keratopathy. *Curr. Opin. Ophthalmol.* **2009**, *20*, 276–281. [CrossRef]
96. Yanai, R.; Nishida, T.; Chikama, T.; Morishige, N.; Yamada, N.; Sonoda, K.H. Potential New Modes of Treatment of Neurotrophic Keratopathy. *Cornea* **2015**, *34* (Suppl. 11), S121–S127. [CrossRef]
97. Bitirgen, G.; Ozkagnici, A.; Malik, R.A.; Kerimoglu, H. Corneal nerve fibre damage precedes diabetic retinopathy in patients with type 2 diabetes mellitus. *Diabet Med.* **2014**, *31*, 431–438. [CrossRef]
98. Barsegian, A.; Lee, J.; Salifu, M.O.; McFarlane, S.I. Corneal Neuropathy: An Underrated Manifestation of Diabetes Mellitus. *J. Clin. Endocrinol. Diabetes* **2018**, *2*. [CrossRef]
99. Zhivov, A.; Winter, K.; Hovakimyan, M.; Peschel, S.; Harder, V.; Schober, H.C.; Kundt, G.; Baltrusch, S.; Guthoff, R.F.; Stachs, O. Imaging and quantification of subbasal nerve plexus in healthy volunteers and diabetic patients with or without retinopathy. *PLoS ONE* **2013**, *8*, e52787. [CrossRef]
100. Schultz, R.O.; Van Horn, D.L.; Peters, M.A.; Klewin, K.M.; Schutten, W.H. Diabetic keratopathy. *Trans. Am. Ophthalmol. Soc.* **1981**, *79*, 180–199.
101. Manaviat, M.R.; Rashidi, M.; Afkhami-Ardekani, M.; Shoja, M.R. Prevalence of dry eye syndrome and diabetic retinopathy in type 2 diabetic patients. *BMC Ophthalmol.* **2008**, *8*, 10. [CrossRef]

102. Burda, N.; Mema, V.; Md, E.M.; Selimi, B.; Zhugli, S.; Lenajni, B.; Bunjaku, I. Prevalence of dry eye syndrome at patients with diabetus melitus tip 2, one year retrospective study May 2011–June 2012. *J. Acute Dis.* **2012**, *1*, 110–114. [CrossRef]
103. Bikbova, G.; Oshitari, T.; Baba, T.; Bikbov, M.; Yamamoto, S. Diabetic corneal neuropathy: Clinical perspectives. *Clin. Ophthalmol.* **2018**, *12*, 981–987. [PubMed]
104. Achtsidis, V.; Eleftheriadou, I.; Kozanidou, E.; Voumvourakis, K.I.; Stamboulis, E.; Theodosiadis, P.G.; Tentolouris, N. Dry eye syndrome in subjects with diabetes and association with neuropathy. *Diabetes Care* **2014**, *37*, e210–e211. [CrossRef] [PubMed]
105. Shih, K.C.; Lam, K.S.; Tong, L. A systematic review on the impact of diabetes mellitus on the ocular surface. *Nutr. Diabetes* **2017**, *7*, e251. [CrossRef] [PubMed]
106. Misra, S.L.; Braatvedt, G.D.; Patel, D.V. Impact of diabetes mellitus on the ocular surface: A review. *Clin. Exp. Ophthalmol.* **2016**, *44*, 278–288. [CrossRef]
107. Tavakoli, M.; Kallinikos, P.; Iqbal, A.; Herbert, A.; Fadavi, H.; Efron, N.; Boulton, A.J.M.; Malik, R.A. Corneal confocal microscopy detects improvement in corneal nerve morphology with an improvement in risk factors for diabetic neuropathy. *Diabet Med.* **2011**, *28*, 1261–1267. [CrossRef]
108. Azmi, S.; Jeziorska, M.; Ferdousi, M.; Petropoulos, I.N.; Ponirakis, G.; Marshall, A.; Alam, U.; Asghar, O.; Atkinson, A.; Jones, W.; et al. Early nerve fibre regeneration in individuals with type 1 diabetes after simultaneous pancreas and kidney transplantation. *Diabetologia* **2019**, *62*, 1478–1487. [CrossRef]
109. Bommer, C.; Heesemann, E.; Sagalova, V.; Manne-Goehler, J.; Atun, R.; Barnighausen, T.; Vollmer, S. The global economic burden of diabetes in adults aged 20–79 years: A cost-of-illness study. *Lancet Diabetes Endocrinol* **2017**, *5*, 423–430. [CrossRef]

Publisher's Note: MDPI stays neutral with regard to jurisdictional claims in published maps and institutional affiliations.

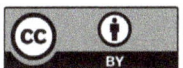

© 2020 by the authors. Licensee MDPI, Basel, Switzerland. This article is an open access article distributed under the terms and conditions of the Creative Commons Attribution (CC BY) license (http://creativecommons.org/licenses/by/4.0/).

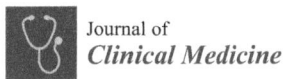

Article

Efficacy and Safety of *Houttuynia* Eye Drops Atomization Treatment for Meibomian Gland Dysfunction-Related Dry Eye Disease: A Randomized, Double-Blinded, Placebo-Controlled Clinical Trial

Zhaolin Liu [1,2,3], Ming Jin [4], Ying Li [5], Jun Liu [6], Xianghua Xiao [7], Hongsheng Bi [8], Zhiqiang Pan [9], Huijun Shi [10], Xiaofeng Xie [8], Minglian Zhang [10], Xuemin Gao [11], Lei Li [11], Weijie Ouyang [1,2,3], Liying Tang [1,2,3], Jieli Wu [1,2,3], Yiran Yang [1,2,3], Jiaoyue Hu [1,2,3] and Zuguo Liu [1,2,3],*

1. Department of Ophthalmology, Xiang'an Hospital of Xiamen University, Fujian Provincial Key Laboratory of Ophthalmology and Visual Science, Xiamen 361102, China; zhaolin@stu.xmu.edu.cn (Z.L.); 24520190154789@stu.xmu.edu.cn (W.O.); liyingtang@stu.xmu.edu.cn (L.T.); 24520180155744@stu.xmu.edu.cn (J.W.); yangyr1026@stu.xmu.edu.cn (Y.Y.); jiaoyuehu@xmu.edu.cn (J.H.)
2. Eye Institute of Xiamen University, School of Medicine, Xiamen University, Xiamen 361102, China
3. Department of Ocular Surface, Xiamen University Affiliated Xiamen Eye Center, Xiamen 361102, China
4. Department of Ophthalmology, China-Japan Friendship Hospital, Beijing100029, China; jinming57@163.com
5. Department of Ophthalmology, Peking Union Medical College Hospital, Beijing 100006, China; liyingpumch@126.com
6. Department of Ophthalmology, Shenzhen Eye Hospital, Shenzhen 518040, China; jiu28@126.com
7. Department of Ophthalmology, Xi'an First Hospital, Shaanxi Eye Research Institute, Shaanxi 710001, China; xianghuaxiao@yeah.net
8. Department of Ophthalmology, Shandong University of Traditional Chinese Medicine Affiliated Eye Hospital, Jinan 250004, China; hongshengbi@126.com (H.B.); yankeboshi@126.com (X.X.)
9. Department of Ophthalmology, Capital Medical University Affiliated Beijing Tongren Hospital, Beijing 100730, China; panyj0526@sina.com
10. Department of Ophthalmology, Hebei Eye Hospital, Xingtai 054001, China; 15631901079@163.com (H.S.); zhmlyk@sohu.com (M.Z.)
11. Technical Center for Drug Research and Evaluation of China Association of Traditional Chinese Medicine, Beijing 100061, China; xuemingao2011@163.com (X.G.); cptlilei@sina.com (L.L.)
* Correspondence: zuguoliu@xmu.edu.cn; Tel./Fax: +86-592-2183761

Received: 15 September 2020; Accepted: 8 December 2020; Published: 12 December 2020

Abstract: Purpose: To evaluate the efficacy and safety of *Houttuynia* eye drops (a Chinese traditional medicine) atomization treatment in meibomian gland dysfunction (MGD)-related dry eye disease (DED) patients. Methods: A total of 240 eligible patients diagnosed with MGD-related DED were assigned either *Houttuynia* eye drops or placebo for atomization once daily for four weeks in a multi-center, randomized, double-blind, placebo-controlled clinical study. Primary outcome evaluations used included eye symptom score (using the Chinese Dry Eye Questionnaire), meibum quality, and tear break-up time (TBUT), while safety evaluations included adverse events (AEs), visual acuity, and intraocular pressure monitoring. Indicators were measured at baseline as well as one week, two weeks, and four weeks after treatment. Results: Primary outcome measures of the *Houttuynia* group were improved compared with their placebo counterparts following four-week treatment. Eye symptom scores were significantly reduced relative to the baseline in the *Houttuynia* group (mean ± standard error of the mean, 9.00 ± 0.61) compared with the placebo group (6.29 ± 0.55; $p = 0.0018$). Reduction in meibum quality score in the *Houttuynia* group (0.91 ± 0.10) was also significantly higher compared with the placebo group (0.57 ± 0.10; $p = 0.0091$), while TBUT in the treatment group (6.30 ± 0.22) was also longer than in the latter (5.60 ± 0.24; $p = 0.0192$). No medication-related adverse events were observed. Conclusions: Atomization treatment with

Houttuynia eye drops is both clinically and statistically effective for the treatment of mild to moderate MGD-related DED patients. This approach is generally safe and was tolerated well by patients.

Keywords: *Houttuynia*; ultrasonic atomization; meibomian gland dysfunction; dry eye

1. Introduction

TFOS DEWS II [1] has defined dry eye is a multifactorial disease of the ocular surface characterized by a loss of homeostasis of the tear film and accompanied by ocular symptoms, in which tear film instability and hyperosmolarity, ocular surface inflammation and damage, and neurosensory abnormalities play etiological roles. The prevalence of dry eye disease (DED) is currently between 5% and 50% globally and particularly high in Asian countries [2–4]. The causes of DED are very complex, including age, systemic immune disease, visual display terminal, and meibomian gland dysfunction (MGD) [1]. MGD is one of the most common causes of DED overall and is also the main underlying factor leading to evaporative dry eye (EDE). Thus, DED caused by MGD is also known as MGD-related DED. Epidemiological investigations showed that 80% of DED patients have either developed this condition from MGD or are also suffering from this affliction [3]. Prevalence rates of MGD-related DED in Asian populations over the age of 40 range between 46.2% and 69.3% [4]. It is clear that MGD-related DED is characterized by terminal duct obstructions and/or qualitative/quantitative changes in glandular secretions; this latter effect reduces lipid secretion to tear film and increases evaporation, resulting in tear hyperosmolarity. These tear changes further induce inflammatory cascade reactions which then cause a series of clinical symptoms. Changes in tear fluid also aggravate destruction of the eyelid margin and meibomian gland, conditions which then go on to develop into a vicious cycle [5–7].

A variety of methods are utilized for the treatment of MGD-related DED, including physical therapies such as meibomian gland massage, intraductal meibomian gland probing, lipiflow, intense pulsed light, and local anti-inflammatory drugs. Although these approaches are all effective to a certain extent, problems remain including the inconvenience of application, high financial costs, insignificant effects, and some side effects [5,8]. It is therefore necessary to consider ways to explore new therapies that are safe, effective, and convenient in order to improve MGD-related DED treatment.

Traditional medicine has often been used for the clinical treatment of DED in China, and a great deal of documentation supports the fact that this approach achieves positive therapeutic effects [9]. Ultrasonic atomization is a method that destroys liquid surface tension and atomizes droplets into fine molecules via ultrasonic vibration. It is the most commonly utilized ophthalmological method in Chinese traditional medicine for DED treatment. This therapy for 20 min enables the drug to fully contact and penetrate the ocular surface and take effect. Stimulation of an atomized steam can promote blood and lymph circulation in eyelid tissue and thus enhance the discharge of meibomian gland secretions [10]. The majority of Chinese hospitals possess specialized ultrasonic atomization units and traditional medicine is the most commonly applied treatment. Although several studies have evaluated the therapeutic effects of ultrasonic nebulization for the treatment of MGD, DED, and MGD-related DED [10–12], clear clinical evidence is lacking from a standardized multicenter, double-blind, randomized, controlled clinical study.

The plant *Houttuynia cordata* is used in traditional Chinese medicine because it induces anti-inflammatory effects. This therapy mainly reduces the levels of inflammation-related cytokines and chemokines by inhibiting the Nuclear Factor Kappa-B (NF-κB)/Mitogen-Activated Protein Kinase (MAPK) pathway, leading to anti-inflammatory effects [13–15]. Thus, *Houttuynia* eye drops have been widely used across China for the treatment of DED. A number of non-double-blind, non-randomized, single-center small sample studies have shown that ultrasonic atomization using *Houttuynia* eye drops is both safe and effective for treating dry eye [16,17]. Therefore, building on this earlier work and in order to evaluate the specific therapeutic effects and safety of ultrasonic-atomized *Houttuynia* eye drops for the treatment of MGD-related DED, the China Association of Traditional Chinese Medicine (CATCM) organized the novel multi-center, randomized, double-blind, placebo-controlled trial reported in this study. So far, this is the first multicenter, randomized, double-blind, placebo-controlled study to evaluate the efficacy and safety of traditional Chinese medicine for the treatment of DED.

2. Methods

This randomized, double-blind, placebo-controlled, multi-center study was conducted at eight centers across China (Table S1) between 31 October 2018 and 29 January 2019. The design of this clinical trial complied with local laws and regulations and was developed in accordance with accepted standards for Good Clinical Practice of Pharmaceutical Products (2003) [18], Provisions of Drug Registration (2007) [19], and the Declaration of Helsinki. Data acquisition and analysis were performed in compliance with protocols approved by the Ethical Committee of Xiamen University and China-Japan Friendship Hospital (*ethical approval number 2018-97-K69*) and were prospectively registered on the Chinese Clinical Trial Registry www.chictr.org.cn (ChiCTR1800018611). All subjects signed informed consent forms prior to study initiation.

2.1. Study Patients

A total of 120 cases were included in the experimental *Houttuynia* group and the control placebo group, respectively, by applying the 1:1 design principle. Patients needed to meet the following inclusion criteria. First, subjects were required to be aged between 18 and 70 years and had to be diagnosed with MGD-related DED. Diagnostic criteria for MGD were according to the "Expert consensus of diagnosis and treatment of meibomian gland dysfunction in China (2017)" [20]. People who had eye symptoms, combined with abnormal eyelid margin and meibomian gland opening, or abnormal meibum secretion, were diagnosed as MGD. Second, diagnostic criteria for DED were according to the "Expert consensus on clinical diagnosis and treatment of dry eye (2013)" [21]. The following examination test criteria were required: 2 mm/5 min < Schirmer I test $\leq$ 10 mm/5 min, 0 s < TBUT $\leq$ 10 s, and corneal fluorescence staining point numbers < 10 points. That is, only patients with mild or moderate dry eye were included because severe dry eye generally needs to be combined with other treatments. Third, patients had to not use, or had to have stopped using, artificial tears for more than seven days. We chose just one eye from each subject for observations; if both eyes met the inclusion criteria, the more severely affected eye was used, while if the condition in both eyes was identical, the right one was used.

Patients were excluded if they had conditions including additional eye diseases such as macular degeneration, glaucoma, keratitis, and retinal vascular embolism, as well as lacrimal passage obstructions, prominent exophthalmos, and severe corneal decompensation. Patients were also excluded if they had undergone eye surgery less than half a year ago, if they had a history of wearing corneal contact lens up to one week prior to enrollment, or if they had suffered from other serious primary diseases including those of the cardiovascular, cerebrovascular, liver, kidney, or hematopoietic systems. Patients were excluded from this trial if they had an allergic constitution or were allergic to experimental drug ingredients. Exclusion also took place if patients had participated in other clinical trials within the last three months, or if individuals were unable to cooperate or were mentally ill.

2.2. Study Design

A double-blind design was used in this study. Thus, the 1:1 ratio between experimental treatment and control groups was used to generate random codes using the statistical software SAS9.4 (SAS Institute Inc., Cary, NC, USA), applying the block randomization method. Subjects were then assigned a medication box labeled with a serial number which contained all medications for the treatment duration. The experimental group used commercially available *Houttuynia* eye drops (specification: 8 mL; national drug approval no. Z20010110; Sichuan Shenghe Pharmaceutical Co. Ltd., China). The exact composition of Houttuynia eye drops was 2-undecanone ($C_{11}H_{22}O$) at the concentration of 9.8 µg/mL, and 2-undecanone was the main effective component of the Houttuynia cordata extract [14,15]. Meanwhile, the control group was treated with a placebo agent (Sichuan Shenghe Pharmaceutical Co. Ltd., Chengdu, China), and the placebo was a 0.72% (g/mL) sodium chloride solution with a pH value of 6.7 and osmotic pressure of 237 mOsmol/kg. Patients were also equipped with handheld ultrasonic nebulizers (product number: HL100A, Yuwell, Jiangsu, China) (Figure S1). The medication application method used in this study was atomizing each eye for 20 min per day with the ultrasonic nebulizer held in front of each eye. The atomizing tube was placed 5–10 cm away from the eye, and the patient kept their eyes wide open, staring in all directions intermittently to ensure that the atomizing agent fully touched the conjunctival sac. Patients used 20 mL houttuynia cordata eye drops or placebo at a time. The temperature of an ultrasonic-atomized aerosol is very close to room temperature, making the therapy induce slight irritation. The treatment course was four weeks with visit points at time zero (baseline) and then after one week, two weeks, and four weeks; treatment efficacy and safety assessments were carried out on-site during these visits. All tests were carried out using the same equipment type. The tester and the statistician were both unaware of patient groupings.

2.3. Outcome Measures

Primary outcomes evaluated included eye symptom score (using the Chinese Dry Eye Questionnaire, which is a dry eye questionnaire that conforms to the use habits of Chinese patients; the clinical diagnosis of dry eye in Chinese patients showed better diagnostic value than the OSDI questionnaire) [22] (Table S2), meibum quality, and tear break-up time (TBUT). Secondary outcomes evaluated included meibum expressibility, meibomian gland dropout, eyelid margin change, conjunctival congestion, corneal staining, and the Schirmer I test [23].

Sodium fluorescein TBUT was measured using a commercial fluorescein strip which was moistened and applied to the lower eyelid conjunctiva. One minute after application, patients were then asked to blink three times and to hold their eyes open. The time between the eyes open and the appearance of the first dark spot on the precorneal film was then measured using a slit lamp with cobalt blue illumination and a yellow-barrier filter. This was repeated three times before an average for each eye was recorded [21].

Meibomian gland functionality was assessed by applying digital pressure to the central (nasal, temporal) third of the lower/upper lids in order to determine MGD extent and severity (i.e., expressibility and meibum quality). Scoring values for meibum quality were as follows: 0, clear (normal); 1, cloudy; 2, cloudy with particles; and 3, inspissated (like toothpaste). Values were recorded for the highest grade encountered from any expressed glands, encompassing a range between 0 and 3. Similarly, meibum expressibility scoring criteria were as follows: 0, all glands expressed; 1, 3–4 glands expressed; 2, 1–2 glands expressed; and 3, no glands expressed. Meibum expressibility was scored based on five glands from the nasal side, while values for the middle and temporal sides of the lower eyelid were also recorded. Total scores for these three parts were recorded at the same time, across a range between 0 and 9 [23].

The eyelid margin change scoring criteria used follow standards set by the international MGD consensus group, while the presence or absence of lid abnormalities were scored via irregularity of the lid margin, lid margin vascular engorgement including plugging of the meibomian orifices, and anterior or retroplacement of the MCJ. These were either scored as present (1) or absent (0), across a range between 0 and 4 [23].

Meibomian gland dropout scoring criteria refer to the loss of acinar tissue detected by meibography. Non-contact meibography using a standard infrared video security camera was examined in patients. Scoring values for meibomian gland dropout were as follows: 0, no gland dropout; 1, between 1% and 33%; 2, between 34% and 66%; and 3, ≥67% dropout. The percentage of partial, or total, gland dropout of the lower lid was recorded across a range between 0 and 3 [23].

The MGD staging was determined according to the score of meibum quality, eyelid margin change, meibomian gland expressibility (middle meibomian gland expression score), and dropout. The higher these index scores were, the more serious the MGD was [20].

The conjunctival congestion scoring criteria used here follow the classification outlined by the Cornea and Contact Lens Research Unit, as follows: 0, no hyperemia; 1, mild hyperemia; 2, moderate hyperemia; and 3, severe hyperemia [24].

The corneal staining scoring criteria involved fluorescein staining that was examined two minutes subsequent to the instillation of sodium fluorescein at the slit lamp using cobalt blue illumination and a yellow-barrier filter. The 12-points method was used to assess the staining degree. Each of the four quadrants of the cornea on a scale ranged between 0 and 3: 0, no staining; 1, between one and 30 dots stained; 2, >30 dots stained without fusion; and 3, corneal diffuse or coalescent punctate staining, corneal filaments, and an ulcer. Scores for the four quadrants were then summed to attain a total score for each eye across a range between 0 and 12 [21].

The Schirmer I test was performed on unanesthetized patients by placing a strip in each eye and recording the wetted length (mm) after five minutes [21].

Eye tolerance, irritant symptoms, and treatment satisfaction values were also incorporated in this analysis.

The safety evaluations included adverse events (AEs), routine eye examinations (including monitoring of uncorrected/corrected visual acuity and intraocular pressure (IOP)), vital signs, and laboratory indicators (including blood and urine routine, liver and kidney function) which were selected according to the requirements of each hospital and the condition of subjects. Artificial tears, anti-inflammatory eye drops, and physical therapies such as eyelid cleaning, the use of hot compresses, meibomian gland massages, acupuncture, and silicone eye masks were prohibited. The comorbidity of patients and the use of any drug or treatment for the comorbidity was recorded, including the drug name (or other treatment), dosage, number, and time of use. If a prohibited drug or treatment was used, the subjects were required to discontinue the study.

2.4. Statistical Methods

A descriptive quantitative statistical analysis was performed encompassing the number of cases, mean, standard error of the mean (SEM), and 95% confidence intervals (CIs). A group *t*-test or a Wilcoxon rank-sum test was then used to make comparisons between groups and covariance analysis was also performed. In the case of qualitative data, a descriptive statistical analysis was carried out on the number of cases in various categories and their percentages. Thus, the chi-squared test alongside the Fisher exact test was used to compare enumerated data between the different treatment groups, while a Wilcoxon rank-sum test was used for comparison amongst treatment groups. A CMH-χ^2 test was used when the center or other factors were considered, while the relationship between a reduction in eye symptom score after four weeks of treatment and baseline scores was analyzed using Spearman's correlation coefficient. The reduction in eyelid margin change score vs. the baseline was also examined using Spearman's correlation coefficient, following the intention-to-treat principle (ITT). The latest observation data were carried forward to the final test result in each case to determine missing values for the main efficacy evaluation index (the last observation carried forward (LOCF) method). The post hoc subgroups were defined according to baseline severity of symptoms (eye symptoms score ≥15 vs. <15) and severity of signs (meibum quality score 0–3, middle meibomian gland expression score 0–3, eyelid margin change score 0–4, conjunctival congestion score 0–2, corneal staining score 0, 1, >1). Tests of interaction were used to evaluate whether the effect of atomization treatment with Houttuynia eye drops and placebo differed among subgroups. The software packages SAS9.4 (SAS Institute Inc., Cary, NC, USA) and GraphPad Prism version 8.2.1 (GraphPad Software, San Diego, CA, USA) were used for all statistical calculations. All tests were two-sided, and $p < 0.05$ was considered significant.

3. Results

A total of 240 selected patients were randomized for double-blind treatment. Two patients in the Houttuynia group did not take medication, thus 120 and 118 patients in the placebo and Houttuynia groups, respectively, were analyzed. A total of 113 and 103 patients completed all study visits, respectively; this means that seven and 13 patients dropped out from each group for various reasons (Figure 1). The data in Table S3 demonstrate patient clinical characteristics at baseline. These data show no significant differences in demographic characteristics between the placebo and Houttuynia groups, comprising about 75% of women with an average age of about 38 years. Results also show no statistical differences in the data at baseline between the two groups in terms of ocular symptoms as well as in signs of MGD and DED.

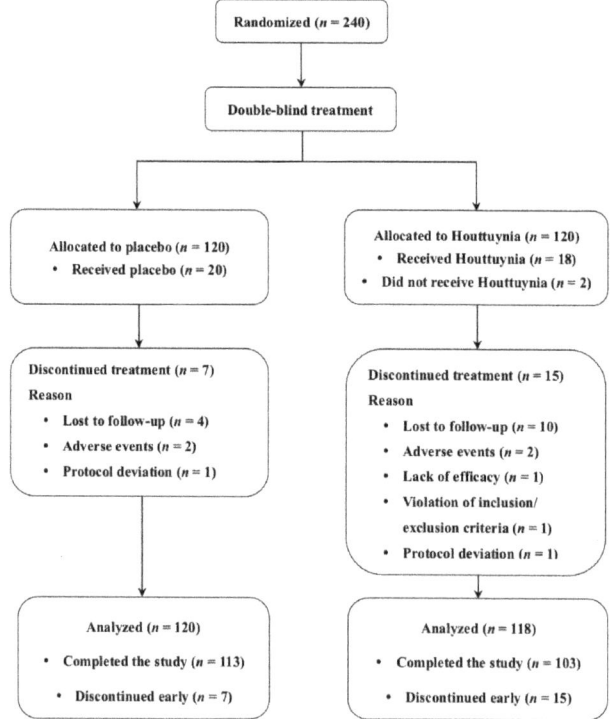

Figure 1. Subject flow chart.

3.1. Efficacy Evaluation

3.1.1. Primary Outcomes

Total and individual ocular symptom scores gradually decreased in both the groups in the following three visits (Figure 2A). There was a statistically significant difference between the two groups in the score reduction of 1 week ($p = 0.0002$) and 2 weeks ($p = 0.0020$); results reveal a 6.29 ± 0.55 ($p < 0.0001$) and 9.00 ± 0.61 ($p < 0.0001$) reduction in total symptom scores after four weeks of atomization treatment compared with baseline in the placebo and *Houttuynia* groups, respectively, as well as a statistically significant difference between the two ($p = 0.0018$) (Table 1). Results for each individual symptom score show that values for the *Houttuynia* group dropped more than in the placebo group, while reduced values for eye dryness, foreign body sensation, and photophobia were statistically different between the two groups (Table S4).

Table 1. Changes in eye symptoms and signs parameters after 4 weeks of treatment.

Variables	Placebo (N = 120)				Houttuynia (N = 118)				p Value for Column Factor (4 Weeks/Change)
	Baseline	After Treatment (4 Weeks)	Change	p Value *	Baseline	After Treatment (4 Weeks)	Change	p Value *	
	Primary outcome								
	Eye symptom score								
Mean ± SEM	15.15 ± 0.78	8.86 ± 0.79	6.29 ± 0.55	<0.0001	15.32 ± 0.74	6.32 ± 0.59	9.00 ± 0.61	<0.0001	0.0152/0.0018
	Meibum quality score								
Mean ± SEM	0.92 ± 0.08	0.56 ± 0.07	0.57 ± 0.10	<0.0001	0.85 ± 0.08	0.31 ± 0.05	0.91 ± 0.10	<0.0001	0.0032/0.0091
	Tear break-up time(s)								
Mean ± SEM	4.00 ± 0.19	5.60 ± 0.24	1.61 ± 0.20	<0.0001	4.33 ± 0.20	6.30 ± 0.22	1.97 ± 0.17	<0.0001	0.0172/0.1648
	Secondary outcome								
	Meibum expressibility score								
Mean ± SEM	2.77 ± 0.21	1.60 ± 0.19	1.67 ± 0.25	<0.0001	2.53 ± 0.20	1.26 ± 0.15	2.06 ± 0.29	<0.0001	0.3535/0.1719
	Eyelid margin change score								
Mean ± SEM	1.65 ± 0.07	1.01 ± 0.08	0.65 ± 0.08	<0.0001	1.56 ± 0.07	0.98 ± 0.08	0.59 ± 0.08	<0.0001	0.7038/0.5411
	Conjunctival congestion score								
Mean ± SEM	0.90 ± 0.06	0.43 ± 0.06	0.62 ± 0.07	<0.0001	0.89 ± 0.06	0.38 ± 0.05	0.67 ± 0.07	<0.0001	0.7089/0.6403
	Corneal staining score								
Mean ± SEM	0.61 ± 0.07	0.34 ± 0.07	0.54 ± 0.14	0.0004	0.59 ± 0.08	0.32 ± 0.06	0.54 ± 0.12	<0.0001	0.9831/0.8253
	Schirmer I test								
Mean ± SEM	5.85 ± 0.19	7.74 ± 0.32	1.88 ± 0.32	<0.0001	5.67 ± 0.20	8.45 ± 0.50	2.77 ± 0.52	<0.0001	0.6298/0.7769
	Meibomian gland dropout score								
Mean ± SEM	0.56 ± 0.07	0.50 ± 0.07	0.16 ± 0.06	0.0313	0.51 ± 0.06	0.40 ± 0.06	0.23 ± 0.08	0.0117	0.2744/0.3069

Change value = post-treatment value—pre-treatment value (tear break-up time, Schirmer I test); change value = pre-treatment value—post-treatment value (eye symptom score, meibum quality score, meibum expressibility score, eyelid margin change score, conjunctival congestion score, corneal staining score, and meibomian gland dropout score). p Value * shows the statistical difference that compared baseline and post-treatment for the same group. p Value for Column Factor shows the statistical difference that compared the placebo group and Houttuynia group. Abbreviations: N, number; SEM, standard error of the mean.

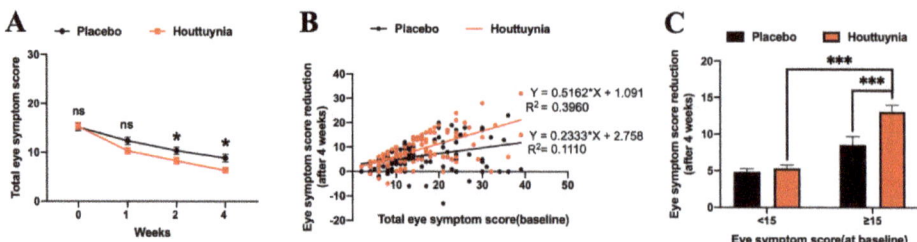

Figure 2. Change in eye symptom score. (**A**) shows eye symptom scores at baseline, one week, two weeks, and four weeks. (**B**) shows the linear correlation between decreases in eye symptom score after four weeks of treatment and scores at baseline. Points represent the values in this figure. The regression line equation and the correlation coefficient R squared value are also shown in this figure. (**C**) highlights the reduction in eye symptom score after four weeks of therapy in scores <15 and ≥15 (at baseline) in two subgroups. Data are presented as mean ± standard error of the mean (SEM). * $p < 0.05$, *** $p < 0.001$. ns, no significance.

Figure 2B reveals a positive linear correlation between eye symptom score reduction after four weeks of treatment and scores at baseline in both groups. Correlation coefficient (r) values were 0.3331 ($p = 0.0002$) and 0.6293 ($p < 0.0001$) in the placebo and *Houttuynia* groups, respectively. We then divided patients into two groups according to the severity of their eye symptoms at baseline (Figure 2C); results show that the reductions in scores after four weeks of therapy in scores < 15 of placebo and *Houttuynia* per group were 4.85 ± 0.45 and 5.32 ± 0.47, respectively, and that there were no statistical differences, while for score ≥ 15, the reductions of placebo and *Houttuynia* group were 8.53 ± 1.14 and 13.07 ± 0.90, respectively. A significant statistical difference was seen between these two groups (95% CI, range between −7.38 and −1.70; $p = 0.0003$) with an interaction p value = 0.0057 (Table 2). These results demonstrate that the group with symptom scores ≥ 15 compared to scores < 15 improved more significantly when treated with *Houttuynia* eye drops.

Results show that both meibum quality and TBUT also improved in both groups (Figure 3). Changes in these two indicators after therapy were also significantly statistically different in the two groups compared with the baseline ($p < 0.0001$) (Table 1). Meibum quality scores decreased after therapy; these reductions were 0.57 ± 0.10 and 0.91 ± 0.10 in the placebo and *Houttuynia* groups after four weeks. There were statistical differences between the Houttuynia and placebo groups in the meibum quality score or the reduction value of the score after four weeks of treatment ($p = 0.0032/0.0091$) (Table 1). Patients were divided into four groups on the basis of meibum quality scores at baseline. Results show that the fall in the *Houttuynia* group was higher amongst each subgroup than in the placebo set (p value for interaction = 0.0282) (Table 2). Values for TBUT in the *Houttuynia* group were always higher than those in the placebo group after treatment over different lengths of time. Indeed, there was a statistically significant difference between the two groups in the TBUT of 1 week ($p = 0.0300$) and 2 weeks ($p = 0.0199$). After four weeks of treatment, TBUT was 5.60 ± 0.24 s and 6.30 ± 0.22 s ($p = 0.0172$) in the placebo and *Houttuynia* groups, respectively.

Table 2. Subgroup analysis.

Variables	Placebo		Houttuynia		Mean Difference (95%CI)	p Value for Interaction
	N	Mean ± SEM	N	Mean ± SEM		
After 4-week therapy						
Primary outcome						
Eye symptom score reduction						0.0057
Score < 15 (at baseline)	73	4.85 ± 0.45	62	5.32 ± 0.47	−0.47 (−2.96 to 2.01)	
Score ≥ 15 (at baseline)	47	8.53 ± 1.14	56	13.07 ± 0.90	−4.54 (−7.38 to −1.70)	

Table 2. Cont.

Variables	N	Placebo Mean ± SEM	N	Houttuynia Mean ± SEM	Mean Difference (95%CI)	p Value for Interaction
Meibum quality score reduction						0.0282
Score = 0 (at baseline)	49	−0.08 ± 0.04	49	−0.02 ± 0.02	−0.06 (−0.41 to 0.29)	
Score = 1 (at baseline)	40	0.35 ± 0.08	43	0.54 ± 0.09	0.18 (−0.57 to 0.20)	
Score = 2 (at baseline)	23	0.96 ± 0.18	21	1.62 ± 0.13	**−0.66 (−1.19 to −0.14)**	
Score = 3 (at baseline)	8	1.38 ± 0.46	5	1.60 ± 0.51	−0.23 (−1.22 to 0.77)	
Secondary outcome						
Middle meibomian gland expression score reduction						0.0051
Score = 0 (at baseline)	42	−0.12 ± 0.06	49	−0.08 ± 0.05	−0.04 (−0.43 to 0.36)	
Score = 1 (at baseline)	52	0.52 ± 0.08	42	0.57 ± 0.10	−0.05 (0.44 to 0.34)	
Score = 2 (at baseline)	23	1.00 ± 0.18	25	1.24 ± 0.18	−0.24 (−0.79 to −0.31)	
Score = 3 (at baseline)	3	1.00 ± 0.58	2	3.00 ± 0.00	**−2.00 (−3.72 to −0.28)**	
Eyelid margin change score reduction						0.0158
Score = 0 (at baseline)	2	−1.00 ± 1.00	3	0.00 ± 0.00	−1.00 (−3.35 to 1.35)	
Score = 1 (at baseline)	57	0.25 ± 0.08	61	0.38 ± 0.09	−0.13 (0.61 to 0.34)	
Score = 2 (at baseline)	46	1.11 ± 0.11	42	1.00 ± 0.13	−0.11 (−0.44 to 0.66)	
Score = 3 (at baseline)	11	1.64 ± 0.24	9	1.78 ± 0.40	−0.14 (−1.30 to 1.02)	
Score = 4 (at baseline)	4	0.75 ± 0.75	3	2.67 ± 1.33	−1.92 (−3.89 to 0.05)	
Conjunctival congestion score reduction						0.6094
Score = 0 (at baseline)	33	−0.06 ± 0.04	32	−0.06 ± 0.04	0.00 (−0.39 to 0.39)	
Score = 1 (at baseline)	66	0.61 ± 0.07	67	0.63 ± 0.06	−0.02 (−0.29 to 0.25)	
Score = 2 (at baseline)	21	0.86 ± 0.17	19	1.05 ± 0.20	−0.20 (−0.69 to 0.30)	
Corneal staining score reduction						0.9723
Score = 0 (at baseline)	65	−0.11 ± 0.05	65	−0.12 ± 0.04	0.02 (−0.32 to 0.35)	
Score = 1 (at baseline)	41	0.56 ± 0.11	45	0.58 ± 0.10	0.02 (−0.39 to 0.42)	
Score > 1 (at baseline)	14	1.07 ± 0.37	8	1.13 ± 0.48	−0.05 (−0.89 to 0.78)	

Score reduction value = pre-treatment value—post-treatment value. Abbreviations: N, number; SEM, standard error of the mean; CI, confidence interval.

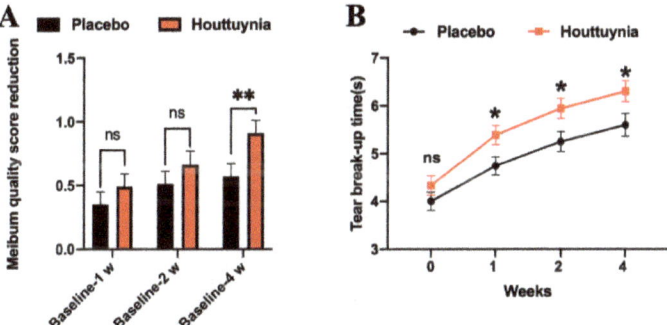

Figure 3. Change in meibum quality and tear break-up time. (**A**) shows the meibum quality score reduction values after one week, two weeks, and four weeks compared with the baseline. (**B**) shows tear break-up time at baseline, one week, two weeks, and four weeks. Data are presented as mean ± SEM. * $p < 0.05$, ** $p < 0.01$, ns, no significance.

3.1.2. Secondary Outcomes

Secondary outcomes in the two groups also improved after four weeks of treatment (Figure 4A–F). Meibum expressibility scores in the *Houttuynia* group subsequent to treatment remained continuously low compared to the placebo group and there were no statistical differences. Patients were then divided into four groups according to their middle meibomian gland expression scores at baseline; this enabled us to demonstrate that decreases in the *Houttuynia* group among each subgroup were higher than those in the placebo group and there were statistical differences for interactions ($p = 0.0051$) (Table 2).

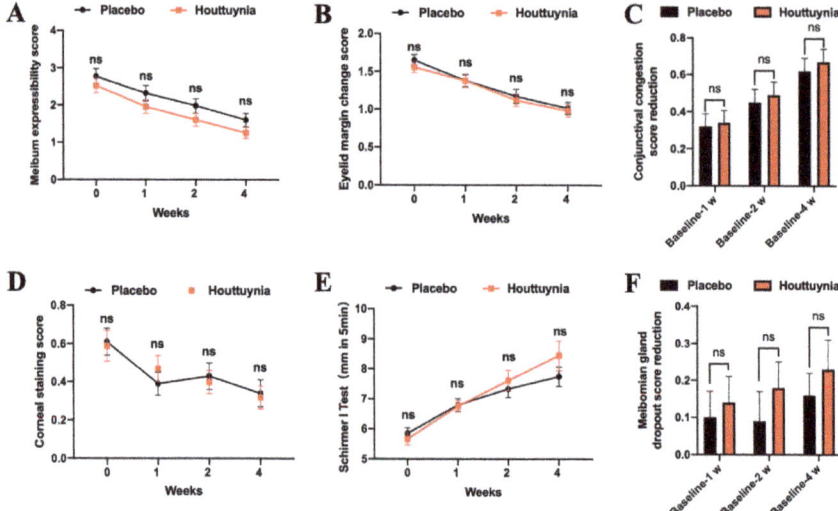

Figure 4. Changes in secondary outcome measures. (**A–E**) illustrate meibum expressibility scores, eyelid margin change, corneal staining, and Schirmer I test results, respectively. These data are shown at baseline as well as after one week, two weeks, and four weeks. (**C,F**) show reduction values for conjunctiva congestion and meibomian gland dropout scores after one week, two weeks, and four weeks compared with the baseline. Data at each point are presented as mean ± SEM. ns, no significance.

Eyelid margin change scores in the *Houttuynia* group were also continuously low compared to the placebo group, although there were no statistical differences. A positive correlation was found between decreases in eyelid margin change scores after four weeks of treatment and these scores at baseline in the two groups. The r-values in this case were 0.7707 ($p = 0.1272$) and 0.9890 ($p = 0.0014$) in the placebo and *Houttuynia* groups, respectively (Table S5). The eyelid margin score reduction of the *Houttuynia* group was more overall than that of the placebo group in each subgroup case, encapsulating a statistically significant interaction difference ($p = 0.0158$) (Table 2).

Results show that conjunctival congestion improved following atomization treatment. Decreased values of the placebo and *Houttuynia* groups were 0.61 ± 0.07 ($p < 0.0001$) and 0.63 ± 0.06 ($p < 0.0001$) in one subgroup (score = 1 at baseline) and 0.86 ± 0.17 ($p < 0.0001$) and 1.05 ± 0.20 ($p < 0.0001$) in another subgroup (score = 2 at baseline) (p value for interaction = 0.6094) (Table 2). The corneal staining score also reduced after treatment: values were 1.07 ± 0.37 and 1.13 ± 0.48 in the placebo and *Houttuynia* groups, respectively. There was no statistical difference in the subgroup at the last visit (corneal staining score > 1 at baseline) (Table 2). Volumes for the Schirmer I test were 7.74 ± 0.32 mm/5 min and 8.45 ± 0.50 mm/5 min (p value for interaction = 0.6298) in the placebo and *Houttuynia* groups, respectively (Table 1). Meibomian gland dropout score reduction gradually increased; score reduction in the *Houttuynia* group was higher than in the placebo group and there was no statistical difference.

Thus, taking all these data together, they suggest that treatment with *Houttuynia* was more effective than treatment with placebo.

3.2. Safety Assessments

Visual acuity and IOP values for the two groups remained basically unchanged following medication. Patients in one center (Peking Union Medical College Hospital) were assessed for blood/urine routines and liver/kidney functions but all indicators remained basically unchanged following medication.

Although some patients exhibited abnormal indicators after medication, there were no clinically significant differences in index values and indicators returned to normal in the follow-up.

The data presented in Table S6 reveal that seven adverse event cases were seen throughout the test. Four of these were in the placebo group (i.e., animal wool allergy, upper respiratory tract infection, blurred vision, and allergic conjunctivitis), and the incidence rate of these events was 2.50%, while three further cases were in the *Houttuynia* group (i.e., upper respiratory tract infection, conjunctivitis, and allergic conjunctivitis). The incidence rate for the cases was 2.54% and data show no statistically significant difference between the two groups. Two subjects in the placebo group and one in the Houttuynia group were withdrawn from the trial due to these adverse events. Indeed, as all adverse event cases either recovered or were relieved, we consider these irrelevant to the experimental treatment.

4. Discussion

The novel results of this strictly randomized, double-blinded, placebo-controlled clinical trial regarding the use of ultrasound-atomized *Houttuynia* eye drops for the treatment of MGD-related DED demonstrate that both the symptoms and signs of this condition are statistically significantly ameliorated from the baseline before treatment. Primary efficacy indicators were significantly enhanced compared with the placebo control group, and differences between the two groups were statistically significant. The specific clinical data were as follows: patients' eye symptom scores decreased by an average of 9 points, meibum quality decreased by nearly 1 point (indicating an improvement of nearly a grade), and TBUT increased to an average of 6.3 s after 4 weeks of treatment. The results of our subgroup analysis also show that the more severe the symptoms and the more turbid the nature of meibomian gland secretions, the better the therapeutic effect of *Houttuynia* eye drops will be. These results suggested that ultrasonically atomized *Houttuynia* eye drops had a clear positive effect on the treatment of MGD-related DED. This therapy can obviously relieve eye-related symptoms, improve meibum quality, and prolong tear break-up time in the clinic.

Inflammation is the main pathological manifestation of DED. This means that anti-inflammatory treatment is the most commonly used therapy for this condition. Inhibiting inflammation can stabilize the tear film and improve the clinical symptoms and signs of DED; indeed, the ultrasonic atomization of *Houttuynia* eye drops can improve both the symptoms and signs of DED, perhaps mainly related to the anti-inflammatory and antibacterial effects of this plant [11–13]. MGD-related DED is characterized by terminal duct obstruction and/or qualitative/quantitative changes in glandular secretions. This is because, on one hand, lipid discharge into the tear film is reduced, causing excessive tear evaporation and tear hyperosmolarity. Tear hyperosmolarity, therefore, also stimulates a cascade in the epithelial cells of the ocular surface, involving MAPK and NF-κB signaling pathways as well as the generation of inflammatory cytokines (i.e., interleukin-1 (IL-1α; IL-1β)), tumor necrosis factor-α (TNF-α)), and proteases. These activate and recruit inflammatory cells, induce inflammatory cascade reactions, and promote inflammation of the meibomian gland, eyelid margin, and ocular surface [25]. On the other hand, meibum stasis inside the gland can promote bacterial proliferation (including *Staphylococcus aureus* and other species); growth of these microorganisms enhances the production of lipid-degrading lipases and esterases that decompose the meibum into toxic mediators including free fatty acids. These toxic mediators increase meibum viscosity and melting temperature and result in tear film instability. Inflammation and the release of inflammatory cytokines can also occur; these phenomena aggravate the destruction of meibomian glands and, again, lead to a vicious circle [7]. The plant *H. cordata* is a traditional Chinese medicine therapy and has been shown to have significant anti-inflammatory and antibacterial effects. Indeed, results show that extracts from this species have anti-inflammatory effects on various cell and animal models. The main anti-inflammatory mechanism in this case acts to reduce the level of inflammation-related cytokines (i.e., TNF-α and IL-1β) and chemokines by inhibiting the NF-κB/MAPK pathway. It is clear that the NF-κB/MAPK pathway is one transduction inflammation pathway caused by MGD-related DED. One in vitro bacteriostatic test showed that *H. cordata* exerts an obvious inhibitory effect on catarrhal bacteria, *S. aureus*, influenza bacillus, and pneumococcus [11,26]. Clinical observations have also shown that this treatment can inhibit bacteria on the ocular surface and can therefore be useful for bacterial conjunctivitis therapy. *Houttuynia* eye drops can inhibit bacterial growth on ocular surfaces and meibomian glands, thereby improving meibum quality.

The results of this study show that patients in the placebo group exhibited improved symptoms as well as all signs after four weeks of treatment. These data were statistically different from those seen before treatment and are mainly related to the ultrasonic atomization treatment method. A number of clinical studies have shown that this method using different liquid can improve meibum expressibility, stabilize the tear film, increase fluid, and mitigate the symptoms and signs of DED [10–12]. The placebo in this study was a sodium chloride solution. A previous study showed that eye atomization treatment with saline alone can also improve the symptoms and signs (including TBUT, corneal fluorescent staining, and Schirmer I test) of dry eye patients. Compared with the artificial tear (0.1% sodium hyaluronate eye fluid of Shentian Pharmaceutical Co., LTD., Shanghai, China) group, the therapeutic effect of the saline atomization group was significantly better ($p < 0.05$) [12]. Ultrasonic atomization makes droplets uniformly, continuously, and comprehensively act on the cornea, conjunctiva, and eyelid, maximizes the contact area between an eye and liquid, and therefore speeds up drug absorption [10]. Therefore, in this study, there was no statistical difference in the change values of TBUT and tear secretion after 4 weeks of treatment, which may be related to the significant improvement effect of ultrasonic atomization on DED. This study has further clarified the effectiveness of this treatment.

Although the experimental group did not exhibit any statistical differences in terms of secondary efficacy indicators in comparison with the placebo group, data on the improvement of symptoms and signs in this former group were better than those in the latter. In addition, post hoc subgrouping analysis was conducted. Due to the limited number of samples, though the subgroup analysis cannot draw accurate conclusions, it can provide potential directions and ideas for the study. Thus, subsequent to grouping secondary indicators according to baseline severity, the data in this study show a statistical difference between the two groups in terms of meibum expressibility and eyelid margin change. This may suggest that patients with more severe meibomian gland blockage and worse eyelid margin state will experience more marked improvements as a result of *Houttuynia* eye drops when compared to the placebo set. This might be due to the therapeutic effects of the ultrasonic atomization method. No statistical differences were seen between conjunctival congestion and corneal fluorescent staining; this may be related to the low occurrence of severe conjunctival congestion and corneal fluorescent staining in the included patients. A further possibility might be that treatment times were not long enough and sample sizes were not big enough; larger samples and longer-term research projects will therefore be needed.

The results of visual acuity, IOP, and laboratory examinations after four weeks of treatment were basically unchanged and there were no adverse events related to the test drug. This shows again that this treatment is safe. Indeed, regarding subjective evaluation results, patients tolerated *Houttuynia* eye drop atomization treatments well, there was little irritation, and individuals were willing to tolerate this approach.

The main limitation of this study was that *Houttuynia* eye drops were not compared with other anti-inflammatory drugs. It is therefore unclear whether, or not, the therapeutic effect of *Houttuynia* eye drops is superior to other anti-inflammatory drugs commonly used in clinical practice. Inflammatory cytokines of tears were not detected during the delivery of this medication, another important indicator that can be used to evaluate eye surface inflammatory state. This is another important indicator that can be used to reflect *Houttuynia* eye drop mechanisms. Another major limitation was that there was missing correction for multiple comparisons. This study tested for multiple hypotheses. The test was considered valid when all three primary indicators were statistically significant. The three indices are independent of each other, and the results of the individual tests are essential, hence we made the decision not to adjust *p* values.

We have shown that treating patients with mild to moderate MGD-related DED for one month via the ultrasonic atomization of *Houttuynia* eye drops can significantly ameliorate the symptoms of eye discomfort, improve meibomian gland function, and stabilize tear films. The results of this study show that this treatment is safe.

Supplementary Materials: The following are available online at http://www.mdpi.com/2077-0383/9/12/4022/s1, Figure S1: The ultrasonic nebulizer, Table S1: Specific distribution of cases at each center, Table S2: Ocular symptom rating scale, Table S3: Characteristics of the patients at baseline, Table S4: Changes in individual eye symptom after 4-week treatment, Table S5: Correlation between indicator change and that at baseline, Table S6: Adverse events during the trial.

Author Contributions: Research design: Z.L. (Zhaolin Liu), M.J., and Z.L. (Zuguo Liu). Data acquisition and/or research execution: Z.L. (Zhaolin Liu), M.J., Y.L., J.L., X.X. (Xianghua Xiao), H.B., Z.P., H.S., X.X. (Xiaofeng Xie), M.Z., X.G., L.L., W.O., L.T., J.W., Y.Y., J.H., and Z.L. (Zuguo Liu). Data analysis: Z.L. (Zhaolin Liu), X.G., and L.L. Data interpretation and writing of the manuscript: Z.L. (Zhaolin Liu) and Z.L. (Zuguo Liu). All authors have read and agreed to the published version of the manuscript.

Funding: This study was supported in part by the grants from China Association of Traditional Chinese Medicine and National Key R&D Program of China (grant number 2018YFA0107304).

Acknowledgments: The authors thank Yueping Zhou from Eye Institute of Xiamen University for his helpful suggestions and guidance.

Conflicts of Interest: The authors report no conflicts of interest in this work. The funders had no role in the design of the study; in the collection, analyses, or interpretation of data; in the writing of the manuscript, or in the decision to publish the results.

Abbreviations

MGD (meibomian gland dysfunction), DED (dry eye disease), TBUT (tear break-up time), AE (adverse event), SEM (standard error of the mean), EDE (evaporative dry eye), CATCM (China Association of Traditional Chinese Medicine), IOP (intraocular pressure), ITT (intention to treat), CI (confidence interval).

References

1. Craig, J.P.; Nichols, K.K.; Akpek, E.K.; Caffery, B.; Dua, H.S.; Joo, C.K.; Liu, Z.; Nelson, J.D.; Nichols, J.J.; Tsubota, K.; et al. TFOS DEWS II Definition and Classification Report. *Ocul. Surf.* **2017**, *15*, 276–283. [CrossRef] [PubMed]
2. Liu, Z.G.; Wang, H. Focusing on the management of chronic dry eye disease. *Zhonghua Yan Ke Za Zhi* **2018**, *54*, 81–83. [CrossRef] [PubMed]
3. Rouen, P.A.; White, M.L. Dry Eye Disease: Prevalence, Assessment, and Management. *Home Healthc. Now* **2018**, *36*, 74–83. [CrossRef] [PubMed]
4. Schaumberg, D.A.; Nichols, J.J.; Papas, E.B.; Tong, L.; Uchino, M.; Nichols, K.K. The international workshop on meibomian gland dysfunction: Report of the subcommittee on the epidemiology of, and associated risk factors for, MGD. *Investig. Ophthalmol. Vis. Sci.* **2011**, *52*, 1994–2005. [CrossRef]
5. Geerling, G.; Baudouin, C.; Aragona, P.; Rolando, M.; Boboridis, K.G.; Benítez-del-Castillo, J.M.; Akova, Y.A.; Merayo-Lloves, J.; Labetoulle, M.; Steinhoff, M.; et al. Emerging strategies for the diagnosis and treatment of meibomian gland dysfunction: Proceedings of the OCEAN group meeting. *Ocul. Surf.* **2017**, *15*, 179–192. [CrossRef]
6. Chhadva, P.; Goldhardt, R.; Galor, A. Meibomian Gland Disease: The Role of Gland Dysfunction in Dry Eye Disease. *Ophthalmology* **2017**, *124*, S20–S26. [CrossRef]
7. Baudouin, C.; Messmer, E.M.; Aragona, P.; Geerling, G.; Akova, Y.A.; Benítez-del-Castillo, J.; Boboridis, K.G.; Merayo-Lloves, J.; Rolando, M.; Labetoulle, M. Revisiting the vicious circle of dry eye disease: A focus on the pathophysiology of meibomian gland dysfunction. *Br. J. Ophthalmol.* **2016**, *100*, 300–306. [CrossRef]
8. Thode, A.R.; Latkany, R.A. Current and Emerging Therapeutic Strategies for the Treatment of Meibomian Gland Dysfunction (MGD). *Drugs* **2015**, *75*, 1177–1185. [CrossRef]
9. Zhou, W.Y.; Li, Y.H. A survey on treatment of dry eye by traditional chinese medicine and integrative chinese and Western medicine. *Chin. J. Integr. Med.* **2006**, *12*, 154–159. [CrossRef]
10. Ma, K.; Li, Q.S.; Zhang, Z.Y.; Xiang, M.H.; Zhao, Y.Q.; Ophthalmology, D.O. Research progress in physical therapy for dry eye. *Int. Eye Sci.* **2018**, *18*, 660–663.

11. Yuqiu Xu, J.C. Research progress of ultrasonic atomization treating dry eye. *Chin. J. Tradit. Chin. Med. Ophthalmol.* **2020**, *30*, 367–370.
12. Zhou, Y. Clinical observation and analysis of dry eye after phacoemulsification and intraocular lens implantation with Traditional Chinese medicine ultrasonic atomization. *J. Hunan Univ. Chin. Med.* **2018**, *A01*, 45–46.
13. Shingnaisui, K.; Dey, T.; Manna, P.; Kalita, J. Therapeutic potentials of Houttuynia cordata Thunb. against inflammation and oxidative stress: A review. *J. Ethnopharmacol.* **2018**, *220*, 35–43. [CrossRef] [PubMed]
14. Muluye, R.A.; Bian, Y.; Alemu, P.N. Anti-inflammatory and Antimicrobial Effects of Heat-Clearing Chinese Herbs: A Current Review. *J. Tradit. Complement Med.* **2014**, *4*, 93–98. [CrossRef] [PubMed]
15. Kumar, M.; Prasad, S.K.; Hemalatha, S. A current update on the phytopharmacological aspects of Houttuynia cordata Thunb. *Pharmacogn. Rev.* **2014**, *8*, 22–35. [PubMed]
16. Chen, Y.Z.; Zhao, X.Q.; Zhang, M.L.; Zeng, L.; Du, S.B.; Wang, F.L. Effect of hyaluronate eye drops combined with houttuynia cordata eye drops on the treatment of dry eye. *Int. J. Ophthalmol.* **2011**, *11*, 704–705.
17. Liang, T.; Lin, H.; Gao, Y.; Zhao, G.Q. Clinical observation of houttuynia cordata eyedrops with artificial tear in the treatment of dry eye. *Int. J. Ophthalmol.* **2010**, *10*, 70–71.
18. National Medical Products Administration. Good Clinical Practice of Pharmaceutical Products. Available online: http://www.nmpa.gov.cn/yaopin/ypfgwj/ypfgbmgzh/20030806010101443.html (accessed on 6 August 2003).
19. National Medical Products Administration. Provisions of Drug Registration. Available online: https://www.nmpa.gov.cn/xxgk/fgwj/bmgzh/20070710010101571.html (accessed on 10 July 2007).
20. China branch of Asian dry eye Association; Ocular Surface and Tear Disease Group of Ophthalmology Specialized Committee of the Cross-Strait Medical Exchange Association. Expert consensus of diagnosis and treatment of meibomian gland dysfunction in China (2017). *Chin. J. Ophthalmol.* **2017**, *53*, 657–661.
21. Department of Ophthalmology, Chinese Academy of Medical Sciences. Expert consensus on clinical diagnosis and treatment of dry eye (2013). *Chin. J. Ophthalmol.* **2013**, *49*, 73–75.
22. Zhao, H.; Liu, Z.; Yang, W.; Xiao, X.; Chen, J.; Li, Q.; Zhong, T. Development and assessment of a dry eye questionnaire applicable to the Chinese population. *Zhonghua Yan Ke Za Zhi* **2015**, *51*, 647–654.
23. Tomlinson, A.; Bron, A.J.; Korb, D.R.; Amano, S.; Paugh, J.R.; Pearce, E.I.; Yee, R.; Yokoi, N.; Arita, R.; Dogru, M. The international workshop on meibomian gland dysfunction: Report of the diagnosis subcommittee. *Investig. Ophthalmol. Vis. Sci.* **2011**, *52*, 2006–2049. [CrossRef] [PubMed]
24. Efron, N.; Morgan, P.B.; Katsara, S.S. Validation of grading scales for contact lens complications. *Ophthalmic Physiol. Opt.* **2001**, *21*, 17–29. [PubMed]
25. Bron, A.J.; de Paiva, C.S.; Chauhan, S.K.; Bonini, S.; Gabison, E.E.; Jain, S.; Knop, E.; Markoulli, M.; Ogawa, Y.; Perez, V.; et al. TFOS DEWS II pathophysiology report. *Ocul. Surf.* **2017**, *15*, 438–510. [CrossRef] [PubMed]
26. Sekita, Y.; Murakami, K.; Yumoto, H.; Mizuguchi, H.; Amoh, T.; Ogino, S.; Matsuo, T.; Miyake, Y.; Fukui, H.; Kashiwada, Y. Anti-bacterial and anti-inflammatory effects of ethanol extract from Houttuynia cordata poultice. *Biosci. Biotechnol. Biochem.* **2016**, *80*, 1205–1213. [CrossRef] [PubMed]

Publisher's Note: MDPI stays neutral with regard to jurisdictional claims in published maps and institutional affiliations.

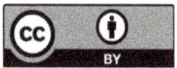

© 2020 by the authors. Licensee MDPI, Basel, Switzerland. This article is an open access article distributed under the terms and conditions of the Creative Commons Attribution (CC BY) license (http://creativecommons.org/licenses/by/4.0/).

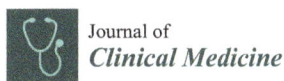

Article

Treatment Response to Gabapentin in Neuropathic Ocular Pain Associated with Dry Eye

Hyeon-Jeong Yoon, Jonghwa Kim and Kyung Chul Yoon *

Department of Ophthalmology, Chonnam National University Medical School and Hospital, 42 Jebong-ro, Dong-gu, Gwangju 61469, Korea; yoonhyeonjeong@hanmail.net (H.-J.Y.); ccaaacc@hanmail.net (J.K.)
* Correspondence: kcyoon@jnu.ac.kr; Tel.: +82-62-220-6741; Fax: +82-62-227-1642

Received: 22 October 2020; Accepted: 19 November 2020; Published: 22 November 2020

Abstract: Purpose: To investigate the response to gabapentin treatment in patients with dry eye (DE) accompanied by features of neuropathic ocular pain (NOP), and to analyze the differences between clinical manifestations of the groups according to treatment response. Methods: We retrospectively reviewed the records of 35 patients with DE accompanied by NOP features and obtained information on their medical history and previous ocular history. The patients underwent clinical examinations of the tear film, ocular surface, and meibomian gland and completed the Ocular Pain Assessment Survey (OPAS). One month after treatment with topical eye drops, add-on of gabapentin treatment was determined according to the Wong–Baker FACES Pain Rating Scale (WBFPS). A reduction of 2 points or more on the WBFPS was considered a positive treatment response. Enrolled patients were divided into three groups according to the treatment response: topical treatment response group (group 1, $n = 11$); gabapentin response group (group 2, $n = 13$); and gabapentin non-response group (group 3, $n = 11$). The medical history, clinical parameters, and OPAS scores were compared between groups. Results: The incidence of systemic comorbidities was higher in group 2 than in other groups. The corneal staining scores were lower in groups 2 and 3 than in group 1. Among the treatment response groups, group 2 showed improvements in OPAS scores of ocular pain severity, pain other than eyes, and quality of life, while group 1 showed improved OPAS scores of ocular pain severity and ocular associated factors. Group 2 exhibited lower scores of pains aggravated by mechanical and chemical stimuli than group 3. Conclusions: Gabapentin could be effective in patients who have systemic comorbidity and less pain evoked by mechanical and chemical stimuli for the treatment of DE patients with NOP, which is refractory to topical treatment.

Keywords: gabapentin; dry eye; neuropathic pain

1. Introduction

Dry eye (DE) is a multifactorial disease of the ocular surface characterized by a loss of homeostasis of the tear film and accompanied by ocular symptoms [1]. The prevalence of DE has increased considerably worldwide over the last three decades [2]. Some patients with DE experience severe pain that reduces their quality of life (QoL) with minimal ocular surface signs [1,3]. Their manifestations include a variety of unpleasant spontaneous ocular sensations, such as burning, aching, and photoallodynia [1,3]. A neurobiological mechanism is known to underline the ocular symptoms of DE [3].

The classification of pain is based on the underlying etiology: nociceptive, neuropathic, and mixed [4]. The primary approach to treating severe ocular pain is to target potential nociceptive factors [5]. Topical treatment could be attempted to lower tear osmolarity and reduce inflammation [6]. If the pain cannot be resolved with the primary approach, neuropathic pain could be considered [5,7,8]. In DE, persistent damage to the ocular surface and nerve endings induced by tear film instability and inflammation can cause peripheral neuronal sensitization. Moreover, repeated peripheral nerve injury can lead to central neuronal sensitization [9–12].

DE and neuropathic pain share several common features, including frequent discordance between the symptoms and signs, abnormal somatosensory testing, accompanying comorbidity, and anatomic nerve injury or somatosensory nerve sensitization [9,13]. Ocular pain symptoms disproportionally outweighing the clinical signs are suggestive of an underlying neuropathic etiology that requires systemic pain management [9,13].

Oral gabapentin is the first-line agent for the treatment of chronic systemic neuropathic pain [14]. Especially, gabapentin could reverse elements of central sensitization in patients with chronic pain [15–17]. This agent has been studied as a therapy for ocular pain after refractive surgery and painful DE [7,18–20]. However, central nervous system (CNS) depression may occur as a side effect [15], and the therapeutic efficacy of gabapentin for neuropathic ocular pain (NOP) has not been verified. Hence, ophthalmologists are less likely to use gabapentin for treating NOP which is refractory to topical agents. In this study, we aimed to investigate the response to gabapentin treatment in DE patients with NOP features and compare the clinical parameters and ocular pain assessment survey (OPAS) scores between groups according to the treatment response.

2. Methods

Ethical approval was obtained from the Chonnam National University Hospital Institutional Review Board, and the study protocol adhered to the guidelines of the Declaration of Helsinki. Data were collected by retrospective review of the patients' medical charts and recorded using electronic case report forms.

2.1. Study Population

Patients with DE accompanied by NOP features, who underwent evaluation between January 2018 and February 2020, were included in the analysis. DE was diagnosed at the first visit, based on an ocular surface disease index (OSDI) score ≥ 13 and tear break-up time (TBUT) ≤ 10 s. The inclusion criteria were as follows: (1) chronic ocular pain lasting for more than 3 months, which was unresponsive to topical lubricants (e.g., sodium hyaluronate, carboxymethylcellulose sodium, carbomer, lanolin ointment, etc.); (2) discordance between the painful DE symptoms and signs; (3) specific descriptors, including spontaneous burning, stinging, photosensitivity, and allodynia; and (4) Wong–Baker FACES Pain Rating Scale (WBFPS) score ≥ 6. The exclusion criteria were as follows: (1) topical anti-inflammatory drug use, including steroids and cyclosporin; (2) use of systemic medications that alter the pain and mood status, including analgesics, antidepressants, and antiepileptics; (3) systemic comorbidities that contraindicate the use of gabapentin, including chronic kidney disease; and (4) follow-up duration of less than 2 months.

2.2. Measurement of Clinical Parameters

The OSDI score, TBUT, Schirmer score, corneal stain score (CSS), and meibomian gland (MG) parameters were evaluated by the same investigator (K.C.Y.). Only the "worse" eye was assessed as follows: (1) eyes with severe CSS, or (2) the right eye if the CSS was the same in both eyes.

The OSDI questionnaire was used to quantify the vision-related QoL and included the following subscales: (1) ocular symptoms (OSDI symptoms); (2) vision-related activities of daily living (OSDI visual function); and (3) environmental triggers (OSDI trigger). The total OSDI score and each subscale score, which ranged from 0 to 100, were analyzed [21].

TBUT was assessed using a moistened fluorescein strip (Haag-Streit, Koeniz, Switzerland), and the time interval between the last complete blink and the first appearance of a dry spot or disruption of the tear film was recorded in seconds. This examination was performed thrice, and the mean TBUT value was used for the analysis. CSSs were obtained through a white light and cobalt blue filter, using the area-density index, scoring area and density of the superficial punctate corneal lesion and multiplying the area and density score [22]. Schirmer score was measured using a calibrated sterile strip (Color Bar Schirmer Tear Test; Eagle Vision Inc., Memphis, TN, USA) under topical anesthesia (0.5% proparacaine chloride). The sterile strips were placed at the lateral canthus away from the cornea and left for 5 min with the eyes closed. Schirmer scores were represented as the length of wetting in millimeters for 5 min.

The MG quality score was graded using a scale ranging from 0 to 3 as follows: grade 0, normal, clear oil expressed; grade 1, opaque, diffusely turbid, normal viscosity; grade 2, opaque, increased viscosity; and grade 3, inspissated (thick, toothpaste-like appearance) meibum or non-expressible glands. The MG expressibility score was graded by counting the central eight expressed MG orifices of the lower lid as follows: grade 0, all glands are expressible; grade 1, 3–4 glands are expressible; grade 2, 1–2 glands are expressible; and grade 3, no gland is expressible [23].

2.3. Assessment of Ocular Pain

The WBFPS was chosen to screen pain severity in patients with DE. We explained to the patients that each face represented a person who had no pain, had some pain, or had severe pain. Patients chose the face that best depicts the pain they were experiencing at that moment [24].

All patients completed the OPAS, which is a validated questionnaire for neuropathic pain that combines patient responses regarding ocular and non-ocular pain intensity, impact on QoL, aggravating factors, associated factors, and symptomatic relief [25]. The questions were divided into sections for analysis: questions 4–9 pertained to eye pain intensity (0 to 60); questions 10–11, pertained to non-eye pain (0 to 20); questions 13–19 (0–10, total score 0 to 60) assessed the QoL (reading and/or computer use; driving and/or watching TV; general activity; mood; sleep; and enjoying life/relations with other people); questions 20–21 (each score 0–1, total score 0 to 2) assessed aggravating factors (mechanical and chemical stimuli); and questions 22–25 (each score 0–1, total score 0 to 4), assessed associated factors (redness; burning; sensitivity to light; and tearing). The section on symptomatic relief was excluded, and only questions 4–25 were analyzed in this study.

2.4. Protocol of Treatment and Grouping

At the first visit, all patients were instructed to instill preservative-free sodium hyaluronate 0.15% (Hyaluni eye drops 0.15%®, Taejoon Pharmaceutical Co., Ltd., Seoul, Korea) 6 times a day, and loteprednol 0.5% (Lotemax®, Bausch & Lomb, Rochester, NY, USA) and cyclosporin A ophthalmic nanoemulsion 0.05% (Cyporin N®, Taejoon, Seoul, Korea) twice a day. After 1 month of treatment, an add-on of gabapentin 600 to 1200 mg/day (Neurontin cap®, Pfizer, New York, NY, USA) was determined according to the WBFPS score. The topical treatment was continued without gabapentin if the WBFPS score decreased by more than 2 points. If not, the add-on gabapentin treatment was administered for 1 month.

Patients were divided into three groups according to the treatment response: group 1 comprised patients who experienced symptomatic relief only with eye drops (topical treatment response group, $n = 11$); group 2 comprised patients who experienced symptomatic relief after the administration of gabapentin (gabapentin response group, $n = 13$); and group 3 comprised patients who were unresponsive to both treatments (gabapentin non-response group, $n = 11$; Figure 1).

2.5. Statistical Analysis

Statistical analyses were conducted using Statistical Package for the Social Sciences, version 22.0, for Windows (SPSS Inc., Chicago, IL, USA). The normality of distribution for all variables was assessed using the Shapiro–Wilk test. Fisher's exact test was used for categorical data. Variables satisfying normal distribution were analyzed using the one-way analysis of variance and independent t-test, and those with non-normal distribution were analyzed with the Mann–Whitney U test. Post hoc analysis was performed after multiple comparison analysis using Tukey's honestly significant difference test and Bonferroni adjustment. The symptom scores obtained before and after treatment were compared using the Wilcoxon signed-rank test, with differences corrected using the Benjamini–Hochberg procedure using false discovery rates of 0.25. p-values less than 0.05 were considered statistically significant.

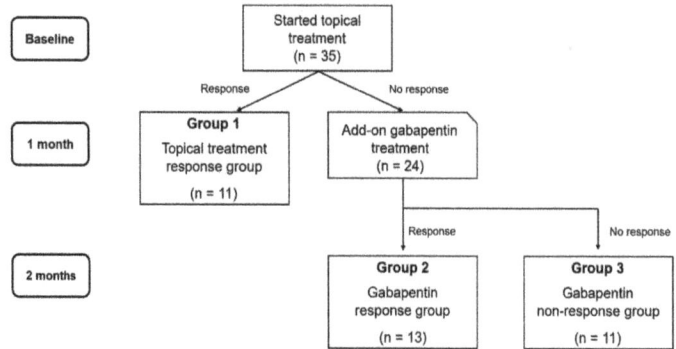

Figure 1. Flowchart of treatment protocol and grouping.

3. Results

This study included 35 patients with DE accompanying NOP features. The mean age was 55.6 ± 11.7 years, and 27 patients (77.1%) were women. There were no differences in baseline characteristics according to sex (data not shown). Only 1 of the 24 patients treated with gabapentin experienced a side-effect (mild tremor).

Table 1 shows the demographics and medical history of the patients enrolled in this study. There was no history of systemic comorbidity, ocular surgery, and trauma in group 1. Systemic comorbidities including rheumatologic, neurologic, and phycological disorders were more frequent in group 2 than in group 3 ($p = 0.034$). No differences were observed between the previous ocular histories of groups 2 and 3.

Table 1. Demographics and personal history of patients with dry eye accompanied by neuropathic ocular pain features.

	Topical Treatment ($n = 11$)	Gabapentin Treatment		p-Value
		Response ($n = 13$)	Non-Response ($n = 11$)	
Demographics				
Age (years)	59.4 ± 11.7	52.5 ± 10.3	55.5 ± 13.2	0.367
Sex (M:F)	3:8	3:10	2:9	0.879
Comorbidities, n	0	7	1	0.010
Rheumatologic disease	0	3	0	
Neurologic disorder	0	2	1	
Psychological disorder	0	2	0	
Previous ocular history, n	0	6	6	0.014
Cataract	0	2	1	
LASIK/LASEK	0	1	3	
Ocular trauma	0	1	1	
Eyelid surgery	0	2	1	
Number of previously used topical agents, n	1.55 ± 0.69	1.77 ± 0.60	1.82 ± 0.75	0.603

M, male; F, female; LASIK, laser-assisted in situ keratomileusis; LASEK, laser-assisted sub-epithelial keratectomy. Compared using Fisher's Exact test.

Table 2 presents the comparisons of the clinical DE and MG parameters of the three groups. The CSS of groups 2 and 3 were lower than those of group 1 ($p = 0.048$ and $p = 0.033$). There were no differences between the CSS and other clinical parameters of groups 2 and 3.

Table 2. Clinical parameters in patients with dry eye accompanied by neuropathic ocular pain features according to the treatment response.

	Topical Treatment (n = 11)	Gabapentin Treatment		p-Value	Post Hoc Analysis		
		Response (n = 13)	Non-Response (n = 11)		Group 1 vs. 2	Group 1 vs. 3	Group 2 vs. 3
OSDI	71.9 ± 7.34	69.2 ± 35.3	74.48 ± 19.1	0.959	0.993	0.994	0.956
Tear film and ocular surface parameters							
TBUT (sec)	4.73 ± 2.28	4.62 ± 1.94	4.00 ± 1.27	0.621	0.988	0.640	0.707
Schirmer test score (mm)	6.73± 5.31	5.85 ± 1.41	7.91 ± 2.98	0.369	0.814	0.712	0.336
CSS (0–9)	1.09 ± 1.04	0.31 ± 0.75	0.27 ± 0.47	0.031	0.048	0.033	0.994
MG parameters							
MG quality (0–3)	0.91 ± 0.83	0.85 ± 0.69	0.82 ± 0.75	0.959	0.977	0.957	0.996
MG expressibility (0–3)	0.55 ± 0.69	0.77 ± 0.60	0.69 ± 0.79	0.712	0.711	0.811	0.988

All values are presented as mean ± SD. OSDI, ocular surface disease index; TBUT, tear break-up time; CSS, corneal staining score; MG, meibomian gland. Comparison using one-way analysis of variance, and post hoc analysis using Tukey's honestly significant difference test with Bonferroni adjustment.

Table 3 shows the changes in the OPAS scores of groups 1 and 2. Improved OPAS scores of ocular pain severity and associating factors were noted after treatment in group 1 (both $p = 0.026$). Group 2 exhibited improved OPAS scores of ocular pain severity, pain other than eyes, and QoL ($p = 0.011$, $p = 0.026$, and $p = 0.011$, respectively).

Table 3. Changes in the Ocular Pain Assessment Survey score in the topical treatment and gabapentin response groups.

	Pre	Post	p-Value
Topical treatment response group			
Eye pain intensity (0–60)	41.0 (22.0–60.0)	29.5 (21.0–38.0)	0.026
Non–eye pain (0–20)	6.0 (5.0–7.0)	13.5 (9.0–18.0)	0.063
Quality of life (0–60)	37.5 (14.0–60.0)	34.8 (23.0–46.6)	0.113
Aggravating factors (0–2)	1.30 (1.00–1.60)	1.35 (0.80–1.90)	0.459
Associated factors (0–4)	2.85 (2.50–3.20)	2.20 (1.60–2.80)	0.026
Gabapentin response group			
Eye pain intensity (0–60)	38.0 (22.0–38.0)	26.0 (21.0–35.0)	0.011
Non–eye pain (0–20)	13.0 (10.0–19.0)	8.0 (6.0–16.0)	0.026
Quality of life (0–60)	43.0 (31.0–53.0)	20.0 (12.0–47.0)	0.011
Aggravating factors (0–2)	0.60 (0.20–1.40)	0.90 (0.80–1.30)	1.000
Associated factors (0–4)	1.50 (1.40–2.60)	0.80 (0.30–3.20)	0.122

All values are presented as median (interquartile range). Comparing using Wilcoxon signed-rank test.

The comparisons of the OPAS scores between groups 2 and 3 are presented in Table 4. The scores of "enjoying life/relations with other people" associated with the QOL and pain aggravated by mechanical and chemical stimuli were lower in group 2 than in group 3 ($p = 0.019$, $p = 0.003$, and $p = 0.004$, respectively).

Table 4. Comparison of the Ocular Pain Assessment Survey score between the gabapentin response and non-response groups.

	Gabapentin Treatment		p-Value
	Response (n = 13)	Non-Response (n = 11)	
Eye pain intensity (0–60)	39.0 (15.0–40.0)	35.0 (19.5–44.5)	0.722 †
Non–eye pain (0–20)	8.0 (0.0–10.0)	4.0 (0.75–11.75)	0.249 †
Quality of life			
Reading and/or computer use (0–10)	0.0 (0.0–8.0)	7.0 (4.25–9.75)	0.254 †
Driving and/or watching TV (0–10)	6.67 ± 1.97	6.20 ± 2.94	0.674 *
General activity (walking, etc.) (0–10)	5.00 ± 3.30	5.40 ± 3.57	0.788 *
Mood (0–10)	1.0 (0.0–7.0)	6.5 (3.25–9.0)	0.456 †
Sleep (0–10)	5.0 (5.0–6.0)	5.0 (0.0–10.0)	0.381 †
Enjoying life/relations with other people (0–10)	4.67 ± 3.06	7.60 ± 2.17	0.019 *
Aggravating factors			
Mechanical stimuli (0–1)	0.42 ± 0.24	0.78 ± 0.28	0.003 *
Chemical stimuli (0–1)	0.40 ± 0.28	0.76 ± 0.22	0.004 *
Associated factors			
Redness (0–1)	0.50 ± 0.35	0.45 ± 0.32	0.628 *
Burning sensation (0–1)	0.50 ± 0.32	0.45 ± 0.42	0.381 *
Sensitivity to light (0–1)	0.60 ± 0.17	0.45 ± 0.33	0.080 *
Tearing (0–1)	0.4 (0.4–0.5)	0.3 (0.03–0.88)	0.123 †

* Compared using independent t-test. † Compared using Mann–Whitney U test.

4. Discussion

Pain is an unpleasant sensory and emotional experience associated with actual or potential tissue damage, or described with respect to such damage, and can be classified into nociceptive and neuropathic pain [26]. Nociceptive pain is caused by actual or threatened damage to tissue due to the activation of nociceptors. In contrast, neuropathic pain is caused by a lesion or disease of the somatosensory nervous system. Repeated peripheral nerve injury can lead to peripheral sensitization, and prolonged peripheral ectopic pain initiates central sensitization [13,26].

DE is a multifactorial disease of the ocular surface, which is accompanied by ocular symptoms [1]. At times, patients experience ocular pain that affects their QoL. The discordance between the ocular symptoms and signs suggest an underlying neuropathic pain etiology; in such cases, ocular pain could be refractory to conventional topical DE treatment [5,8,13]. Gabapentin is the first-line treatment for systemic neuropathic pain in conditions such as fibromyalgia, postherpetic pain, and diabetic neuropathy [14]. It is an anti-convulsant drug that reduces the release of multiple excitatory neurotransmitters by acting on the α2δ subunit of the voltage-gated calcium channels, thus decreasing central sensitization [7,15].

However, limited data are available to support the use of systemic neuropathic pain medication for NOP associated with DE. A prospective, placebo-controlled study demonstrated that gabapentin reduced postoperative pain after photorefractive keratectomy [27]. However, a recent randomized pilot study showed that pregabalin, which has a similar mechanism with gabapentin, failed to prevent DE symptoms after laser-assisted in situ keratomileuses [28]. Ongun et al. [19] showed that gabapentin was more effective for the treatment of severe DE with NOP compared to topical treatment. In the present study, we aimed to analyze the differences in the clinical manifestations between groups according to treatment response in patients with DE accompanied by NOP features.

Our results showed that the frequency of other comorbidities such as rheumatologic, neurologic, and psychological disorders was higher in the gabapentin response group. Gabapentin has pharmacologic characteristics, binding to voltage-sensitive calcium channels at the α2δ subunit, affecting their function as well as influencing receptor trafficking [15]. It can secondarily influence gamma-aminobutyric acid and glutamate tone and activity via this mechanism [15]. Therefore, gabapentin can relieve not only neuropathic pain but also general systemic symptoms, such as mood, sleep, vasomotor symptoms, etc. [15,29]. This explanation corresponds to the results seen in Table 4, i.e., the significant improvement in non-ocular pain and QoL.

In contrast, the topical treatment response group had no ocular history including surgery and trauma, with more severe CSS compared to the other groups. The sensory neurons of the ocular surface and nociceptors could actually be injured in patients who had ocular surgery and trauma leading to neuroinflammation associated with peripheral and central sensitization [5,8,13]. Topical anti-inflammatory agents such as topical steroids and cyclosporin could decrease the release of proinflammatory neuropeptides and cytokines from injured nerves, affecting nociceptive pain and peripheral sensitization [9]. However, improvement of corneal nerve morphologic status and central sensitization has not been demonstrated. Therefore, patients with previous ocular history, including surgery and trauma, may not respond to topical treatment and require systemic NOP treatment.

The evoked pain in response to chemical and mechanical stimulation tended to be greater in the gabapentin non-response group than in the gabapentin response group. Evoked pain, including allodynia and hyperalgesia, is provoked or increased pain in response to stimulation [26]. These manifestations are common clinical characteristics of neuropathic pain; however, their underlying mechanisms are complex and diverse depending on the provoking stimulus [30]. The efficacy of gabapentin for the alleviation of systemic neuropathic pain was proven by several randomized, double-blind placebo-controlled studies [14]. Nevertheless, few studies have specifically focused on the treatment of evoked pain. Furthermore, one study showed that mechanical allodynia was a negative predictor of the overall effect of pregabalin in patients with postherpetic neuralgia [30,31].

Dieckmann et al. [9] suggested the proparacaine challenge test for differentiating between peripheral and central neuropathic pain and proposed a corresponding treatment strategy for DE patients with neuropathic pain etiology. The results of our study showed that the treatment response was related not only to the degree of central sensitization before treatment, but also to the patients' systemic comorbidity, ocular history, ocular surface status, and presence of evoked pain. Gabapentin can cause side effects including CNS depression (drowsiness, dizziness, headache, etc.) and mood problems; thus, consultation with a neuropsychiatrist may be needed [15]. In this study, only one patient experienced a mild tremor as a side-effect for gabapentin treatment. Therefore, we believe gabapentin may be tolerable in DE patients associated with NOP. In addition, our results will help clinicians predict in which DE patients associated with NOP gabapentin treatment will be more effective.

Our study had some limitations. First, it was designed retrospectively and the sample size was small. Patients were recruited from a single tertiary center; thus, the findings may not be representative of the general DE population. Further prospective and longitudinal studies with a large sample size are required in the future. Second, the threshold value for determining the group classification may not have been a representative value. We classified patients with an improvement of 2 or more points on the WBFPS as the treatment response group; however, this might be not a standardized cut-off value. Moreover, we did not analyze the results of the proparacaine challenge test. It was difficult to classify the enrolled patients based on the central or peripheral phenotype of pain, since the majority of participants showed a mixed phenotype. Third, the extent of actual nerve damage was not measured using in vivo confocal microscopy. However, to the best of our knowledge, this was the first study to analyze the differences in the clinical manifestations between groups according to treatment response in DE patients with NOP features.

In conclusion, gabapentin could be successful for the treatment of DE patients with NOP features who have systemic comorbidities including rheumatological, neurological, and psychological disorders, and less evoked pain in response to mechanical and chemical stimuli. Topical treatment for DE with NOP features could be successful for patients who have a corneal staining and no ocular history including surgery and trauma.

Author Contributions: Conceptualization, K.C.Y.; methodology, H.-J.Y., J.K.; software, H.-J.Y.; validation, H.-J.Y., K.C.Y.; formal analysis, H.-J.Y.; investigation, H.-J.Y.; resources, H.-J.Y., J.K.; data curation, H.-J.Y., J.K.; writing—original draft preparation, H.-J.Y.; writing—review and editing, H.-J.Y., K.C.Y.; visualization, H.-J.Y.; supervision, K.C.Y.; project administration, K.C.Y.; funding acquisition, K.C.Y. All authors have read and agreed to the published version of the manuscript.

Funding: This study was supported by a grant of the Korea Health Technology R&D Project through the Korea Health Industry Development Institute (KHIDI), funded by the Ministry of Health and Welfare, Republic of Korea (HR20C0021050020) and the Chonnam National University Hospital Biomedical Research Institute (BCRI 20072).

Conflicts of Interest: The authors declare no conflict of interest.

References

1. Craig, J.P.; Nichols, K.K.; Akpek, E.K.; Caffery, B.; Dua, H.S.; Joo, C.-K.; Liu, Z.; Nelson, J.D.; Nichols, J.J.; Tsubota, K.; et al. TFOS DEWS II Definition and Classification Report. *Ocul. Surf.* **2017**, *15*, 276–283. [CrossRef] [PubMed]
2. Stapleton, F.; Alves, M.; Bunya, V.Y.; Jalbert, I.; Lekhanont, K.; Malet, F.; Na, K.-S.; Schaumberg, D.; Uchino, M.; Vehof, J.; et al. TFOS DEWS II Epidemiology Report. *Ocul. Surf.* **2017**, *15*, 334–365. [CrossRef] [PubMed]
3. Belmonte, C.; Nichols, J.J.; Cox, S.M.; Brock, J.A.; Begley, C.G.; Bereiter, D.A.; Dartt, D.A.; Galor, A.; Hamrah, P.; Ivanusic, J.J.; et al. TFOS DEWS II pain and sensation report. *Ocul. Surf.* **2017**, *15*, 404–437. [CrossRef] [PubMed]
4. Nicholson, B. Differential Diagnosis: Nociceptive and Neuropathic Pain. *Am. J. Manag. Care* **2006**, *12*, 7.
5. Dermer, H.; Lent-Schochet, D.; Theotoka, D.; Paba, C.; Cheema, A.A.; Kim, R.S.; Galor, A. A Review of Management Strategies for Nociceptive and Neuropathic Ocular Surface Pain. *Drugs* **2020**, *80*, 547–571. [CrossRef] [PubMed]
6. Jones, L.; Downie, L.E.; Korb, D.; Benitez-Del-Castillo, J.M.; Dana, R.; Deng, S.X.; Dong, P.N.; Geerling, G.; Hida, R.Y.; Liu, Y.; et al. TFOS DEWS II Management and Therapy Report. *Ocul. Surf.* **2017**, *15*, 575–628. [CrossRef] [PubMed]
7. Small, L.R.; Galor, A.; Felix, E.R.; Horn, D.B.; Levitt, R.C.; Sarantopoulos, C.D. Oral Gabapentinoids and Nerve Blocks for the Treatment of Chronic Ocular Pain. *Eye Contact Lens* **2019**. [CrossRef]
8. Galor, A.; Levitt, R.C.; Felix, E.R.; Martin, E.R.; Sarantopoulos, C.D. Neuropathic ocular pain: An important yet underevaluated feature of dry eye. *Eye* **2015**, *29*, 301–312. [CrossRef]
9. Dieckmann, G.; Goyal, S.; Hamrah, P. Neuropathic Corneal Pain. *Ophthalmology* **2017**, *124*, S34–S47. [CrossRef]
10. Baron, R.; Binder, A.; Wasner, G. Neuropathic pain: Diagnosis, pathophysiological mechanisms, and treatment. *Lancet Neurol.* **2010**, *9*, 807–819. [CrossRef]
11. Kalangara, J.P.; Galor, A.; Levitt, R.C.; Felix, E.R.; Alegret, R.; Sarantopoulos, C.D. Burning Eye Syndrome: Do Neuropathic Pain Mechanisms Underlie Chronic Dry Eye? *Pain Med.* **2016**, *17*, 746–755. [CrossRef] [PubMed]
12. Peirs, C.; Seal, R.P. Neural circuits for pain: Recent advances and current views. *Science* **2016**, *354*, 578–584. [CrossRef] [PubMed]
13. Galor, A.; Moein, H.-R.; Lee, C.; Rodriguez, A.; Felix, E.R.; Sarantopoulos, K.D.; Levitt, R.C. Neuropathic pain and dry eye. *Ocul. Surf.* **2018**, *16*, 31–44. [CrossRef] [PubMed]
14. Attal, N.; Cruccu, G.; Baron, R.; Haanpää, M.; Hansson, P.; Jensen, T.S.; Nurmikko, T. European Federation of Neurological Societies EFNS guidelines on the pharmacological treatment of neuropathic pain: 2010 revision. *Eur. J. Neurol.* **2010**, *17*, 1113-e88. [CrossRef] [PubMed]
15. Kukkar, A.; Bali, A.; Singh, N.; Jaggi, A.S. Implications and mechanism of action of gabapentin in neuropathic pain. *Arch. Pharmacal. Res.* **2013**, *36*, 237–251. [CrossRef] [PubMed]
16. Castel, A.; Vachon, P. Gabapentin reverses central pain sensitization following a collagenase-induced intrathalamic hemorrhage in rats. *J. Pain Res.* **2013**, *7*, 5–12. [CrossRef] [PubMed]
17. Gottrup, H.; Juhl, G.; Kristensen, A.D.; Lai, R.; Chizh, B.A.; Brown, J.; Bach, F.W.; Jensen, T.S. Chronic oral gabapentin reduces elements of central sensitization in human experimental hyperalgesia. *Anesthesiology* **2004**, *101*, 1400–1408. [CrossRef] [PubMed]
18. Michael, R.; Jeffers, J.V.; Messenger, W.; Aref, A.A. Gabapentin for presumed neuropathic ocular pain. *Am. J. Ophthalmol. Case Rep.* **2020**, *19*. [CrossRef]

19. Ongun, N.; Ongun, G.T. Is gabapentin effective in dry eye disease and neuropathic ocular pain? *Acta Neurol. Belg.* **2019**. [CrossRef]
20. Woreta, F.A.; Gupta, A.; Hochstetler, B.; Bower, K.S. Management of post-photorefractive keratectomy pain. *Surv. Ophthalmol.* **2013**, *58*, 529–535. [CrossRef]
21. Schiffman, R.M.; Christianson, M.D.; Jacobsen, G.; Hirsch, J.D.; Reis, B.L. Reliability and validity of the Ocular Surface Disease Index. *Arch. Ophthalmol.* **2000**, *118*, 615–621. [CrossRef] [PubMed]
22. Miyata, K.; Amano, S.; Sawa, M.; Nishida, T. A novel grading method for superficial punctate keratopathy magnitude and its correlation with corneal epithelial permeability. *Arch Ophthalmol.* **2003**, *121*, 1537–1539. [CrossRef] [PubMed]
23. Tomlinson, A.; Bron, A.J.; Korb, D.R.; Amano, S.; Paugh, J.R.; Pearce, E.I.; Yee, R.; Yokoi, N.; Arita, R.; Dogru, M. The international workshop on meibomian gland dysfunction: Report of the diagnosis subcommittee. *Investig. Ophthalmol. Vis. Sci.* **2011**, *52*, 2006–2049. [CrossRef] [PubMed]
24. Wong-Baker FACES Foundation. Available online: https://wongbakerfaces.org/ (accessed on 20 October 2020).
25. Qazi, Y.; Hurwitz, S.; Khan, S.; Jurkunas, U.V.; Dana, R.; Hamrah, P. Validity and Reliability of a Novel Ocular Pain Assessment Survey in Quantification and Monitoring of Corneal and Ocular Surface Pain. *Ophthalmology* **2016**, *123*, 1458–1468. [CrossRef]
26. Loeser, J.D.; Treede, R.-D. The Kyoto protocol of IASP Basic Pain Terminology. *Pain* **2008**, *137*, 473–477. [CrossRef]
27. Pakravan, M.; Roshani, M.; Yazdani, S.; Faramazi, A.; Yaseri, M. Pregabalin and gabapentin for post-photorefractive keratectomy pain: A randomized controlled trial. *Eur. J. Ophthalmol.* **2012**, *22* (Suppl. 7), S106–S113. [CrossRef]
28. Galor, A.; Patel, S.; Small, L.R.; Rodriguez, A.; Venincasa, M.J.; Valido, S.E.; Feuer, W.; Levitt, R.C.; Sarantopoulos, C.D.; Felix, E.R. Pregabalin Failed to Prevent Dry Eye Symptoms after Laser-Assisted in Situ Keratomileusis (LASIK) in a Randomized Pilot Study. *JCM* **2019**, *8*, 1355. [CrossRef]
29. Rowbotham, M.; Harden, N.; Stacey, B.; Bernstein, P.; Magnus-Miller, L. Gabapentin for the treatment of postherpetic neuralgia: A randomized controlled trial. *JAMA* **1998**, *280*, 1837–1842. [CrossRef]
30. Jensen, T.S.; Finnerup, N.B. Allodynia and hyperalgesia in neuropathic pain: Clinical manifestations and mechanisms. *Lancet Neurol.* **2014**, *13*, 924–935. [CrossRef]
31. Stacey, B.R.; Barrett, J.A.; Whalen, E.; Phillips, K.F.; Rowbotham, M.C. Pregabalin for postherpetic neuralgia: Placebo-controlled trial of fixed and flexible dosing regimens on allodynia and time to onset of pain relief. *J. Pain* **2008**, *9*, 1006–1017. [CrossRef]

Publisher's Note: MDPI stays neutral with regard to jurisdictional claims in published maps and institutional affiliations.

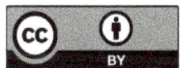

© 2020 by the authors. Licensee MDPI, Basel, Switzerland. This article is an open access article distributed under the terms and conditions of the Creative Commons Attribution (CC BY) license (http://creativecommons.org/licenses/by/4.0/).

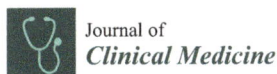

Brief Report

Topical TRPM8 Agonist for Relieving Neuropathic Ocular Pain in Patients with Dry Eye: A Pilot Study

Hyeon Jeong Yoon [1], Jonghwa Kim [1], Jee Myung Yang [2], Edward T. Wei [3], Seong Jin Kim [4,*] and Kyung Chul Yoon [1,*]

1. Department of Ophthalmology, Chonnam National University Medical School and Hospital, 42 Jebong-ro, Dong-gu, Gwangju 61469, Korea; yoonhyeonjeong@hanmail.net (H.J.Y.); ccaaacc@hanmail.net (J.K.)
2. Department of Ophthalmology, Asan Medical Center, University of Ulsan College of Medicine, 88, Olympic-Ro 43 Gil, Songpa-gu, Seoul 05505, Korea; jeemang87@gmail.com
3. School of Public Health, University of California, Berkeley, CA 94720, USA; koolicin@yahoo.com
4. Department of Dermatology, Chonnam National University Medical School and Hospital, 42 Jebong-ro, Dong-gu, Gwangju 61469, Korea
* Correspondence: seongkim@chonnam.ac.kr (S.J.K.); kcyoon@jnu.ac.kr (K.C.Y.)

Received: 1 December 2020; Accepted: 10 January 2021; Published: 12 January 2021

Abstract: Background: Activation of TRPM8, a cold-sensing receptor located on the cornea and eyelid, has the potential to relieve the neuropathic ocular pain (NOP) in dry eye (DE) by inhibiting other aberrant nociceptive inputs. We aimed to investigate the effect of a topical TRPM8 agonist, cryosim-3 (C3), on relieving DE-associated NOP. Methods: We conducted a prospective pilot study of 15 patients with DE-associated NOP. These patients applied topical C3 to their eyelid, 4 times/day for 1 month. The patients underwent clinical examinations. They also completed the Ocular Pain Assessment Survey (OPAS), which is a validated questionnaire for NOP, at baseline, 1 week, and 1 month after treatment. Result: At 1 week, the OPAS scores of eye pain intensity, quality of life (driving/watching TV, general activity, sleep, and enjoying life/relations with other people), and associated factors (burning sensation, light sensitivity, and tearing) improved. The total OPAS scores of eye pain intensity, quality of life, and associated factors remained improved at 1 month. The Schirmer test scores also improved at 1 month. Conclusion: TRPM8 agonist (C3) could be a novel agent for treating patients with DE-associated NOP who are unresponsive to conventional treatments.

Keywords: TRPM8 agonist; cryosim-3; dry eye; neuropathic pain

1. Introduction

Dry eye (DE) is a multifactorial disease of the ocular surface characterized by a loss of homeostasis of the tear film and accompanying ocular symptoms [1]. It has a prevalence of 10% to 70% [1]. Some patients with DE experience severe pain that reduces their quality of life (QoL) with minimal ocular signs [1]. Topical agents could be applied as a part of DE treatment to reduce inflammation and tear film osmolality [2]. Generally, if the ocular pain cannot be resolved with topical treatment, other specific causes should be suspected, in particular, neuropathic pain could be the underlying cause [3,4]. In DE, ocular pain disproportionally outweighing the clinical signs is suggestive of underlying neuropathic ocular pain (NOP) nature [4].

Transient receptor potential (TRP) cation channels are associated with the perception of chemical and temperature stimulations [5]. Within the TRP family, TRPM8 is a cold-sensing receptor located on nerve endings of the ophthalmic branch of the trigeminal nerve [6]. Since the activation of TRPM8 can inhibit other aberrant nociceptive inputs, agents for targeting this channel might have the potential to relieve the NOP in DE [7,8]. In particular, TRPM8 is distributed in not only cornea but also eyelid; therefore, it can be activated using topical agents that are applied onto the eyelid without directly instilling eye drops to the cornea [6,9,10]. In our previous study, we revealed the effectiveness of topical cryosim-3 (C3)—a water-soluble and selective TRPM8 agonist—in the treatment of DE by increasing basal tear secretion and alleviating ocular discomfort without any complications [9]. In this pilot study, we aimed to investigate the effect of the topical TRPM8 agonist (C3) on relieving NOP in patients with DE.

2. Methods

This prospective nonrandomized pilot study was conducted in accordance with the tenets of the Declaration of Helsinki. Ethical approval was obtained from the Chonnam National University Hospital Institutional Review Board (CNUH-2018-274). Informed consent was obtained from all included patients. The sample size was calculated using the G*Power software (version 3.1.9.4; Heinrich-Heine University, Germany) with a level of $\alpha = 0.05$ and a power of 95% to detect a 2-point difference in pain scales. Accordingly, a total sample size of 13 patients was found sufficient.

Patients with DE accompanied by NOP features, who underwent evaluation between January and December in 2018, were enrolled. DE was diagnosed based on ocular surface disease index (OSDI) score ≥ 13 and tear break-up time (TBUT) ≤ 7 s. The inclusion criteria were as follows: (1) chronic ocular pain that was unresponsive to conventional topical agents (i.e., lubricants, anti-inflammatories, and secretagogues) for >3 months; (2) discordance between the painful DE symptoms and signs and specific descriptors, including burning or stinging; and (3) a Wong–Baker FACES Pain Rating Scale (WBFPS) score ≥ 4. Patients who had a history of ocular diseases other than DE and those receiving systemic medications that alter the pain and mood statuses were excluded.

The patients were treated with add-on C3 while undergoing conventional topical treatment. C3 samples (2 mg/mL) were diluted in purified water, soaked in gauze, and packaged using automated equipment. The patients applied topical C3 by wiping the gauze on the closed eyelid margin, 4 times/day for 1 month (Figure 1B).

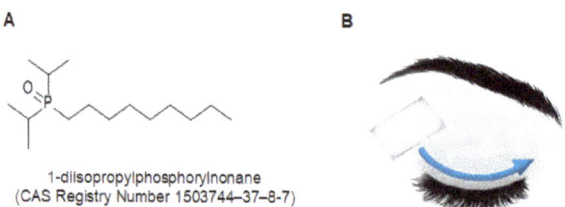

Figure 1. Chemical structure of cryosim-3 (**A**) and the method of topical application of the gauze containing cryosim-3, which targets TRPM8 on the eyelid margin (**B**).

The OSDI questionnaire, which ranged from 0 to 100, was used to quantify the vision-related QoL. TBUT, the time interval between the last complete blink and the first appearance of disruption of the tear film, was measured thrice, and the mean value was used for analysis. Corneal staining scores were assessed using the area-density index, by multiplying the area and density score. The Schirmer test score represented the length of wetting, and was measured using a calibrated sterile strip placed at the lateral canthus for 5 min under topical anesthesia (0.5% proparacaine). Only the score of the right eye was assessed.

The WBFPS was chosen to screen the pain severity in the patients with DE. The patients chose the face that best depicted the pain they were experiencing. At baseline, 1 week, and 1 month after treatment, the patients also completed the OPAS, which is a validated questionnaire for neuropathic pain as previously described [11]. The questions were divided into sections for analysis: questions 4–9 pertained to eye pain intensity (0 to 60); questions 10–11 pertained to non-eye pain (0 to 20); questions 13–19 (0–10, total score 0 to 60) assessed the QoL (reading and/or computer use, driving and/or watching TV, general activity, mood, sleep, and enjoying life/relations with other people); questions 20–21 (each score 0–1, total score 0–2) assessed aggravating factors (mechanical and chemical stimuli); questions 22–25 (each score 0–1, total score 0–4) assessed associated factors (redness, burning, sensitivity to light, and tearing). The section on symptomatic relief of the OPAS was excluded, and only questions 4–25 were analyzed. The questions were divided into 5 sections as follows: eye pain intensity, non-eye pain, QoL, aggravating factors, and associated factors.

Statistical analyses were conducted using PASW Statistics for Windows, Version 18.0 (SPSS Inc., Chicago, IL, USA). The normality of distribution was assessed using the Shapiro–Wilk test. The Wilcoxon signed-rank test and repeated-measures analysis of variance with Bonferroni's post hoc test were used for comparing parameters before and after treatment. A p-value <0.05 was considered statistically significant.

3. Results

This study enrolled 20 patients with DE accompanying NOP features. Five patients (25.0%) discontinued the treatment because of drug ineffectiveness or intolerance. The remaining 15 patients (75.0%) were included in the analysis. Their mean age was 59.5 ± 13.0 years, and nine patients (60.0%) were women. Five patients had a history of intraocular surgery, and one patient had a history of ocular trauma.

At 1 week after treatment, eye pain intensity, QoL (driving/watching TV, general activity, sleep, and enjoying life/relations with other people), and associated factors (burning sensation, light sensitivity, and tearing) were improved. The total Ocular Pain Assessment Survey (OPAS) scores of eye pain intensity, QoL (sleep), and associated factors (burning sensation and light sensitivity) remained improved at 1 month. However, the score of non-eye pain and aggravating factors did not change after treatment (Table 1). Among the clinical DE parameters, OSDI and Schirmer test score were improved at 1 month after treatment (Table 2). There were no significant differences in pain scores according to previous medications (Supplementary Table S1).

Table 1. Changes in the Ocular Pain Assessment Survey scores after the application of cryosim-3 for 1 month.

	Baseline [a]	1 Week [b]	1 Month [c]	p-Value *		
				a vs. b	a vs. c	b vs. c
Eye pain intensity (0–60)	30.60 ± 12.84	26.47 ± 11.45	21.53 ± 10.84	0.009	0.015	0.073
Non-eye pain (0–20)	7.67 ± 6.22	6.73 ± 6.18	5.47 ± 5.62	0.999	0.435	0.409
Quality of life (total 0–60)	33.53 ± 14.24	27.60 ± 15.49	27.17 ± 16.06	0.003	0.022	0.743
Reading and/or computer use (0–10)	7.79 ± 1.76	7.14 ± 2.48	6.93 ± 2.59	0.120	0.054	0.272
Driving and/or watching TV (0–10)	6.80 ± 2.31	5.27 ± 2.52	5.60 ± 2.90	0.002	0.070	0.417
General activity (walking, etc.) (0–10)	4.00 ± 3.18	3.27 ± 2.71	3.20 ± 2.86	0.016	0.138	0.843
Mood (0–10)	5.40 ± 2.77	4.53 ± 2.50	4.40 ± 2.47	0.121	0.177	0.769
Sleep (0–10)	4.27 ± 3.81	2.93 ± 3.67	2.73 ± 3.81	0.027	0.049	0.486
Enjoying life/relations with other people (0–10)	5.07 ± 2.84	4.33 ± 2.97	4.27 ± 3.03	0.036	0.068	0.806
Aggravating factors (total 0–2)	1.11 ± 0.49	0.87 ± 0.56	0.88 ± 0.57	0.113	0.132	0.077
Mechanical stimuli (0–1)	0.63 ± 0.29	0.47 ± 0.25	0.47 ± 0.26	0.068	0.086	0.999
Chemical stimuli (0–1)	0.47 ± 0.35	0.41 ± 0.35	0.41 ± 0.32	0.363	0.432	0.872
Associated factors (total 0–4)	2.09 ± 0.76	1.55 ± 0.85	1.58 ± 0.93	0.006	0.046	0.835
Redness (0–1)	0.41 ± 0.32	0.41 ± 0.30	0.39 ± 0.30	0.094	0.104	0.080
Burning sensation (0–1)	0.57 ± 0.37	0.40 ± 0.33	0.29 ± 0.29	0.007	0.002	0.015
Sensitivity to light (0–1)	0.76 ± 0.24	0.57 ± 0.26	0.59 ± 0.28	0.005	0.030	0.663
Tearing (0–1)	0.36 ± 0.29	0.17 ± 0.18	0.21 ± 0.27	0.013	0.197	0.578

All values are presented as mean ± SD. * Compared using repeated measures analysis of variance with Bonferroni's post hoc test. (a) means "baseline", (b) means "1-week", and (c) means "1-month"

Table 2. Changes in clinical parameters after the application of cryosim-3 for 1 month.

	BASELINE	1 Month	Z	p-Value
Ocular surface disease index	57.5 ± 13.8	40.2 ± 12.6	−3.41	0.001
Tear break-up time (s)	4.13 ± 0.83	4.00 ± 0.85	−0.82	0.414
Schirmer test score (mm)	7.07± 2.76	8.47 ± 2.80	−3.02	0.003
Corneal staining score (0–9)	0.60 ± 0.91	0.13 ± 0.35	−1.82	0.068

All values are presented as mean ± SD. Compared using the Wilcoxon signed rank test.

4. Discussion

DE is a multifactorial disease of the ocular surface that is accompanied by ocular symptoms [1]. The prevalence of DE has increased considerably worldwide over the last three decades [1]. Some patients with DE experience ocular pain that affects their QoL without any specific abnormal ocular signs [1]. The classification of pain is based on the underlying etiology: (1) nociceptive pain caused by actual or threatened damage to tissues due to the activation of nociceptors, and (2) neuropathic pain caused by a lesion or disease of the somatosensory nervous system [12]. Repeated peripheral nerve injury can lead to peripheral sensitization, and prolonged peripheral ectopic pain initiates central sensitization [4]. Ocular pain symptoms disproportionally outweighing the clinical signs are suggestive of an underlying NOP that might require specific management including systemic treatment [4].

However, chronic NOP associated with DE is a challenging clinical problem that is difficult to treat with conventional medications [4,13]. Conventional topical agents such as cyclosporine A could decrease the release of proinflammatory neuropeptides and cytokines from injured nerves, thereby affecting nociceptive pain and peripheral sensitization [13]. However, these topical treatments appear to have limitations in producing an improvement in the corneal nerve morphologic status and central sensitization in patients with chronic NOP. Current systemic medication mainly includes oral antidepressants, anticonvulsants, or gabapentinoid; however, these systemic treatments have several limitations, such as delayed onset, variable efficacy, and unacceptable side effects [4,13,14]. In addition, limited data are available to support the use of systemic neuropathic pain medications for NOP associated with DE [14–16]. In this regard, topical agents that are rapid acting, effective, and safe are needed for treating the NOP in DE.

Several members of the TRP super family have emerged as important targets for pain control owing to their critical role in nociception, especially, in chronic states [5]. TRP receptors have been identified in the cornea (TRPV1-4, TRPA1, TRPC4, and TRPM8), conjunctiva (TRPV1, TRPV2, and TRPV4), and eyelid (TRPM8) [6]. In addition, many studies have reported an association between the dysfunction of TRP channels and DE [3,6,17]. TRPM8 is the principal receptor associated with sensing coolness and regulates lacrimal function via response to evaporative cooling and hyperosmolar stimuli [10,18–20]. Several studies have showed that cooling the periocular area with an ice pack or instilling cold artificial tears into the eye could relieve ocular pain after surgery [21,22]. Both TRPM8 agonists and antagonists are considered therapeutic agents for pain control [5–7,23]. TRPM8 antagonists were shown to improve acute and chronic pain such as cold allodynia [23,24]. However, TRPM8 antagonists can reduce basal tear secretion as an undesirable side effect in DE, as shown in the result of experiments using TRPM8 knock-out mice [20]. TRPM8 agonist could present significant anti-allodynic activity through an excessive activation of TRPM8, leading to its downregulation [25]. Furthermore, TRPM8 agonists have been found to have analgesic effects on neuropathic pain, such as chemotherapy-induced neuropathic pain [8,26,27].

This pilot study showed that the topical application of a TRPM8 agonist (C3) to the eyelid was safe and effective in relieving NOP in patients with DE. We previously showed that the topical application of C3 stimulates basal tear secretion and relieves ocular discomfort in patients with mild DE [9]. The sensory fibers of TRPM8, which innervate the upper eyelid and cornea, are located in the ophthalmic branch of the trigeminal nerve [6]. We speculated in this study that TRPM8 signaling via the eyelid margins may be perceived in the brain as signals from not only the cornea but also the entire ocular surface [9]. Activation of TRPM8 leads to the central synaptic release of glutamate, which then suppresses the injury-activated nociceptive afferent neurotransmission through inhibitory receptors at nerves ending (Figure 2) [8]. In addition, a hypothesis suggests that these actions attenuate neuropathic sensitization on the dorsal horn [8]. In addition, OSDI and Schirmer test scores improved, but TBUT and corneal staining scores remained unchanged after C3 treatment. TRPM8 agonist is known to increase the basal tear secretion and reduce ocular discomfort via neuronal action, but it does not have direct effect on the tear film [6,9]. These results were consistent with our previous study [9].

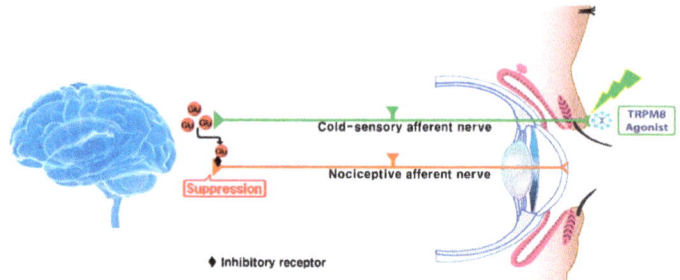

Figure 2. Schematic illustrating the mechanism of action of the TRPM8 agonist in relieving ocular pain in patients with dry eye.

Topical delivery of C3 to the eyelid margins could minimize corneal exposure that induces side effects, such as discomfort or paradoxical ocular pain [9]. In addition, the wiping of C3 was more comfortable for patients than conventional instillation of eye drops, and produced a painless cooling sensation lasting approximately 40 min [9]. The OPAS scores also decreased at 1 week after treatment, indicating that the topical drug produces effect faster than systemic drugs do [14]. Moreover, although the effect was temporary, C3 was particularly effective when the patients experienced severe pain due to DE, such as when driving or sleeping, thereby resulting in an improved QoL.

This study included a short follow-up period of 1 month and a small sample size. In our study, 15 patients who were included in the analysis showed improved symptoms after treatment; however, a larger sample size would have yielded a more accurate response rate. The number of enrolled patients was too small to perform a subgroup analysis. This was a single-center study, and hence, the findings should be verified in future multicenter prospective randomized control studies evaluating the objective signs.

In addition, we did not strictly control for previous medications for DE when enrolling the patients. This might have induced a bias during analysis. However, patients in our study did not respond to conventional treatment for a long period of time (122.7 days), but they showed an improvement of ocular pain within 1 week after C3 treatment. This improvement suggests a direct effect of C3 treatment rather than a delayed effect of previous conventional treatment. We believe that including patients with varying histories of medical treatments may likely emulate the actual use of this drug. Despite the aforementioned limitations, the TRPM8 agonist (C3) could be a novel agent for treating NOP in patients with DE who are unresponsive to conventional topical treatment.

Supplementary Materials: The following are available online at http://www.mdpi.com/2077-0383/10/2/250/s1, Table S1: Previous topical treatment and Wong-Baker FACES Pain Rating Scale (WBFPS) score in enrolled patients.

Author Contributions: Conceptualization, K.C.Y., E.T.W., S.J.K.; methodology, H.J.Y., J.K., E.T.W., S.J.K.; software, H.J.Y., J.K., J.M.Y.; validation, H.J.Y., J.M.Y., K.C.Y.; formal analysis, H.J.Y.; investigation, H.J.Y., J.K.; resources, H.J.Y., J.K.; data curation, H.J.Y., J.K.; writing—original draft preparation, H.J.Y.; writing—review and editing, H.J.Y., K.C.Y.; visualization, H.J.Y.; supervision, K.C.Y.; project administration, K.C.Y.; funding acquisition, K.C.Y. All authors have read and agreed to the published version of the manuscript.

Funding: This study was partially supported by the Technology Innovation Program (20009481) funded By the Ministry of Trade, Industry & Energy (MOTIE, Korea), a grant of the Korea Health Technology R&D Project through the Korea Health Industry Development Institute (KHIDI), funded by the Ministry of Health and Welfare, Republic of Korea (HR20C0021050020), and the Chonnam National University Hospital Biomedical Research Institute (BCRI 20072).

Institutional Review Board Statement: Ethical approval was obtained from the Chonnam National University Hospital Institutional Review Board (CNUH-2018-274).

Informed Consent Statement: Informed consent was obtained from all included patients.

Data Availability Statement: The data presented in this study are available on request from the corresponding author. The data are not publicly available due to ethical issue.

Conflicts of Interest: E.T.W. is listed on a patent application on the use of C3 for eye discomfort and nasal congestion (Di-Isopropyl-phosphinoyl-alkane (DIPA) compounds as topical agents for the treatment of sensory discomfort). World Intellectual Property Organization, WO2015059432, 30 April 2015). The other authors declare no conflict of interest.

References

1. Craig, J.P.; Nichols, K.K.; Akpek, E.K.; Caffery, B.; Dua, H.S.; Joo, C.-K.; Liu, Z.; Nelson, J.D.; Nichols, J.J.; Tsubota, K.; et al. TFOS DEWS II Definition and Classification Report. *Ocul. Surf.* **2017**, *15*, 276–283. [CrossRef] [PubMed]
2. Jones, L.; Downie, L.E.; Korb, D.; Benitez-Del-Castillo, J.M.; Dana, R.; Deng, S.X.; Dong, P.N.; Geerling, G.; Hida, R.Y.; Liu, Y.; et al. TFOS DEWS II Management and Therapy Report. *Ocul. Surf.* **2017**, *15*, 575–628. [CrossRef] [PubMed]
3. Belmonte, C.; Nichols, J.J.; Cox, S.M.; Brock, J.A.; Begley, C.G.; Bereiter, D.A.; Dartt, D.A.; Galor, A.; Hamrah, P.; Ivanusic, J.J.; et al. TFOS DEWS II Pain and Sensation Report. *Ocul. Surf.* **2017**, *15*, 404–437. [CrossRef] [PubMed]
4. Galor, A.; Moein, H.-R.; Lee, C.; Rodriguez, A.; Felix, E.R.; Sarantopoulos, K.D.; Levitt, R.C. Neuropathic Pain and Dry Eye. *Ocul. Surf.* **2018**, *16*, 31–44. [CrossRef]
5. Brederson, J.-D.; Kym, P.R.; Szallasi, A. Targeting TRP Channels for Pain Relief. *Eur. J. Pharmacol.* **2013**, *716*, 61–76. [CrossRef]
6. Yang, J.M.; Wei, E.T.; Kim, S.J.; Yoon, K.C. TRPM8 Channels and Dry Eye. *Pharmaceuticals* **2018**, *11*, 125. [CrossRef]
7. Fernández-Peña, C.; Viana, F. Targeting TRPM8 for Pain Relief. *TOPAINJ* **2013**, *6*, 154–164. [CrossRef]
8. Proudfoot, C.J.; Garry, E.M.; Cottrell, D.F.; Rosie, R.; Anderson, H.; Robertson, D.C.; Fleetwood-Walker, S.M.; Mitchell, R. Analgesia Mediated by the TRPM8 Cold Receptor in Chronic Neuropathic Pain. *Curr. Biol.* **2006**, *16*, 1591–1605. [CrossRef]
9. Yang, J.M.; Li, F.; Liu, Q.; Rüedi, M.; Wei, E.T.; Lentsman, M.; Lee, H.S.; Choi, W.; Kim, S.J.; Yoon, K.C. A Novel TRPM8 Agonist Relieves Dry Eye Discomfort. *BMC Ophthalmol.* **2017**, *17*, 101. [CrossRef]
10. Wei, E.T. Improving Brain Power by Applying a Cool TRPM8 Receptor Agonist to the Eyelid Margin. *Med. Hypotheses* **2020**, *142*, 109747. [CrossRef]
11. Qazi, Y.; Hurwitz, S.; Khan, S.; Jurkunas, U.V.; Dana, R.; Hamrah, P. Validity and Reliability of a Novel Ocular Pain Assessment Survey in Quantification and Monitoring of Corneal and Ocular Surface Pain. *Ophthalmology* **2016**, *123*, 1458–1468. [CrossRef] [PubMed]
12. Loeser, J.D.; Treede, R.-D. The Kyoto Protocol of IASP Basic Pain Terminology. *Pain* **2008**, *137*, 473–477. [CrossRef] [PubMed]
13. Dieckmann, G.; Goyal, S.; Hamrah, P. Neuropathic Corneal Pain. *Ophthalmology* **2017**, *124*, S34–S47. [CrossRef] [PubMed]
14. Yoon, H.-J.; Kim, J.; Yoon, K.C. Treatment Response to Gabapentin in Neuropathic Ocular Pain Associated with Dry Eye. *JCM* **2020**, *9*, 3765. [CrossRef] [PubMed]
15. Ongun, N.; Ongun, G.T. Is Gabapentin Effective in Dry Eye Disease and Neuropathic Ocular Pain? *Acta Neurol. Belg.* **2019**. [CrossRef]
16. Galor, A.; Patel, S.; Small, L.R.; Rodriguez, A.; Venincasa, M.J.; Valido, S.E.; Feuer, W.; Levitt, R.C.; Sarantopoulos, C.D.; Felix, E.R. Pregabalin Failed to Prevent Dry Eye Symptoms after Laser-Assisted in Situ Keratomileusis (LASIK) in a Randomized Pilot Study. *J. Clin. Med.* **2019**, *8*, 1355. [CrossRef]

17. Arcas, J.M.; González, A.; Gers-Barlag, K.; González-González, O.; Bech, F.; Demirkhanyan, L.; Zakharian, E.; Belmonte, C.; Gomis, A.; Viana, F. The Immunosuppressant Macrolide Tacrolimus Activates Cold-Sensing TRPM8 Channels. *J. Neurosci.* **2019**, *39*, 949–969. [CrossRef]
18. Knowlton, W.M.; Palkar, R.; Lippoldt, E.K.; McCoy, D.D.; Baluch, F.; Chen, J.; McKemy, D.D. A Sensory-Labeled Line for Cold: TRPM8-Expressing Sensory Neurons Define the Cellular Basis for Cold, Cold Pain, and Cooling-Mediated Analgesia. *J. Neurosci.* **2013**, *33*, 2837–2848. [CrossRef]
19. Quallo, T.; Vastani, N.; Horridge, E.; Gentry, C.; Parra, A.; Moss, S.; Viana, F.; Belmonte, C.; Andersson, D.A.; Bevan, S. TRPM8 Is a Neuronal Osmosensor That Regulates Eye Blinking in Mice. *Nat. Commun.* **2015**, *6*, 7150. [CrossRef]
20. Parra, A.; Madrid, R.; Echevarria, D.; del Olmo, S.; Morenilla-Palao, C.; Acosta, M.C.; Gallar, J.; Dhaka, A.; Viana, F.; Belmonte, C. Ocular Surface Wetness Is Regulated by TRPM8-Dependent Cold Thermoreceptors of the Cornea. *Nat. Med.* **2010**, *16*, 1396–1399. [CrossRef]
21. Fujishima, H.; Yagi, Y.; Toda, I.; Shimazaki, J.; Tsubota, K. Increased Comfort and Decreased Inflammation of the Eye by Cooling after Cataract Surgery. *Am. J. Ophthalmol.* **1995**, *119*, 301–306. [CrossRef]
22. Fujishima, H.; Yagi, Y.; Shimazaki, J.; Tsubota, K. Effects of Artificial Tear Temperature on Corneal Sensation and Subjective Comfort. *Cornea* **1997**, *16*, 630–634. [CrossRef] [PubMed]
23. De Caro, C.; Russo, R.; Avagliano, C.; Cristiano, C.; Calignano, A.; Aramini, A.; Bianchini, G.; Allegretti, M.; Brandolini, L. Antinociceptive Effect of Two Novel Transient Receptor Potential Melastatin 8 Antagonists in Acute and Chronic Pain Models in Rat. *Br. J. Pharmacol.* **2018**, *175*, 1691–1706. [CrossRef] [PubMed]
24. Fakih, D.; Baudouin, C.; Réaux-Le Goazigo, A.; Mélik Parsadaniantz, S. TRPM8: A Therapeutic Target for Neuroinflammatory Symptoms Induced by Severe Dry Eye Disease. *Int. J. Mol. Sci.* **2020**, *21*, 8556. [CrossRef] [PubMed]
25. De Caro, C.; Cristiano, C.; Avagliano, C.; Bertamino, A.; Ostacolo, C.; Campiglia, P.; Gomez-Monterrey, I.; La Rana, G.; Gualillo, O.; Calignano, A.; et al. Characterization of New TRPM8 Modulators in Pain Perception. *Int. J. Mol. Sci.* **2019**, *20*, 5544. [CrossRef]
26. Fallon, M.T.; Storey, D.J.; Krishan, A.; Weir, C.J.; Mitchell, R.; Fleetwood-Walker, S.M.; Scott, A.C.; Colvin, L.A. Cancer Treatment-Related Neuropathic Pain: Proof of Concept Study with Menthol—A TRPM8 Agonist. *Support Care Cancer* **2015**, *23*, 2769–2777. [CrossRef]
27. Tamamoto-Mochizuki, C.; Murphy, K.M.; Olivry, T. Pilot Evaluation of the Antipruritic Efficacy of a Topical Transient Receptor Potential Melastatin Subfamily 8 (TRPM8) Agonist in Dogs with Atopic Dermatitis and Pedal Pruritus. *Vet. Dermatol.* **2018**, *29*, 29-e14. [CrossRef]

Publisher's Note: MDPI stays neutral with regard to jurisdictional claims in published maps and institutional affiliations.

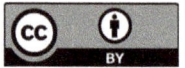

© 2021 by the authors. Licensee MDPI, Basel, Switzerland. This article is an open access article distributed under the terms and conditions of the Creative Commons Attribution (CC BY) license (http://creativecommons.org/licenses/by/4.0/).

MDPI
St. Alban-Anlage 66
4052 Basel
Switzerland
Tel. +41 61 683 77 34
Fax +41 61 302 89 18
www.mdpi.com

Journal of Clinical Medicine Editorial Office
E-mail: jcm@mdpi.com
www.mdpi.com/journal/jcm

www.ingramcontent.com/pod-product-compliance
Lightning Source LLC
LaVergne TN
LVHW070619100526
838202LV00012B/682